Get ready. Get set. Get moving!

Access to exercise videos included with any new book.

Start getting fit today! REGISTER NOW!

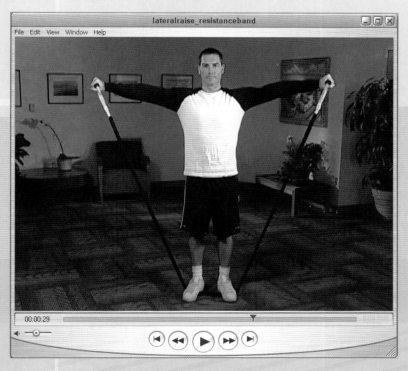

lateralraise_resistanceband

File   Edit   View   Window   Help

00:00:29

Registration will let you:

- Access over 80 exercise demonstration videos

- Select from resistance band, free weight, machine, stability ball, and flexibility exercises

- Exercise at your own pace, in the comfort of your own home

- View safety tips

www.aw-bc.com/hopson

TO REGISTER

1. Go to www.aw-bc.com/hopson

2. Click "Exercise Videos."

3. Click "Register."

4. Follow the on-screen instructions to create your login name and password.

Your Access Code is:

Note: If there is no silver foil covering the access code, it may already have been redeemed, and therefore may no longer be valid.

TO LOG IN

1. Go to www.aw-bc.com/hopson

2. Click "Exercise Videos."

3. Enter your login name and password.

Remember to bookmark the site after you log in.

http://247pearsoned.custhelp.com

PRE-COURSE/POST-COURSE ASSESSMENT

Name:_____ Date(s): _____

As you complete the key fitness/wellness lab assessments in this course, record your results in the "Pre-Course Assessment" column. At the end of the course, re-do the labs, record your results in the "Post-Course Assessment" column, and see the progress you have made!

Lab	Pre-Course Assessment	Post-Course Assessment
Lab 2.2: Using a Pedometer	Average steps taken per day: _____	Average steps taken per day: _____

Lab 4.2: Assessing Your Cardiorespiratory Fitness Level	**3-minute step test**
	  1 minute recovery HR: _____ (bpm)
	  Fitness rating: _____
	1-mile walk test
	  VO$_2$max: _____ Fitness rating: _____
	1.5-mile run test
	  VO$_2$max: _____ Fitness rating: _____
		3-minute step test
		  1 minute recovery HR: _____ (bpm)
		  Fitness rating: _____
		1-mile walk test
		  VO$_2$max: _____ Fitness rating: _____
		1.5-mile run test
		  VO$_2$max: _____ Fitness rating: _____

Lab 5.1: Assessing Your Muscular Strength	**Bench press**
	  S/BW ratio: _____ Rating: _____
	Leg press
	  S/BW ratio: _____ Rating: _____
		Bench press
		  S/BW ratio: _____ Rating: _____
		Leg press
		  S/BW ratio: _____ Rating: _____

Lab 5.2: Assessing Your Muscular Endurance	**20RM assessment**
	  Bench press 20RM weight lifted: _____
	  Leg press 20RM weight lifted: _____
	Push-up assessment
	  Repetitions: _____ Rating: _____
	Curl-up assessment
	  Repetitions: _____ Rating: _____
		20RM assessment
		  Bench press 20RM weight lifted: _____
		  Leg press 20RM weight lifted: _____
		Push-up assessment
		  Repetitions: _____ Rating: _____
		Curl-up assessment
		  Repetitions: _____ Rating: _____

Lab 6.1: Assessing Your Flexibility	**Sit-and-reach test**
	  Reach distance (inches): _____
	  Rating:_____
		Sit-and-reach test
		  Reach distance (inches): _____
		  Rating:_____

Lab 7.1: How to Calculate Your BMI	BMI: _____ kg/m^2 Weight classification: _____	BMI: _____ kg/m^2 Weight classification: _____
Lab 7.2: How to Measure and Evaluate Your Body Circumferences	Waist: _____ Hip: _____ Upper arm: _____ (right) _____ (left) Forearm: _____ (right) _____ (left) Thigh: _____ (right) _____ (left) Calf: _____ (right) _____ (left) Neck: _____ Waist-to-hip ratio: _____ Disease risk rating: _____	Waist: _____ Hip: _____ Upper arm: _____ (right) _____ (left) Forearm: _____ (right) _____ (left) Thigh: _____ (right) _____ (left) Calf: _____ (right) _____ (left) Neck: _____ Waist-to-hip ratio: _____ Disease risk rating: _____
Lab 7.3: Estimate Your Percent Body Fat (Skinfold Test)	Sum of 3 skinfolds: _____ Percent body fat estimate: _____ Rating: _____	Sum of 3 skinfolds: _____ Percent body fat estimate: _____ Rating: _____
Lab 8.2: Keeping a Food Diary and Analyzing Your Daily Nutrition *and* Lab 8.3: Improving Your Nutrition	Milk intake: _____ cups Meat and beans intake: _____ oz. Vegetables intake: _____ cups Fruits intake: _____ cups Grains intake: _____ oz.	Milk intake: _____ cups Meat and beans intake: _____ oz. Vegetables intake: _____ cups Fruits intake: _____ cups Grains intake: _____ oz.
Lab 9.1: Calculating Energy Balance and Setting Energy Balance Goals	Estimated calorie intake: _____ Total energy expenditure (EE): _____ Calories	Estimated calorie intake: _____ Total energy expenditure (EE): _____ Calories
Lab 9.3: Your Weight Management Plan	% body fat: _____ Weight: _____ lb. BMI: _____ kg/m^2	% body fat: _____ Weight: _____ lb. BMI: _____ kg/m^2
Lab 10.1: How Stressed Are You?	Sum of negative scores: _____ Interpretation: _____	Sum of negative scores: _____ Interpretation: _____
Lab 11.1: Understanding Your CVD Risk	Family risk for CVD, total points: _____ Lifestyle risk for CVD, total points: _____ Additional risks for CVD, total points: _____	Family risk for CVD, total points: _____ Lifestyle risk for CVD, total points: _____ Additional risks for CVD, total points: _____

Behavior Change Contract

Choose a health behavior that you would like to change, starting this quarter or semester. Sign the contract at the bottom to affirm your commitment to making a healthy change and ask a friend to witness it.

My behavior change will be:

_____

My long-term goal for this behavior change is:

_____

Barriers that I must overcome to make this behavior change are   (things that I am currently doing or situations that contribute to this behavior or make it harder to change):

    1. _____

    2. _____

    3. _____

The strategies I will use to overcome these barriers are:

    1. _____

    2. _____

    3. _____

Resources I will use to help me change this behavior include:

    a friend/partner/relative: _____

    a school-based resource: _____

    a community-based resource: _____

    a book or reputable website: _____

In order to make my goal more attainable, I have devised these short-term goals

short-term goal	target date	reward
short-term goal	target date	reward
short-term goal	target date	reward

When I make the long-term behavior change described above, my reward will be:

_____ target date: _____

I intend to make the behavior change described above. I will use the strategies and rewards to achieve the goals that will contribute to a healthy behavior change.

Signed: _____   Witness: _____

GET FIT, STAY WELL!

Janet L. Hopson, M.A.
San Francisco State University

Rebecca J. Donatelle, Ph.D.
Oregon State University

Tanya R. Littrell, Ph.D.
Portland Community College

Benjamin Cummings

San Francisco   Boston   New York
Cape Town   Hong Kong   London   Madrid   Mexico City
Montreal   Munich   Paris   Singapore   Sydney   Tokyo   Toronto

Acquisitions Editor: *Sandra Lindelof*
Development Manager: *Barbara Yien*
Development Editor: *Cathy Murphy*
Art Development Editor: *Laura Southworth*
Assistant Editor: *Jacob Evans*
Managing Editor: *Deborah Cogan*
Production Supervisor: *Beth Masse*
Production Management and Compositor:
   Progressive Information Technologies
Senior Art Editor: *Donna Kalal*
Cover and Interior Designer: *Yvo Riezebos*
Illustrator: *Dragonfly Media Group*
Photo Researcher: *Kristin Piljay*
Senior Manufacturing Buyer: *Stacey*
   Weinberger
Marketing Manager: *Neena Bali*
Market Development Manager: *Josh Frost*
Text Printer: *Worldcolor Dubuque*
Cover Printer: *Phoenix Color*
Cover Photo Credits: *© Getty Images / Blasius*
   Erlinger, © Getty Images / Photodisc, © 2007
   Masterfile

ISBN-10: 0-321-57657-8 (Student edition)
ISBN-13: 978-0-321-57657-6 (Student edition)
ISBN-10: 0-321-59492-4 (Brief edition)
ISBN-13: 978-0-321-59492-1 (Brief edition)
ISBN-10: 0-321-58703-0 (Professional copy)
ISBN-13: 978-0-321-58703-9 (Professional copy)

Benjamin Cummings
is an imprint of

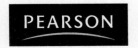

www.pearsonhighered.com

2 3 4 5 6 7 8 9 10—**V042**—14 13 12 11 10

To the memory of Ruth and David Hopson, who taught me, by example and encouragement, to love fitness activity.—**JLH**

To the strong, intelligent, loving, and hard-working women who have motivated me and taught me to care about the important things—especially my mom, Agnes E. Donatelle.—**RJD**

To my mom, whose continued unconditional support and encouragement of her children is an inspiration.—**TRL**

JANET L. HOPSON, M.A.

A full-time author, Janet L. Hopson has written or co-authored nine books, including two popular nonfiction books on human pheromones and human brain development, and six textbooks on general biology for college and high school students. Ms. Hopson currently teaches science writing at San Francisco State University and has taught the subject at two campuses of the University of California. She holds B.A. and M.A. degrees from Southern Illinois University and the University of Missouri. She has won awards for magazine writing, and her articles have appeared in *Smithsonian, Psychology Today, Science Digest, Science News, Outside,* and others. She is married and enjoys competitive tennis, raising horses, golfing, swimming, reading, and traveling.

REBECCA J. DONATELLE, PH.D.

Dr. Rebecca (Becky) J. Donatelle is an Associate Professor of Health Promotion and Behavior in the Department of Public Health at Oregon State University in Corvallis, Oregon. She teaches courses in Health Behaviors, Infectious Diseases, Chronic Disease Prevention and Control, and Violence and Public Health, and has taught thousands of students in health-related fields over the years. As a researcher and behavioral scientist with an emphasis on intervention science, much of her work has focused on women's health and the health of elderly populations. Her research has been published in numerous journals, and she has been a guest speaker and presenter at professional conferences throughout the country. Dr. Donatelle is also the author of the highly successful introductory health textbooks *Access to Health* and *Health: The Basics,* published by Benjamin Cummings. These texts are internationally well-regarded and have been adopted by hundreds of colleges and universities around the world.

TANYA R. LITTRELL, PH.D.

Dr. Tanya R. Littrell is a full-time faculty member in Fitness Technology and Physical Education at Portland Community College in Portland, Oregon. Dr. Littrell worked as a fitness director for many years before attending graduate school at Oregon State University, where she earned both a master's degree in Human Performance/Exercise Physiology and a doctoral degree in Exercise Science/Exercise Physiology. Dr. Littrell has been teaching lifetime fitness classes for undergraduates since 1998. When she is not teaching, preparing to teach, or writing, you can find Dr. Littrell on the trails running or mountain biking, rock climbing, traveling, or spending quality time with her family.

CONTENTS

DETAILED CONTENTS

BOXES

LABS

PREFACE

You may have noticed that health, fitness, and wellness are highly popular topics! Open a newspaper, turn on the TV, or surf the Internet and you will undoubtedly find articles about the benefits of exercise, the health risks associated with obesity, or the results of a recent nutritional study. At the same time, if you are a college student taking a fitness and wellness course, you may feel a sense of disconnect between those stories and your own life. You might wonder: What has any of this got to do with me?

Our primary goal in writing this textbook was simple: to get students to realize that the lifestyle choices you make now—regardless of your current age—have real and lasting effects on your lifelong wellness. How often you exercise, the types of food you eat, how well you manage your stress levels, whether or not you abuse drugs and alcohol—all of these factors can affect your health in profound and long-term ways.

We also wanted to write a textbook that takes into account the many challenges facing today's students. Perhaps you want to begin a fitness program, but don't live near a gym, or don't know where to start. Maybe you've tried to lose weight in the past, only to gain all of it back—or tried to quit smoking, only to relapse within a month. Perhaps you're a "nontraditional" college student with a family to support, and little time for exercise or stress management. We have written this book with you in mind—to offer you maximum flexibility and options for creating a fitness and wellness program that you can personalize for your own goals and time demands.

Finally, we wanted this textbook to address a common fact of life: the gap between knowing what we *ought* to do (for example, exercise more, eat healthier foods, quit smoking, etc.) and actually *doing it*. Throughout this textbook, we emphasize that effective behavior change is a gradual process, based on having realistic expectations and setting achievable short-term and long-term goals. We offer numerous strategies for overcoming obstacles to behavior change, as well as tools for taking active measures to live a healthier lifestyle.

With these goals in mind, the following are some of the unique features you'll find in this textbook.

KEY FEATURES OF THIS TEXT

- **Case Studies** presented at the beginning of each chapter introduce an engaging "character" who reflects the concerns and questions that readers are likely to have themselves. Questions listed at the end of the case studies are designed to test your recall of the material, to encourage critical thinking, and to help you apply the chapter's topics to your own life.

- **Labs are designed to teach skills, assess your current fitness/wellness, and commit to lasting behavior change.** The book includes three types of labs: 1) a skill-acquisition lab, 2) a self-assessment lab, and 3) an action-plan lab. Together, the labs teach you how to assess your current level of fitness/wellness, introduce practical lifelong skills, and encourage real behavior change. *You'll find online versions of all of the labs for* Get Fit, Stay Well! *at the book's website at:* **www.aw-bc.com/hopson.** *We also offer many additional labs online, designed to accommodate varying skill levels, differing access to equipment, and the specific needs of students with disabilities.*

- **The most modern presentation of strength-training techniques available** includes over 70 photos of strength-training and flexibility exercises, featuring actual college students, modern gym equipment, and options for students with limited access to equipment (such as resistance band exercises). We organize the exercises by muscles worked so that exercisers can make apples-to-apples comparisons and choose the most appropriate exercise for their individual needs. We also include orientation diagrams alongside exercise photos to show exactly which muscle groups benefit. *You can find videos of many*

exercises, as well as many alternate exercises, at **www.aw-bc.com/hopson.**

- **A separate chapter on diabetes** (and other chronic diseases) provides valuable, up-to-date information about one of today's national health epidemics—and what you can do today to avoid chronic health problems in the future.

- **A strong emphasis on behavior change.** *Try it Now!* boxes provide suggestions for immediate action (such as logging on to *MyPyramid.com* for an analysis of your daily diet and physical activity). *Tools for Change* boxes provide tools for longer-term change (such as how to make healthy choices while dining out). "Plan for Change" labs allow you to write out and commit to action plans for behavior change. This textbook also comes automatically packaged with the *Behavior Change Logbook,* which provides numerous strategies for making healthy lifestyle decisions with staying power.

- **Facts and Fallacies** boxes investigate common questions and controversies relevant to chapter topics. Topics covered include "Does Spot Reduction Work?" (p. 118), "Can You Be Overweight and Fit?" (p. 205), and "Is it Safe to Eat Fish?" (p. 233).

- **Understanding Diversity** boxes address topics relevant to diverse student populations—acknowledging that age, race, gender, disability, and individual life circumstances can result in specific fitness and wellness needs. Topics covered include "Women and Weight Training" (p. 114), "Do You Have Special Vitamin and Mineral Needs?" (p. 236), "Getting Active Despite Disability" (p. 42), and "Stress in Traditional and Nontraditional Students" (p. 303).

- **Spotlight** boxes highlight interesting or current topics related to the chapter at hand, including "Tracking Your Fitness Program Online," (p. 62), "Sleep,

Performance, and Stress" (p. 306), and "An Example of the Stretch Reflex" (p. 162).

- **A running glossary** helps you easily review and master key terms.

- **End-of-chapter review questions and critical thinking questions** encourage you to review and evaluate material you've just read.

- **Research citations** demonstrate the accuracy, currency, and scientific grounding for information presented in the text.

- **A pre- and post-course progress worksheet** at the beginning of the book allows you to assess your progress on key fitness/wellness assessments, before and after you implement a fitness/wellness program.

- **Sample fitness programs** in Appendix B provide templates for fitness programs designed for beginning exercisers.

INSTRUCTOR SUPPLEMENTS

This textbook comes with unparalleled supplemental resources to assist instructors with classroom preparation and presentation.

TEACHING TOOL BOX

Save hours of valuable planning time with one comprehensive course planning kit. Adjuncts, part-time, and full-time faculty alike will find in one box a wealth of supplements and resources that reinforce key learning from the text and suit virtually any teaching style. The Teaching Tool Box includes:

- A comprehensive Media Manager which provides **all art, photos, and tables from the text; PowerPoint lecture presentations; a computerized test bank; ABC**

News videos on health/fitness topics; PRS-enabled Active Lecture (clicker) Questions; Quiz Show Game questions; and over 80 exercise demonstration videos.

- **Full-color transparency acetates** that include all art and tables, as well as selected photos from the book.

- **Instructor's Resource Manual/Test Bank** that includes detailed chapter summaries, suggested readings, a video list, and over 1600 test bank questions in multiple-choice, true/false, matching, and short-essay formats.

- Access to **MyFitnessLab** course management website (see detailed description below)

- **Fitness Support Manual** including first-time teaching tips, chapter outlines, and sample syllabi.

- **Great Ideas: Active Ways to Teach Health and Wellness** is loaded with teaching tips from instructors on how to make class come alive, including collaborative and active learning techniques and effective use of technology in the classroom.

- **Take Charge of Your Health Worksheets** contain 50 self-assessment worksheets covering a wide variety of topics.

- **Course-at-a-Glance Reference Guide** is your roadmap to the many assets in the Teaching Tool Box. Resources are organized chapter by chapter so you can easily see the assets available for each chapter in the book.

MYFITNESSLAB
www.aw-bc.com/myfitnesslab
This online course management program is loaded with valuable teaching resources that

make it easy to give assignments and track student progress. Powered by CourseCompass™, the preloaded content in MyFitnessLab includes **unsurpassed resources for teaching online or hybrid courses,** including:

- Audio/visual lectures that students can view online

- Lab worksheets from the book in online format

- Many additional labs, designed and adapted for students with varying levels of fitness, differing levels of access to equipment, and those with disabilities

- ABC News Lecture Launcher video clips

- Over 80 exercise demonstration videos in downloadable format, focusing on strength training and flexibility exercises. Many of these exercises can be done at home with readily available equipment such as resistance bands, free weights, and stability balls

- Online quizzes and test bank

- A robust, annotatable E-book version of *Get Fit, Stay Well!*

STUDENT SUPPLEMENTS

COMPANION WEBSITE FOR *GET FIT, STAY WELL!*

www.aw-bc.com/hopson

The *Get Fit, Stay Well!* companion website offers students hundreds of practice quiz questions, online labs, 50 health self-assessment worksheets, web links to fitness/wellness-related topics, glossary/flashcards to review key terms, and over 80 exercise demonstration videos.

NEW LIFESTYLES DIGITAL FIVE-STEP PEDOMETER

This digital pedometer includes a time clock and measures number of steps taken, distance covered (in miles), activity time, and calories burned. For information about packaging the pedometer with student texts, please contact your local Pearson sales representative.

BEHAVIOR CHANGE LOG BOOK AND WELLNESS JOURNAL

Automatically packaged with student copies of the textbook, this booklet helps students track their daily exercise and nutritional intake and create a personalized long-term nutrition and fitness program. It also includes a behavior change contract and topics for journal-based activities.

LIVE RIGHT! BEATING STRESS IN COLLEGE AND BEYOND

This booklet gives students useful tips for coping with stressful life challenges both during college and throughout life. Topics include sleep, managing finances, time management, coping with academic pressure, and relationships.

EAT RIGHT! HEALTHY EATING IN COLLEGE AND BEYOND

This handy, full-color booklet provides students with practical guidelines, tips, shopper's guides and recipes that turn healthy eating principles into blueprints for action. Topics include healthy eating in the cafeteria, dorm room, and fast-food restaurants; planning meals on a budget; weight management; vegetarian alternatives; and the effects of alcohol on health.

MYDIETANALYSIS

Powered by ESHA Research, Inc., MyDietAnalysis features a database of nearly 20,000 foods. This easy-to-use program allows students to track their diet and activity for up to three profiles and to assess the nutritional value of their food consumption.

MYFITNESSLAB

www.aw-bc.com/myfitnesslab
Powered by CourseCompass™, the preloaded content in MyFitnessLab includes **unsurpassed resources for students taking online or hybrid courses,** including:

- Audio/visual lectures that students can view online

- Lab worksheets from the book in online format

- Many additional labs, designed and adapted for students with varying levels of fitness, differing levels of access to equipment, and those with disabilities

- ABC News Lecture Launcher video clips

- Over 80 exercise demonstration videos in downloadable format, focusing on strength training and flexibility exercises. Many of these exercises can be done at home with readily available equipment, such as resistance bands, free weights, and stability balls

- Online practice quizzes

- An annotatable E-book version of *Get Fit, Stay Well!*

ACKNOWLEDGMENTS

From Janet Hopson

Preparing and releasing a new book such as *Get Fit, Stay Well!*—along with its accompanying study and instructional materials—is an enormous undertaking. The authors' efforts are just part of a complex, well-integrated team effort. We would like to thank the following members of the Benjamin Cummings book team: Barbara Yien, who so ably, tirelessly, and cheerfully coordinated and managed this huge program; Frank Ruggirello, Sandra Lindelof, and Deirdre Espinoza, who all championed this book in its early stages; Cathy Murphy and Laura Southworth, our text and art development editors; Beth Masse, Linda Kern, and Heather Meledin, our production coordinators; art editor Donna Kalal; photo researcher Kristin Piljay; Yvo Riezebos, who is responsible for this book's striking and dynamic design; Susan Scharf, who prepared and coordinated the many excellent print ancillaries that accompany the book; Erik Fortier, who managed the superb web/multimedia supplements; ancillaries authors Natalie Rose, Teresa Snow, Laura Bonazzoli, and Elizabeth O'Neill; and Neena Bali and Josh Frost, who handled the important task of making sure this book's development was informed by extensive instructor and student feedback. We would also like to thank the following individuals who each played important roles along the way: CJ Jones, Elena Dorfman, Betsy Roll, Marcy Lunetta, Laura Stone, Elisa Rassen, Deborah Cogan, Claire Alexander, Mark Wales, and Jacob Evans. Without all of you, there would be no *Get Fit, Stay Well!,* and any success the book may have in reaching and helping students belongs to the entire team.

From Rebecca Donatelle

After working on several college textbooks over the years, one thing has become very clear to me: the publishing house you choose to work with is the single most important factor in producing a quality textbook that is going to be successful in the marketplace. Benjamin Cummings has assembled a truly remarkable group of top-notch acquisition, editorial, production, marketing, sales, and ancillary staff to help "birth" and nurture a text through development and ultimate growth. I am fortunate to have had the opportunity to work with individuals who worry the details and possess an incredible degree of creativity and professionalism. You are truly THE BEST . . . thank you so much to each and every one of you. Additionally, I would like to thank my co-authors, Jan and Tanya. From conceptualization to final product, this text would not have happened without your efforts.

From Tanya Littrell

I could not have even entertained the idea of working on this project without the support of my husband, Erik Offner, and my son, Garen Marter. These two have lived with me through the ups and downs, the deadlines, the stress, and the great feeling of completion. I love you both and could not have done it without you. I would also like to thank fellow faculty members at Portland Community College who have been supportive throughout this project; in particular, Janeen Hull, a faculty peer and friend who was always there to talk, read text, and "check-in" about anything. My graduate work and teaching at Oregon State University really set the stage for my work on this project, and so I would like to thank Anthony Wilcox, department chair of Nutrition and Exercise Sciences, for having faith in me as an instructor and giving me teaching and supervisory experience that lead to this opportunity.

REVIEWERS, CLASS TESTERS, AND FOCUS GROUP PARTICIPANTS

We would like to thank the hundreds of instructors and students who reviewed, class-tested, and/or participated in focus groups for earlier drafts of this text. Your feedback was instrumental to this book's development!

REVIEWERS

John Acquaviva, Northern Virginia Community College–Annandale
Helaine Alessio, Miami University
Tom Altena, Missouri State University–Springfield
Kym Atwood, University of West Florida
Christina Beaudoin, University of Southern Maine
Carol Biddington, California University of Pennsylvania
Robert Bowen, Northern Michigan University
Ron Carda, University of Wisconsin–Madison
Tony Caterisano, Furman University
Curt Cattau, Concordia University–Irvine
Deborah Cavion, Mount San Antonio College
Trey Cone, University of Central Oklahoma
J. Sunshine Cowan, University of Central Oklahoma
Richard DeMarco, Greenville Technical College

Mandi Dupain, Millersville University
Michael Dupper, The University of Mississippi
Nancy Estes, Broward Community College
Tammy Evetovich, Wayne State College
Kelly Frazier, Furman University
Ken Grace, Chabot College
Melissa Haithcox, Edinboro
Jeffrey Hallam, The University of Mississippi
Karen Hand, Northern Illinois University
Kevin Harper, University of Texas–Arlington
Ronnie Harris, Jacksonville State University
Amy Howton, Kennesaw State University
Erica Jackson, Kennesaw State University
Sandy Kimbrough, Texas A&M University–Commerce
Garry Ladd, Southwestern Illinois College
Rosemary Lindle, University of Maryland–College Park
Julie Lombardi, Millersville University
Dennis Mishko, Keystone College
Scott Murr, Furman University
Elizabeth O'Neill, Central Connecticut State University
Kelly Quick, University of Sioux Falls
Charles Pelitera, Canisius College
Julian Reed, Furman University
Betsy Reeder, Harford Community College
Matthew Rothbard, Towson University
Amy Rowland, City University of New York
Carl Runk, Towson University
Tammy Sabourin, Valencia Community College–East
Barbara Shewfelt, Foothill College
Jacob Silvestri, Hudson Valley Community College

Jason Slack, Utah Valley State College
Kenneth Sparks, Cleveland State University
Sean Stickney, Kennesaw State University
Deborah Stone, Louisiana State University
Linda Tiedt, St. Louis Community College–Meramec
Kelly Van Gorden, Bloomsburg University
Barbara Walker, St. Ambrose University
Jennifer White, University of Wisconsin–Whitewater
Andrea Willis, Abraham Baldwin Agricultural College

CLASS TESTERS

Abraham Baldwin Agricultural College: Andrea Willis
Anderson University: James R. Scott, Becky Hull
Arkansas State University: Janet Benight, Pam Burke
Auburn University: Jared Russell, Justin Shroyer
Augusta State University: Lurelia Hardy, Shirley Darracott, Charles Darracott
Bloomsburg University: Kelly VanGorden, Andrea Fradkin
Brigham Young University–Hawaii: Donna Chun
Broward Community College: Ibis Dominguez, Sharon Rifkin, Nancy Estes, Lisa Bernstein
California Baptist University: Nicole MacDonald
California State University, Fresno: Mark Baldis, Felicia Greer
California University of Pennsylvania: Chris Harman
Cameron University: Joe Jones
Canisius College: Charles Pelitera
Cape Fear Community College: Donald "Doc" Wilson
Chabot College: Jeffrey Drouin
Coastal Carolina University: Christine Rockey
College of San Mateo: Tania Beliz
Concordia College: Marion Askegaard

East Central University: Kent Franz
Edinboro University of Pennsylvania: George Roberts
El Camino College: Tom Storer
Florida International University: Laura Blitzer
Furman University: Scott Murr, William Pierce, Alicia Powers
Greenville Technical College: Melissa Adrian
Harding University: Kenneth Turley
Illinois State University: Karen Kae Dennis
Indiana University: Susan Simmons
Jacksonville State University: Donna Hey
Kennesaw State University: Amy Howton, Natalie Rose
Keystone College: Dorothy Anthony, Dennis Mishko
LeTourneau University: Wayne Jacobs
Lock Haven University: Martha Rowedder
Mercer County Community College: John Kalinowski
Miami University: Randal Claytor
Midwestern State University: Julie Wood
Missouri State University: Gayle Runke
Montgomery County Community College: Anne Livezey, Georgette Howell
Moraine Valley Community College: Cathy Nolan
Northern Virginia Community College–Annandale: John Acquaviva, Gamal Aboshadi
Pacific Lutheran University: Bradford Moore, Stephanie Kerr, Allison Stringer
Penn State University: Megan Schuchert
Raritan Valley Community College: Augie Eosso, Linda Romaine
Salem State College: George Abboud
St. Ambrose University: Jason Vorwerk
Tarleton State University: Lance Drake, Penny Wright
Tarrant County College, Northeast: Donna Gardner
Texas A&M University–Kingsville: Judy Bloomquist

Texas A&M University–Commerce: Sandy Kimbrough
Truckee Meadows Community College: Andrea Simone-Call
Truman State University: Evonne Bird
University of Central Oklahoma: J. Sunshine Cowan
University of Mississippi: Jeffrey Hallam
University of Nebraska: Christina Perry
University of Sioux Falls: Kelly Quick, Rebecca Schultz
University of Texas–Pan American: Marcelo Schmidt
University of West Florida: Kym Atwood
University of Wisconsin–Madison: Ronnie Carda
Valdosta State University: Jennifer Sue Head
Valencia Community College–East: Tammy Sabourin
Western Carolina University: William Papin
Western Michigan University: Carol Weideman
York College of CUNY: Nancy Palladino

FOCUS GROUP/FORUM PARTICIPANTS

John Acquaviva, Northern Virginia Community College–Annandale
Dorothy Anthony, Keystone College
Michael Bird, Truman State University
Ron Carda, University of Wisconsin
Donna Chun, Brigham Young University–Hawaii
Donna Cobb, University of Central Oklahoma
Trey Cone, University of Central Oklahoma
Joel Dering, Cameron University

Laura Dillman, Abilene Christian University
Mandi Dupain, Millersville University
John Downing, Missouri State University
Nancy Estes, Broward Community College
Patrick Gelinas, Dutchess Community College
Melissa Haithcox, Edinboro University
Abdelhadi Halawa, Millersville University
David Harackiewicz, Central Connecticut State University
Chris Harman, California University of Pennsylvania
Kevin Harper, Tarrant County College–Northeast
Ronnie Harris, Jacksonville State University
Amy Howton, Kennesaw State University
Miranda Kaye, Pennsylvania State University
Julie Lombardi, Millersville University
Jay Merhoff, East Central College
Amy McKay, Tarleton State University
Natalie Rose, Kennesaw State University
Gayle Runke, Missouri State University
Tammy Sabourin, Valencia Community College–East
Cara Sidman, University of Wisconsin–Whitewater
Teresa Snow, Georgia Institute of Technology
Marilyn Strawbridge, Butler University
Scott Strohmeyer, University of Central Missouri
Carol Weideman, Western Michigan University
Susan Whitlock, Kennesaw State University

Many thanks to all!

GET FIT, STAY WELL!

Brief Edition

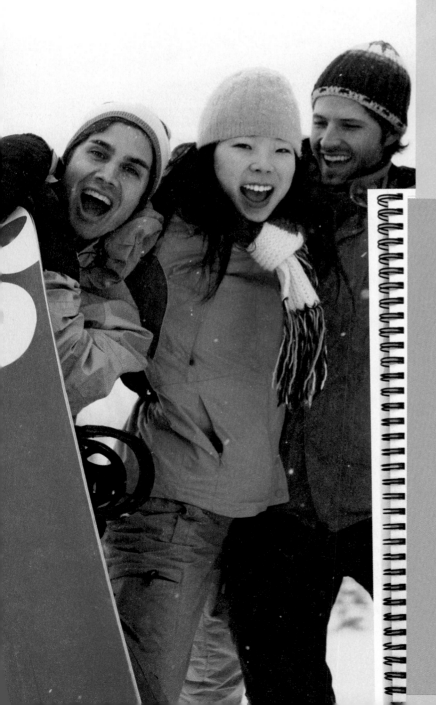

CHAPTER 1

Making Personal Wellness Choices

OBJECTIVES

Describe the six dimensions of wellness.

Explain the benefits of wellness for individuals and for society as a whole.

Identify six basic wellness behaviors.

Identify the typical stages of the behavior change process.

Create a plan for changing a specific behavior.

Carlos

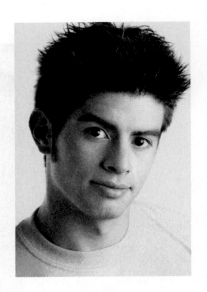

"Hi, I'm Carlos. I just started my freshman year in college. It's my first time living away from home, and there are a lot of new things to get used to. I know my family sacrificed a lot for me to be here, so I feel pressure to do well. I also miss my girlfriend, Liz—she has one year of high school left, and it's been really hard being away from her. I like my classes so far, but I am never caught up with my reading, and I haven't had a good night's sleep in about three weeks. To top it all off, I caught a cold that has been going around, and I feel miserable! What can I do to better manage my life?"

Can you relate to any of Carlos's problems? If so, you are not alone. A majority of college students report that stress, depression, inadequate sleep, frequent colds, and relationship problems are all factors that negatively affect their academic performance (Figure 1.1).[1] When asked to rate their overall **wellness,** at least one-third of college students described it as only fair or poor.

Wellness is an optimal soundness of body and mind. To understand wellness, it helps to first consider the concept of *health*. While historically the term "health" meant merely the absence of disease, experts today view it as a much more inclusive term that encompasses everything from environmental health to the health of populations. The term *wellness* conveys a more distinct, personalized definition of health. It is the achievement of the highest level of health possible in physical, social, intellectual, emotional, environmental, and spiritual dimensions. It describes a vibrant state in which a person enjoys life to the fullest, adapts relatively easily to life's many challenges, feels that life is meaningful, and functions effectively in society. Wellness behaviors include healthy eating, regular exercise, weight management, and stress manage-

wellness The achievement of the highest level of health possible in physical, social, intellectual, emotional, environmental, and spiritual dimensions

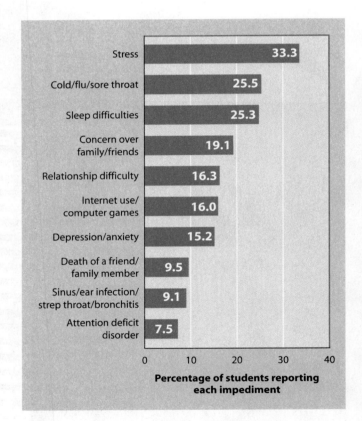

FIGURE 1.1

The top 10 impediments to academic performance, as reported by students.

Data from: American College Health Association, "National College Health Assessment, Reference Group Executive Summary, Fall 2006" (Baltimore: American College Health Association, 2007).

UNDERSTANDING DIVERSITY

NONTRADITIONAL STUDENTS AND WELLNESS

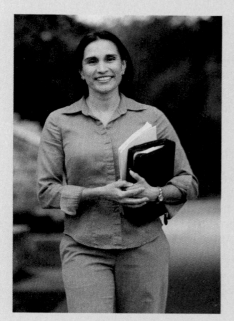

Since the 1980s, there has been a steady decline in the percentages of *traditional students* at colleges and universities—that is, 18- to 24-year-olds who go right on to college after high school with financial support from their parents.[1] During the same time period, schools have welcomed more and more *nontraditional students*—those who are 25 or older and who have spent time working, doing military service, or engaging in other activities before returning to post–high school education, full- or part-time. Nontraditional students represent at least 40 percent of today's college students, and they broaden our discussion of student wellness.

Nontraditional students are usually employed, self-supporting, and are often married with children; thus, their wellness needs differ from those of younger students. Because many of them juggle work, school, and family, they often need and derive special benefit from stress management skills.[2] Many find less time for exercise and benefit from encouragement and new ideas for increasing activity. Nontraditional students make meals for themselves and for children more often than do traditional students and thus have broader nutritional considerations. Nearly two-thirds of nontraditional students are women and can participate in screenings and programs for women's and children's medicine.[3]

Nontraditional students also tend to partake more in career counseling programs, but less in social support services than do younger traditional students. Many see themselves as unprepared for vigorous college work and are more likely to be stressed and insecure about their academic performance.[4] As a result, they tend to seek psychological and career counseling more often than traditional students as a support for staying in school. At the same time, most nontraditional students report having strong social support from family and friends, and thus appear to be richer in social wellness than younger students.

Sources:
1. Laura Gail Lunsford, "Post Secondary Education for Non-Traditional Students— The New Majority," North Carolina State University, January 2003.
2. Jane E. Myers and A. Keith Mobley, "Wellness of Undergraduates: Comparisons of Traditional and Non-traditional Students," *Journal of College Counseling 7* (April 2004).
3. Susan Molstad, and others, "Health Concerns and Needs of Nontraditional Women Students at a Rural Southern University," *College Student Journal* (September 2001).
4. Stephanie San Miguel Barriman, and others, "Non-Traditional Student's Service Needs and Social Support Resources. A Pilot Study," *Journal of College Counseling 7* (April 2004).

ment. In this book, we will sometimes use the terms *health* and *wellness* interchangeably, but wellness always refers to a more individualized, dynamic concept, requiring significant personal effort, but with the potential to bring great rewards.

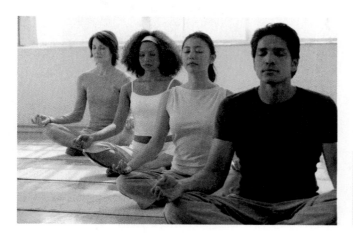

Central to wellness is **physical fitness,** or simply *fitness,* the ability to perform moderate to vigorous levels of physical activity without undue fatigue. Fitness is just one dimension of wellness, but we give it special attention in this book because it influences so many of the other dimensions and because the tools for improving fitness are readily available while you are a college student—a period in your life when you can establish personal habits that will benefit you for a lifetime.

physical fitness The ability to perform moderate to vigorous levels of physical activity without undue fatigue

No single college course can address every health concern or guarantee a lifetime of wellness. Your age, personal history, genetic susceptibility to medical conditions, and the environment you live in all affect your wellness, as do access to high-quality medical care, nutritious food, exercise facilities, and social support networks. Nevertheless, this book will provide effective tools to help you achieve an optimal level of wellness, including:

- information based on a solid foundation of health science and the most current scientific research;
- self-assessments that allow you to carefully examine your health behavior and make positive changes;
- strategies for fitness training, choosing nutritious food, and relieving stress;
- techniques for breaking harmful habits;
- guidance in setting personal goals for wellness behavior;
- reliable resources to assist you in health/wellness decision making.

Improving your wellness is an ambitious but highly achievable goal. The wellness patterns you establish in this course can change how you live each day and can positively affect your quality of life for years to come. We will provide the tools; the rest depends on your own motivation and efforts.

WHAT IS WELLNESS?

You may have healthy relationships, but no fondness for exercise. Perhaps your spiritual life is rich, but you have trouble juggling academic demands. Virtually everyone is stronger in some dimensions of wellness than others. Let's look at the six dimensions of wellness and how each contributes to optimal well-being.

physical wellness A state of physical health and well-being that includes body size and shape, body functioning, measures of strength and endurance, and resistance to disease

social wellness A person's degree of social connectedness and skills, leading to satisfying interpersonal relationships

WELLNESS HAS MANY DIMENSIONS

We can think of wellness as consisting of six dimensions: physical, social, intellectual, emotional, environmental, and spiritual (Figure 1.2). Wellness is a process, and at times you may experience faster growth in one dimension than in others. The dimensions are interconnected, however, so positive effort in one area can help you make progress in others and move you toward greater overall health and well-being.

Physical Wellness **Physical wellness** encompasses all aspects of a sound body, including body size and shape; sensory sharpness and responsiveness; body functioning; physical strength, flexibility, and endurance; resistance to diseases and disorders; and recuperative abilities. The physical state we call *fitness* includes measures of physical wellness and allows a person to exert physical effort without undue stress, strain, or injury. Many of your day-to-day choices and habits can support or undermine your physical wellness, including your diet; amount and types of exercise; sleep patterns; level of stress; use of tobacco, drugs, or alcohol; participation in unsafe sex; observance of traffic laws and wearing helmets and seat belts; daily hygiene (e.g., flossing and brushing teeth); and access to quality medical attention (e.g., regular checkups, vaccinations, and treatment).

Social Wellness **Social wellness** is the ability to have satisfying interpersonal relationships and

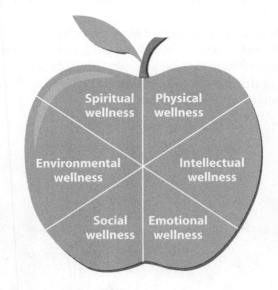

FIGURE 1.2

Wellness is an optimal level of health in six interconnected dimensions of human experience.

FACTS AND FALLACIES

CAN MONEY BUY HAPPINESS?

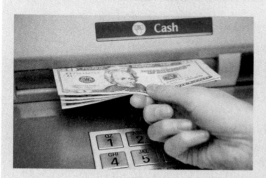

Like many Americans, many students are convinced that money can buy happiness. Debt from large student loans and credit card bills, however, can bring stress and anxiety. These, in turn, can affect academic performance and diminish physical and emotional wellness. Researchers have found that the most materialistic people they studied (those who desired the most money and possessions) reported more foul moods and fewer good moods than less materialistic people.[1] Their relationships are often distant and unfulfilling, and their money-making activities bring materialistic people less pleasure than pursuits such as socializing or volunteering. Most significantly, they tend to be dissatisfied with their amount of money and possessions, no matter how much they have.

The critical factor in materialism appears to be *why* one wants wealth. If a person's reasons for wanting money are mainly to overcome self-doubt, to gain power over others, or to win the race for bigger, better "toys," wealth is unlikely to bring happiness. However, if people want wealth to gain freedom or security, to feel self-pride, or to help others through altruistic giving, then money can indeed bring happiness and satisfaction. Money *can* buy happiness, researchers conclude, but only if you want it for the right reasons.[2]

Sources:
1. Bruce Bower, "Buyer Beware: Some Psychologists See Danger in Excessive Materialism," *Science News* 164 (September 6, 2003): 152–53.
2. A. Srivastava, E. A. Locke, and K. M. Bartol, "Money and Subjective Well-Being: It's Not the Money, It's the Motives," *Journal of Personal and Social Psychology* 80, no. 6 (June 2001): 959–71.

maintain social connectedness. This means you can successfully interact with others, adapt to a variety of social situations, and act appropriately in various settings. Whether you are shy and introverted or outgoing and extroverted, social wellness includes the ability to communicate clearly and effectively; the capacity to establish intimacy through trust and acceptance; a willingness to ask for and give support; an ability to maintain friendships over time; and skills for interacting within groups, such as on the job or in the community.

Intellectual Wellness

Intellectual wellness is the ability to use your brain power effectively to solve problems and meet life's challenges. It allows you to think clearly, quickly, creatively, and critically; use good reasoning and make careful decisions; continually learn from your successes and mistakes; organize and streamline your tasks; maintain a sense of humor; and manage your finances responsibly (see the box **Facts and Fallacies: Can Money Buy Happiness?**).

Emotional Wellness

Emotional wellness means being able to control your emotions and express them appropriately at the right times. Social and emotional problems—such as stress, anxiety, depression, and relationship problems—are increasingly common on college campuses and can impede academic success. Improving emotional wellness requires developing good self-esteem; gaining self-confidence; being able to cope with sadness, anger, resentment, or negativity; and developing an appropriate balance of emotional dependence and independence.

Environmental Wellness

Our home, work, community, and school environments can be relaxing, safe havens or toxic, threatening, and stressful places to be. **Environmental wellness**

intellectual wellness The ability to think clearly, reason objectively, analyze, and use your brain power to solve problems and meet life's challenges

emotional wellness The ability to control emotions and express them appropriately at the right times; includes self-esteem, self-confidence, self-efficacy, and other emotional qualities

environmental wellness An appreciation of the external environment and an understanding of the role one plays in preserving, protecting, and improving the world and its dwindling resources

| Irreversible damage | Chronic illness | Signs of illness | Average wellness | Increased wellness | Optimum wellness |

FIGURE 1.3
The double-headed arrow depicts the continuum of wellness states.

entails understanding how the environment can positively or negatively affect you; the role you play in preserving, protecting, and improving the world around you; and what you can do to conserve dwindling resources for future generations. Environmental wellness also encompasses occupational wellness—that is, access to a safe and healthy workplace.

Spiritual Wellness For some people, **spiritual wellness** may involve a belief in a supreme being or a way of life prescribed by a particular religion. For others, spiritual wellness is a feeling of unity or oneness with others and with nature, as well as having a sense of meaning or value in life. Developing greater spiritual wellness may deepen one's understanding of life's purpose; allow a person to feel a part of a greater spectrum of existence; and promote feelings of love, joy, peace, contentment, and wonder over life's experiences.

THE WELLNESS CONTINUUM

Striving for improvement in all six wellness dimensions is a lifelong process. One good approach is to concentrate on those dimensions that present the most pressing need, while working on the others in a steady but relaxed and motivated way. Most people progress at different speeds in different wellness areas. Over time, a balance of work on all the dimensions—one or two now, others later—will eventually promote overall wellness. Your brain and

body, your thoughts and emotions, your actions and reactions, your relationship to yourself and others—all are interconnected and integrated. Likewise, the dimensions of wellness are interrelated. Eating a nutritious diet, for example, will help you maintain your weight within a recommended range for your height. This, in turn, will benefit your physical fitness. Increasing exercise and general activity, even in the absence of better diet, will also help you manage stress, mood, and body weight. Taken together, your levels of wellness in each dimension place you along a continuum of greater or lesser total wellness (Figure 1.3). Understanding where you are on the **wellness continuum** is a good start to achieving new wellness goals.

Lab1.1 and *Lab1.2* at the end of the chapter will help you assess your current place on the wellness continuum and analyze areas that need improvement.

spiritual wellness A feeling of unity or oneness with people and nature and a sense of life's purpose, meaning, or value; for some, a belief in a supreme being or religion

wellness continuum A spectrum of wellness states from average to optimal in one direction and from average to premature death in the opposite direction

CASE STUDY

Carlos

"I know that my life is pretty good. I'm in college, studying what interests me, and I'm excited about the future. I just constantly feel behind. I'm falling asleep in class, eating a lot of junk food, and not exercising—who has time? Then I got this cold, partly because I have been stressed out and not sleeping much. I've made some friends in my dorm, and it helps to know that a lot of them are going through the same thing. Talking to Liz every night on the phone helps."

1. In which dimensions of wellness could Carlos be stronger? Where would you place him on the wellness continuum?

2. How do you compare to Carlos? In which dimensions of wellness do you feel strongest? In which dimensions could you improve?

WHY DOES WELLNESS MATTER?

Wellness has many benefits for individuals, as well as for society as a whole.

GOOD WELLNESS HABITS CAN HELP YOU LIVE A LONGER, HEALTHIER LIFE

In the United States, the average life expectancy at birth for males is 75 years, and for females it is 80 years (Table 1.1).[2] The average *healthy life expectancy*—the years a person can expect to live without disability or major illness—is 67 for males and 71 for females.[3] Maintaining good wellness habits can help extend your overall life expectancy, as well as your *healthy* life expectancy.

Consider the leading causes of death among Americans ages 20–24 (Figure 1.4).[4] Note that accidents kill more young adults than almost all the other causes combined. By making better wellness choices—such as wearing seat belts and bike helmets, and avoiding dangerous behaviors such as driving under the influence of drugs or alcohol—you can reduce your risk of premature death in an accident.

Among Americans of all ages, the leading causes of death are heart disease and cancer (Figure 1.5).[5] Adults contribute greatly to their own risk for these diseases through poor diets, inactivity, and smoking.[6] By eating a healthy diet, exercising,

TABLE 1.1

Life Expectancy and Healthy Life Expectancy by Country and Gender

Country	Healthy Life Expectancy—Males	Healthy Life Expectancy—Females	Life Expectancy—Males	Life Expectancy—Females
Zimbabwe	34	33	37	34
Somalia	36	38	43	45
India	53	54	61	63
Russia	53	64	59	72
Bangladesh	55	53	62	63
Brazil	57	62	67	74
Argentina	62	68	71	78
China	63	65	70	74
Mexico	63	68	72	77
Kuwait	67	67	76	78
United States	67	71	75	80
France	69	75	76	83
Greece	69	73	77	82
United Kingdom	69	72	76	81
Canada	70	74	78	83
Germany	70	74	76	82
Spain	70	75	77	83
Italy	71	75	78	84
Japan	72	78	79	86
Sweden	72	75	78	83

Source: World Health Organization, World Health Statistics 2007.

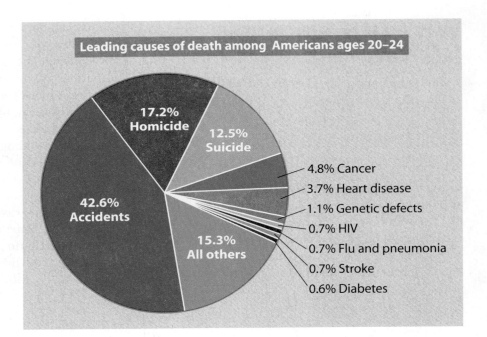

FIGURE **1.4**

The leading causes of death among Americans ages 20–24.

Source: *National Vital Statistics Reports* 55, no. 10 (March 15, 2007).

Leading causes of death among Americans ages 20–24

17.2% Homicide
12.5% Suicide
4.8% Cancer
3.7% Heart disease
1.1% Genetic defects
0.7% HIV
0.7% Flu and pneumonia
0.7% Stroke
0.6% Diabetes
42.6% Accidents
15.3% All others

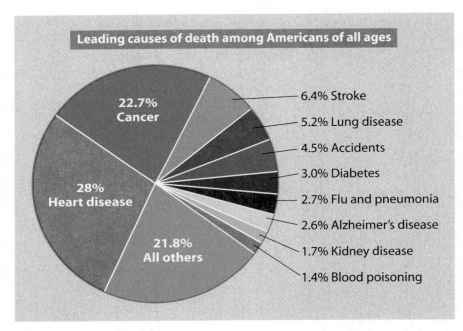

Leading causes of death among Americans of all ages

22.7% Cancer
6.4% Stroke
5.2% Lung disease
4.5% Accidents
3.0% Diabetes
2.7% Flu and pneumonia
2.6% Alzheimer's disease
1.7% Kidney disease
1.4% Blood poisoning
28% Heart disease
21.8% All others

FIGURE **1.5**

The leading causes of death among Americans of all ages.

Source: *National Vital Statistics Reports* 55, no. 10 (March 15, 2007).

and avoiding smoking, you can reduce your risk of developing these diseases. Figure 1.6 shows some of the *modifiable* risk factors for heart disease—that is, risk factors that are within your control. High blood pressure, tobacco use, alcohol use, high cholesterol, obesity, low fruit and vegetable intake, and physical inactivity are all risk factors that, to some extent, are within your power to change.

sedentary Physically inactive; exerting physical effort only for required daily tasks and not for leisure-time exercise

The role of physical activity in decreasing your risk of developing disease is especially compelling. Researchers have shown in hundreds of studies that the vast majority of all illnesses of middle age and later years (including heart disease, cancer, and type-2 diabetes) are related to, and exacerbated by, a lack of physical exercise.[7] Living a **sedentary** life also increases the danger of *hypokinetic diseases*— conditions that can be triggered or worsened by too little movement or activity, such as obesity, back pain, and high blood pressure. Figure 1.7 illustrates some of the health benefits of regular physical activity.

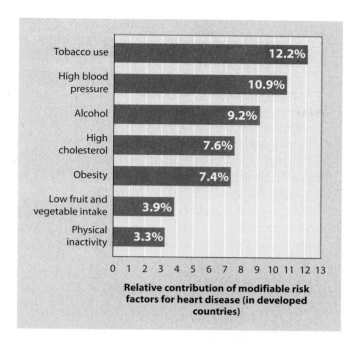

FIGURE 1.6

Tobacco use, alcohol use, and physical inactivity are among the preventable behaviors that contribute to the development of heart disease.

Data from: World Health Organization.

In 1996, the U.S. Surgeon General released a report highlighting the role of physical fitness in overall wellness, and emphasized that most Americans are too inactive.[8] Since that early report, several national agencies have surveyed Americans' activity, diet, and weight patterns. The conclusion: We are one of the most sedentary and overweight nations on earth.[9] Both the American Heart Association and the American College of Sports Medicine now recommend that all healthy adults between the ages of 18 and 65 strive for at least 30 minutes of moderate exercise five days a week, or at least 20 minutes of vigorous exercise three days a week.[10] We will discuss these recommendations in more detail in Chapter 2.

GOOD WELLNESS HABITS BENEFIT SOCIETY AS A WHOLE

A population with high levels of wellness is happier, more productive, and spends less money on health care. Accordingly, achieving better wellness and combating today's chronic diseases are important national priorities.

The Office of the Surgeon General cites six major public health priorities related to disease

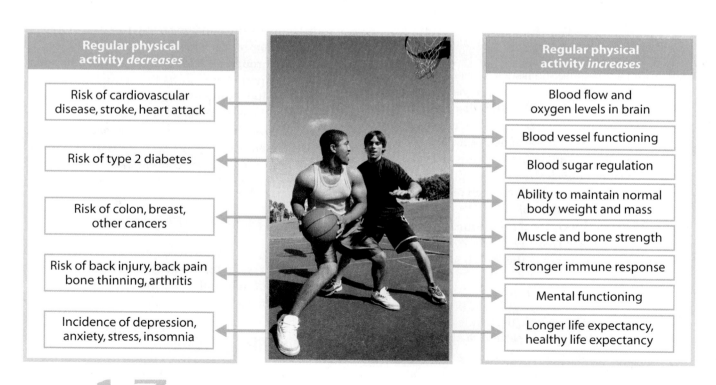

FIGURE 1.7
Regular physical activity results in many health benefits.

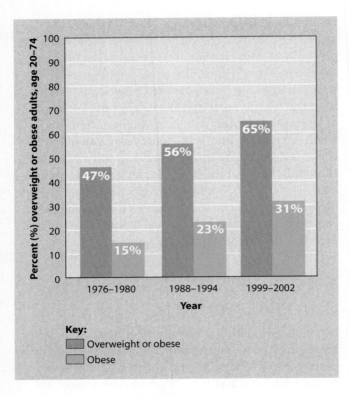

1.8

Overweight and obese adults are now the clear majority, with percentages rising steadily in the past 30 years.

Source: National Center for Health Statistics, based on data from the 1999–2002 National Health and Nutrition Examination Survey (NHANES).

prevention: addressing the issues of overweight and obesity (see Figure 1.8), increasing physical activity, preventing the spread of HIV/AIDS, discouraging tobacco use, preventing birth defects, and preventing injury.[11] In order to address some of these priorities, the Surgeon General advises Americans to eat healthier, be more physically active, not smoke, limit alcohol, and avoid drugs—all of which are wellness behaviors. Other national public health priorities cited by the Surgeon General are summarized in a set of objectives titled *Healthy People 2010*, which has two broad goals: to increase the length and quality of

behavior change An organized, deliberate effort to alter or replace an existing habit or pattern of activity

stages of behavior change From the transtheoretical model, a set of states most people pass through in their awareness of, determination to alter, and efforts to replace existing habits or actions

life, and to eliminate health disparities between different groups based on race, gender, ethnicity, and income.

The high cost of health care and health insurance is a major concern for Americans. In 2005, Americans spent $2 trillion on health care, or 16 percent of the gross domestic product (GDP).[12] Employer health insurance premiums increased by 7.7 percent in 2006, at twice the rate of inflation.[13] Nearly 47 million Americans do not have health insurance, largely due to the high cost of coverage—making them less likely to seek preventive care and adopt wellness behaviors early enough to prevent illness down the line.[14]

WHAT ARE THE STAGES OF BEHAVIOR CHANGE?

Nearly every topic in this textbook requires some shift in old habits to make way for new wellness behaviors—new ways of thinking and acting. Despite good intentions, many people fail to accomplish the changes they want, at least the first time around. That's partly because we tend to see change as a singular *event* instead of a *process* that requires preparation, has several stages, and takes time to succeed. It's very common, for example, for a person to "go cold turkey" on smoking or drinking or being a couch potato. Changes initiated on the spur of the moment, however, seldom work. Classic research shows that we must go through a series of mental and emotional stages over a period of months to adequately prepare ourselves for **behavior change**.[15]

The transtheoretical model of behavior change, developed by psychologists James Prochaska and Carlo DiClemente, delineates six **stages of behavior change:** precontemplation, contemplation, preparation, action, maintenance, and termination.

PRECONTEMPLATION

People in the precontemplation stage have no current intention of changing. They may have tried to change an old habit and given up, or they may be in denial and unaware of the problem.

CONTEMPLATION

In this stage, people recognize that they have a problem and begin to contemplate the need to change within 6 months or so. People can languish in this stage for months or years, however, realizing that they have a negative wellness pattern, such as smoking, poor nutrition, or too little exercise but lacking the time, energy, or commitment to make the change.

PREPARATION

Most people at this stage are within a month or so of taking action. They have thought about what they might do and may even have come up with a plan. Rather than thinking about why they can't begin, they have started to focus on what they can do.

ACTION

In this stage, people begin to execute their action plans. Unfortunately, many people try to take shortcuts; they start behavior change here rather than going through the earlier stages. However, without making a plan, publicly stating the desire to change, enlisting other people's help, and setting realistic goals, they are likely to fail.

MAINTENANCE

In the maintenance stage, people work to prevent a relapse into old habits through a conscious application of wellness tools and techniques. Maintenance requires vigilance, attention to detail, and long-term commitment. You are in the maintenance stage after you have incorporated the new action and have continued it for 6 months or longer without relapse into old habits. Common causes of relapse include overconfidence, daily temptations, stress or emotional distractions, and putting yourself down. It is important to guard against relapse by getting help

from a support group or campus resources when needed.

TERMINATION

At the termination stage, the new behavior is ingrained. This is the last step in the stages of behavior change.

HOW CAN YOU CHANGE YOUR BEHAVIOR?

If you are like most people, you have made a New Year's resolution on January 1, worked hard to adopt some new behavior until about the 10th, started slipping back to your old habits by the 15th, and forgotten about the whole thing by the 31st. Your resolution may well have been a new wellness behavior—lots of resolutions are. Perhaps it was an easy one like "eat more fruit," and you succeeded. More likely, it was a harder one like "start lifting weights three times a week," or "lose 20 pounds," or "give up junk food"—and despite your good intentions, it just didn't stick.

The transtheoretical model we just discussed shows that changing behaviors usually involves a gradual process of awareness, preparation, and *then* action. Understanding this process can help you proceed more deliberately to identify and successfully change a problem behavior. The rest of this chapter takes you through a series of practical steps inspired by the transtheoretical model. Keep in mind that these steps are not linear: People often start one, achieve certain parts of it, and then

CASE STUDY

Carlos

"Here are all of the things I'd like to do in an ideal world: sleep eight hours a night, eat less junk food, exercise more, ace all of my exams, and still have a social life! But I know I can't just snap my fingers and make all of that happen right away. Right now, my main priority is to try to manage my stress level better. I *really* have to get more sleep—it doesn't do me any good to stay up all night studying and then fall asleep in class. Some of my friends take 'power naps' in the afternoon. I might try that! I'm also thinking of signing up for a gym class next

quarter. That way I can be sure to work some exercise into my schedule. Beyond that—well, I think I should probably take things one at a time."

1. What are Carlos's main wellness goals? Where is he in the stages of behavior change for each of them?

2. Name a wellness behavior that you would like to change. In what stage of behavior change would you categorize yourself?

backtrack to work longer on aspects of earlier steps that are more difficult for them. These steps do get easier with practice. They are:

Step 1: Learn about basic wellness behaviors.

Step 2: Prepare to change a behavior.

Step 3: Acquire specific skills that support successful change.

Step 4: Apply what you have learned to change a specific behavior.

Let's examine each of these steps in more detail.

STEP ONE: LEARN ABOUT BASIC WELLNESS BEHAVIORS

The basic wellness behaviors are simple: Strive for fitness. Eat well. Manage your weight. Manage your stress level. Get enough rest to refresh and restore your energy. Avoid tobacco, drugs, and too much alcohol. Practice accident, injury, and disease prevention.

Stay Physically Fit Nowhere does the phrase "Use it or lose it" apply more fully than to your physical fitness. Much of the decline people expect with advancing age is, in fact, a reflection of inactivity and its toll on the body. Staying active every day is probably the single most important wellness behavior you can adopt. This book will encourage you to develop active habits—such as walking and taking the stairs instead of driving and riding the elevator—and make them part of your daily life. Chapters 2–7 will specifically guide you in developing a fitness program that is tailored to your needs.

What motivates some people to exercise but not others? The box **Tools for Change: What Moves You?** explores recent research on exercise motivation in students.

Eat Healthily The American diet tends to be light on nutrition and heavy on calories. Consider this fact: people who move to the United States from other countries often gain weight and develop chronic diseases at elevated rates compared to residents of those other countries.[16] Most Americans consume more calories than we burn off each day. We also tend to eat too much protein, salt, sugar, animal fat, and solidified vegetable oils (*trans* fats). We consume too little fiber and too few helpings of fruits and vegetables.[17] Chapter 8 discusses nutrition and its many benefits, including more energy,

greater stamina, better weight management, stronger disease resistance, and reduced risk of chronic illness.

Manage Your Weight Some people are naturally slim, while others inherit genes for easy weight gain or difficult weight loss. Nevertheless, four factors you *can* control are just as important: your activity level, exercise habits, eating habits, and stress management. As we saw in Figure 1.8, over 60 percent of American adults have a body weight and mass (fat-to-lean ratio) above recommended ranges. Overweight and obesity are correlated with arthritis, bone and joint problems, back pain, decreased physical performance, more chronic illness, and a shorter life expectancy.

Manage Your Stress Most students find college stressful.[18] Research shows that high levels of unrelieved stress can disrupt thinking and memory, disturb sleep, increase depression, impair our immunity to infections, and even contribute to weight gain and abdominal fat. Over many years, unrelieved stress can also contribute to higher blood pressure, premature aging, and increased risk for chronic illnesses.

Chapter 10 describes the toll stress takes on wellness. It shows some of the common but ineffective ways people try to relieve stress, such as drinking alcohol, taking drugs, eating high-calorie "comfort foods," and skipping exercise to save time. It also explains how you can learn to control stress levels effectively, through physical activity, social support, relaxation breathing, and other techniques.

Avoid Smoking, Drugs, and Alcohol Abuse Smoking, drinking, and taking drugs are all ways of manipulating the brain chemically. Unfortunately, they carry high risks for illness and injury.

Practice Accident, Injury, and Disease Prevention *Prevention* has several practical meanings for wellness behavior. It can mean preventing injuries and the accidents that account for most deaths among young adults by reducing alcohol consumption, not drinking and driving, wearing seat belts and helmets, getting enough sleep, and using common sense. It can mean self-care such as daily dental hygiene and regular prostate or breast self-exams. And it can mean preventing disease

TOOLS FOR CHANGE

WHAT MOVES YOU?

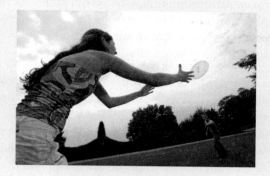

Like many students, you may need powerful motivation to start a fitness program and follow it through. Researchers have discovered several interesting facets of student motivation to be active and fit that you can apply to your own wellness plan.

Studies have found that college students who participated in repetitive exercises such as weight lifting, swimming laps, or jogging around the track usually had *external* motivations for their participation. Many, but not all, tended to focus on their appearance, weight, or stress management and on the improvements that exercise could promote.[1] Conversely, college students who participated in recreational sports such as tennis, softball, and rowing usually had *internal* motivations for participating. They tended to focus on enjoyment and challenge.

If you have trouble sticking with exercise programs, you might find fitness easier if you choose a sport—even a mildly aerobic one such as badminton, horseback riding, Ping-Pong, or bowling—that provides social opportunities and fun as well as physical activity. As long as you spend enough hours at an activity each week, you will benefit. Having fun is simply the insurance that you will put in enough activity time to gain fitness and wellness benefits.

Researchers have confirmed that the social aspect of sports and activities is key for most people. A sense of belonging is central to both fitness and wellness perceptions and efforts. Women who feel connected to a group of others see themselves as healthier than those not connected. Men with similar connections report fewer symptoms of ill health.[2] Many people find that joining something—a team, a gym, a group of friends for a bike ride or a game of Frisbee in the park—helps them enjoy fitness activities and stick with them.

Switching from an inactive to an active lifestyle takes time and the right kind of plan for behavioral change. The same is true for changing risky or unhealthy behaviors to ones that promote wellness. Behavior change is part science, part art, and part effort. What are your motivations for fitness and physical activity? Do you participate in sports? Why or why not? Do you like exercising? Which of your activities are the most fun, and what makes them so?

Sources:
1. M. Kilpatrick, E. Hebert, and J. Bartholomew, "College Students' Motivation for Physical Activity: Differentiating Men's and Women's Motives for Sport Participation and Exercise," *Journal of American College Health* 54, no. 2 (September 2005): 87–94.
2. C. J. Hale, J. W. Hannum, and D. L. Espelage, "Social Support and Physical Health: The Importance of Belonging," *Journal of American College Health* 53, no. 6 (May–June 2005): 276–84.

---

through medical checkups and vaccinations. Adopting behaviors that promote fitness and wellness is the core of prevention and often requires a change in old habits or habit patterns.

STEP TWO: PREPARE TO CHANGE A BEHAVIOR

Habits are usually deeply ingrained, and even minor habits can be surprisingly hard to change. As we have discussed, research has confirmed that people are more successful when they prepare for change emotionally and mentally rather than starting right in on the change itself. Preparations can include examining your current patterns, identifying your beliefs and attitudes, solidifying your motivation, predicting possible barriers to change, making a firm commitment, and choosing a realistic target for change efforts.

Examine Current Habits and Patterns

What current behavior should you work on changing? The assessment in Lab 1.1 will help you identify habits (such as being sedentary or eating junk food) that lower wellness. When considering a habit, ask yourself the following:

- How long has it been going on?

- How often does it happen?

- How serious are the consequences of the habit or problem?

- What are some of your reasons for continuing this problematic behavior?

- What kinds of situations trigger the behavior?

- Are other people involved in this habit? If so, in what way?

Habits involve elements of deliberate choice but are also influenced by demographics, personal

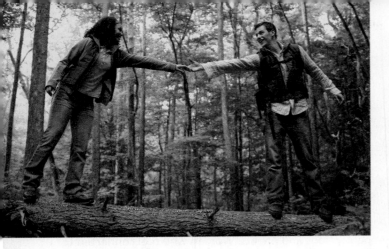

attitudes and beliefs, and many other factors. Age, sex, race, income, family background, education, and access to health care all increase or decrease the likelihood of developing certain health habits. If your parents smoke, for instance, you are 90 percent more likely to start smoking than someone whose parents don't smoke.[19] If your peers smoke, you are 80 percent more likely to smoke. Identifying factors that may encourage negative behaviors or block positive ones can help you prepare for behavior change.

Various factors can reinforce current habits. If you decide to stop smoking but your family and friends keep smoking around you, you may be tempted to start again. Their behavior reinforces your smoking habit. Berating yourself for backsliding can also work against you. Conversely, if you lose a few pounds and your friends tell you how terrific you look, their praise can reinforce your new eating habits. Analyzing the factors that reinforce your current habit pattern can help you understand why you developed and maintained unwanted habits and where you need to make changes in order to succeed.

Assess Current Beliefs and Attitudes

Your attitudes about health and wellness affect your daily choices. When reaching for another cigarette,

motivation One's inducement to do something such as change a current behavior

self-efficacy The degree to which you believe in your own ability to achieve something

locus of control Your belief in whether control over your life events and changes comes primarily from outside of yourself (external locus of control) or from within yourself (internal locus of control)

smokers, for example, sometimes tell themselves, "I'll stop tomorrow" or "They'll have a cure for lung cancer by the time I get it." These beliefs allow them to continue smoking. One model suggests that several factors must be in place before you successfully change a habit that diminishes wellness.[20] Among these factors are the following:

- You must believe that your current pattern could lead you to a serious problem. The more severe the consequences, the more likely you are to change the behavior. For example, smoking can cause cancer and emphysema and promote heart disease—all of which can be disabling and deadly. The fear of developing those diseases can help a person stop smoking.

- You must believe that you personally are quite susceptible to developing the health problem. For example, losing two parents to lung cancer could make a person work harder to stop smoking.

What beliefs underlie your current pattern of wellness habits, both positive and negative?

Assess Your Motivation

What is your **motivation,** or inducement, to change a wellness behavior? For some, a rewarding result, such as looking better, can motivate change. For others, a feeling of accomplishment or just feeling better every day may do it. Strengthening your motivations is an important part of preparing to change, because even if you backslide, your original reasons and motivations can help you recommit.

Motivations can be external (come from someone or something else) or internal (come from inside yourself) but in either case are part of your sense of self. The degree to which you believe in your own abilities is your **self-efficacy.** Your conviction that you can control events and factors in your life is your **locus of control.** An internal locus of control usually gives you a strong belief in your ability to effect change. An external locus of control usually leads you to see other people and things as controlling what you do and whether you can change. A person's locus of control is usually somewhere between fully external and fully internal. A person with a strong sense of self-efficacy and a largely internal locus of control has a better chance of following through with a decision to change wellness behavior. If you want to quit smoking simply because someone is pressuring you to do so, your chances of success may not be as good as if you quit smoking because of a strong personal desire to do so.

Anticipate and Overcome Barriers to Change

Anticipating **barriers to change,** or possible stumbling blocks, will help you prepare for behavior change. A majority of students, for example, want to lose or gain weight but have failed to do so permanently.[21] Diet failure is based on several barriers to change, including internal drives to eat high-calorie foods and external temptations such as snacks and fast foods on sale in most campus buildings. The following are a few general barriers to wellness change:

- Overambitious goals can derail behavior change. Most people cannot lose weight, stop smoking, and begin running 3 miles a day all at the same time. Wanting to achieve dramatic change within unrealistically short time frames—such as losing 20 pounds in 1 month—tends to be equally unsuccessful. Habits are best changed one at a time, taking small, progressive steps; rewarding successes; and being patient with yourself.

- Self-defeating beliefs and attitudes can impede successful change. Believing that you are too young to worry about fitness and wellness can bar you from making a solid commitment to change. Likewise, thinking you are helpless to change your weight, smoking, or fitness habits could undermine your efforts. Greater self-efficacy and more positive expectations may help.

- Failing to accurately assess your current state of wellness could block progress. You might assume that you are strong and flexible, for example, when you are actually below average for your age. Failing to gather enough data on wellness risks and benefits can also be a barrier that leaves you with weakened motivation and commitment.

- Lack of support and guidance can act as a barrier. Supportive friends are a good start. You should also seek guidance from your fitness and wellness instructor; from counselors and other campus resources; from up-to-date, trusted health sources on the Internet (see the box **Spotlight: Wellness Sources You Can Trust**); and from health professionals such as those at your student health center.

Commitment

The more strongly you state an intention to change a wellness habit, either verbally or on paper, the more likely you will succeed. A public statement of commitment to become more physically active, for example, along with the support and encouragement of friends and family can help you stick with your plans to change.

Try it NOW! Ask yourself where your locus of control is. • Is it internal or external? • Are your motivations for behavior change based on pressure from other people in your life, or do they come from within you?

Target Behaviors

The last preparatory step is to choose one well-defined habit, or **target behavior,** as your initial focus for change. Starting small and building on success is a much better strategy than trying for too much and failing.

STEP THREE: ACQUIRE SPECIFIC SKILLS THAT SUPPORT SUCCESSFUL CHANGE

Various kinds of skills support a program of change once you've prepared yourself mentally and emotionally. These skills will help you identify your old pattern, visualize a new one, choose a realistic goal, and help yourself achieve it.

See Yourself Honestly and Clearly

To overcome an unhealthy habit, it helps to be honest with yourself about how you established that habit to begin with. Did you start eating a lot of fast food because it was a way to save money? Did you stop exercising because school ended and you were no longer part of a team sport? Truly acknowledging the underlying reasons for your habits can help you take steps to address them (and change the unhealthy behavior).

Visualize New Behavior

Athletes often use a form of mental practice called *imagined rehearsal* or simply *visualization* to reach their performance goals. Picturing themselves accomplishing an

barrier to change A stumbling block you may face in your efforts to alter a current behavior

target behavior One well-defined habit chosen as your primary focus for change

WELLNESS SOURCES YOU CAN TRUST

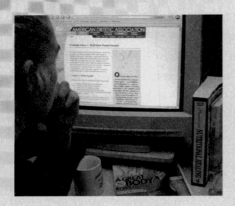

Fitness and wellness are important American preoccupations—and major industries as well. Because so many people sell products and services that purport to improve your health, it is often hard to distinguish legitimate information from thinly disguised advertising. Here are some general tips and specific sources of reliable information.

Look for organizations without a direct interest in your wallet. Examples are health-related agencies of the state and federal government (e.g., CDC or FDA); major colleges and universities; big-name hospitals and medical centers (e.g., Mayo Clinic or Cooper Institute); and well-known nonprofit organizations (e.g., American College of Sports Medicine or American Medical Association). Cross-check any information you gather from other sources against these kinds of known and reliable sources to see if facts and figures are consistent.

Get names of periodicals and lists of websites from approved sources. The American Accreditation Health Care Commission, for example, judges health-related websites and recommends dozens for their credibility and reliability (see www.urac.org). In addition, a website called Quackwatch (www.quackwatch.org) lists dozens of magazines, journals, newsletters, and newspapers that consumers should avoid because they promote misinformation, use unreliable sources for their own articles, or carry advertising for questionable products or services.

If a newspaper or magazine quotes a research report, look up the research itself to see what the authors concluded. Look at details of the study, noting whether the researcher works for a large, recognizable university, government agency, or research institute; whether the study had human subjects or inferred conclusions from lab animals; and whether the conclusions were based on dozens or hundreds of research subjects or just a few.

Take fitness or wellness advice only from experts who represent reliable sources. Your fitness and wellness course materials should be in this category. Well-meaning friends often have misinformation, and promoters of products and services are usually strongly biased.

Read consumer health newsletters published by distinguished universities, research institutes, or nonprofit organizations. Here are some examples of newsletters that discuss both fitness and wellness topics: *Harvard Health Letter; Health News: Straight Talk on the Medical Headlines* (published by the *New England Journal of Medicine); Johns Hopkins Health Insider; Mayo Clinic Health Letter; Nutrition Action Health Letter; U.C. Berkeley Wellness Letter; Tufts Health and Nutrition Letter; Consumer Reports on Health.*

Finally, use approved websites such as the following to learn more about fitness and wellness topics:

CDC Wonder (wonder.cdc.gov)

Mayo Clinic (www.mayoclinic.com)

National Center for Health Statistics (www.cdc.gov/nchs)

National Health Information Center (www.health.gov/nhic)

Harvard School of Public Health, World Health News (www.worldhealthnews.harvard.edu)

American Heart Association (www.americanheart.org)

American Medical Association (www.ama-assn.org)

Healthy People 2010 (www.healthypeople.gov)

U.S. Department of Health and Human Services (www.healthfinder.gov)

American College of Sports Medicine (www.acsm.org)

President's Council on Physical Fitness and Sports (www.fitness.gov)

FDA Information for Consumers (www.fda.gov/opacom/morecons.html)

Note: Web links are always subject to change. Visit this book's website at www.aw-bc.com/hopson to view updated Web links for each chapter.

---

action in their minds ahead of time helps prepare them for real competition. Visualization can help you imagine the way a current negative behavior unfolds, and then allows you to practice in advance what you will say and do to counter it.

For example, suppose you want to quit smoking but know that seeing a friend light up and smelling the smoke will make you grab for a cigarette, too. You could visualize this and then add an alternate ending: using a nicotine replacement

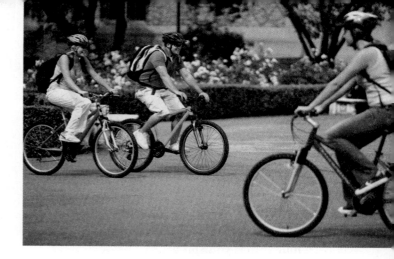

patch and reaching for a piece of sugar-free gum when you have a craving. This kind of careful mental and verbal rehearsal can improve your likelihood of success.

Observe Role Models
Watching others successfully change their behavior can give you ideas and encouragement for your own changes. This process of *modeling,* or learning from role models, can be very helpful. Suppose you have trouble talking to strangers or new acquaintances and want to improve your communication skills. Try observing friends whose social skills you admire and note how they make conversation. Do they talk more or listen more? What techniques help make them successful communicators? If you see behaviors that work well, separate their components so you can model your behavior change on a proven approach.

Learn to "Counter"
Countering is another term for substituting a desired behavior for an undesirable one. You may want to stop eating junk food, for example, but "cold turkey" just isn't realistic—unless the turkey is on a sandwich! Instead, compile a list of substitute foods and places to get them and have this ready before your mouth starts watering at the smell of burgers and fries.

Set Realistic Goals and Objectives
Your wellness goals and objectives should be both *achievable for you* and *in line with what you truly want.*[22] Achievable, truly desired goals increase motivation, and this, in turn, leads to a better chance of success at behavior change.

To set successful goals, try using the *SMART* system. SMART goals are <u>s</u>pecific, <u>m</u>easurable, <u>a</u>ction-oriented, <u>r</u>ealistic, and <u>t</u>ime-oriented. A vague goal would be "Get into better shape by exercising more." A SMART goal would be *specific*—"Start weight training"; *measurable*—"Increase the amount of weight I can safely lift"; *action-oriented*—"I'll go to the gym three times per week"; *realistic*—"I'll increase the weight I can lift by 20 percent (not 200 percent)"; and *time-oriented*—"I'll try my new weight program for 8 weeks, then reassess."

Practice "Shaping"
Shaping is a stepwise process of making a series of small changes.

Suppose you want to start jogging 3 miles every other day, but right now you get tired and winded after half a mile. Shaping would dictate a process of slow, progressive steps such as walking 1 hour every other day at a slow, relaxed pace for the first week; walking for an hour every other day but at a faster pace that covers more distance the second week; and speeding up to a slow run the third week.

Regardless of the change you plan, remember that current habits did not develop overnight, and they will not change overnight, either.

- Start slowly to avoid hurting yourself or causing undue stress.
- Keep the steps of your program small and achievable.
- Be flexible and ready to change your original plan if it proves to be uncomfortable.
- Master one step before moving on to the next.

Control Your Environment
If you are trying to quit drinking, going to a bar could trigger a serious backslide (assuming you are even of legal age to be drinking). Going to dinner and a movie with a sympathetic friend, on the other hand, could help reinforce your abstinence. Think about which people and settings tend to trigger your unwanted behavior, then stay away from them as much as possible and set up supportive situations instead.

Reward Yourself
Setting up a system of rewards can help you keep new behavior on track. What feels like a special reward to you? Every few times you accomplish a new habit or avoid an old one, reward yourself.

countering Substituting a desired behavior for an undesirable one

Rewards can be *consumable,* like cookies or gourmet meals. They can be *active,* like going to a concert or playing Frisbee. They can be *possessional,* like getting a new MP3 player or buying a new CD. A reward can be an *incentive,* like cooking dinner for someone who avoids cigarettes for a week. It can be *social,* like giving someone praise or a hug. And it can be *intrinsic,* meaning a new behavior feels so enjoyable it becomes its own reward.

Think about rewards that would help motivate you to change your behavior and build a few (but not too many) into your program.

Change Your Self-Talk

Your *self-talk*—that is, the way you think and talk to yourself—matters. Think about what you say to yourself when something goes badly or when something succeeds. Purposely blocking or stopping negative thoughts and replacing them with positive ones can help you change a habit. To reinforce new study habits, for example, replace self-talk like this: "I can't believe I flunked that easy exam. I'm so stupid," with a positive message like this: "If I had studied more, I could have gotten at least a C, maybe a B. I just need to start earlier and study harder for the next test."

Use Writing as a Wellness Tool

Throughout the labs in this textbook, you will examine your current wellness habits and analyze them through writing. **Journaling,** or writing personal experiences, interpretations, and results in a journal or notebook, is an important skill for behavior change. Journaling can help you monitor your daily efforts, measure how much you have learned, record how you feel about your progress, and note ideas for improving your program.

---

journaling Keeping a personal journal

behavior change contract A formal document that clarifies the goals and steps you plan to take to change a current habit or habit pattern

---

One extension of journaling is a formal written document called the **behavior change contract.** This functions as a promise to yourself

- as a public declaration of intent
- as an organized plan that lays out start and end dates and daily actions
- as a listing of barriers or obstacles you may encounter
- as a place to brainstorm strategies for overcoming those impediments
- as a collected set of sources of support, and
- as a reminder of the rewards you plan to give yourself for sticking with the program.

Writing a behavior change contract will help you clarify your goals, make a commitment to change, and, if you wish, announce your intentions to supportive friends and family. In *Lab1.3* you will create a behavior change contract as part of your plan for wellness behavior change.

STEP FOUR: APPLY WHAT YOU HAVE LEARNED TO CHANGE A SPECIFIC BEHAVIOR

After you acquire the skills to support successful behavior change, it is time to apply those skills to a specific behavior.

Start by reviewing the material on wellness dimensions in this chapter. Choose a dimension that concerns you, and then select an issue from that dimension that you want to learn more about. For instance, if you're shy, you might want to strengthen your social wellness dimension to develop more close friendships.

Understanding that change is a long-term process, reread the information about the phases of change. Determine your current phase for the wellness dimension you want to enhance. Are you in the contemplation stage or the action stage? What must you still do to prepare for change?

Complete Lab 1.1 and Lab 1.2, which will help you identify habits and behaviors that undermine your fitness and wellness. Then fill out the Behavior Change contract in Lab 1.3. Post the contract where you will see it every day and where you can refer to it as you work through the chapters in this text.

REVIEW QUESTIONS

1. How does *wellness* differ from *health*?
   a. Wellness is the absence of disease
   b. Wellness is the achievement of the highest level of health possible in physical, social, intellectual, emotional, environmental, and spiritual dimensions
   c. Wellness and health are equivalent
   d. Health is a more individualized, dynamic concept than wellness

2. Which dimension of wellness includes good organizational skills and careful financial management?
   a. Social
   b. Intellectual
   c. Emotional
   d. Environmental

3. Modifiable risk factors for disease include all of the following EXCEPT:
   a. Tobacco use
   b. Alcohol use
   c. Genetics
   d. Physical inactivity

4. The American College of Sports Medicine recommends that all healthy adults between the ages of 18 and 65 strive for
   a. At least 30 minutes of moderate exercise five days a week *or* at least 20 minutes of vigorous exercise three days a week
   b. 30 minutes of exercise once a week
   c. 30 minutes of vigorous exercise once a week
   d. 20 minutes of walking once a week

5. Which of the following is *not* one of the top causes of death among Americans 20 to 24?
   a. Accidents
   b. Homicide
   c. Suicide
   d. Hepatitis

6. All of the following are stages of the Transtheoretical Model of Behavior Change EXCEPT:
   a. Pre-contemplation
   b. Preparation
   c. Action
   d. "Cold turkey"

7. What is meant by the term *healthy life expectancy*?
   a. How many years a person can expect to live
   b. How many years a person can expect to live without disability or major illness
   c. A realistic attitude toward how long a person can expect to live
   d. How many years a person believes he or she has to live

8. Which step to behavior change includes visualizing, countering, and rewarding?
   a. Step 1: Learn about basic wellness behaviors
   b. Step 2: Prepare to change a behavior
   c. Step 3: Acquire specific skills that support succesful change
   d. Step 4: Apply what you've learned to change a specific behavior

9. What is "shaping"?
   a. A stepwise process of change, designed to change one small piece of a target behavior at a time
   b. A model of behavior change that uses mental imaging to reshape the brain's signals
   c. A journaling strategy
   d. A way of learning behaviors by watching others perform them

10. How does journaling help with behavior change?
   a. It helps you monitor your daily efforts
   b. It helps you measure how much you have learned
   c. It helps you record how you feel about your progress
   d. All of the above

CRITICAL THINKING QUESTIONS

1. What does it mean to be well? What are the benefits of wellness?

2. Name the dimensions of wellness and assign yourself a score (1 to 5) for your degree of wellness in each dimension. Identify your place on the wellness continuum in Figure 1.3.

3. Which risk-lowering choices do you incorporate into your lifestyle? Take two or three of them and discuss the personal attitudes and beliefs that underlie your present behavior.

4. Using the stages of change (transtheoretical) model, discuss what you might do (in stages) to help a friend stop smoking. Why is it important that a person be ready to change before trying to change?

5. Which habits (wellness-related or not) have you tried to change in the past? Why do you think your efforts succeeded or failed? Using the skills for behavior change from this chapter, write a plan that will help you approach each habit more successfully.

ONLINE RESOURCES

See the Spotlight box on page 16. Also, please visit this book's website at **www.aw-bc.com/hopson** to access additional links related to topics in this chapter.

REFERENCES

1. American College Health Association, "National College Health Assessment. Reference Group Executive Summary Fall 2006" (Baltimore: American College Health Association, 2007).

2. World Health Organization, "World Health Statistics 2006: Mortality." www.who.int/whosis/ whostat2006 (accessed 2007).

3. Ibid.

4. Centers for Disease Control and Prevention, "National Vital Statistics Reports," 55, no. 10 (March 15, 2007).

5. Ibid.

6. Centers for Disease Control and Prevention, "Nationwide Trend," Health-Related Quality of Life; National Center for Chronic Disease Prevention and Health Promotion, www.cdc.gov/hrqol (accessed October 29, 2007).

7. World Health Organization, "Diet and Physical Activity: A Public Health Priority," Global Strategy on Diet, Physical Activity and Health, www.who.int/ dietphysicalactivity (accessed October 29, 2007).

8. Centers for Disease Control and Prevention, "Physical Activity and Health: A Report of the Surgeon General," www.cdc.gov/nccdphp/ sgr/sgr.htm (1999).

9. Centers for Disease Control and Prevention, "Behavioral Risk Factor Surveillance System (BRFSS)." www.cdc.gov/brfss; National Center for Health Statistics, "National Health and Nutrition Examination Survey (NHANES)," www.cdc.gov/ nchs/nhanes.htm (2003–2004).

10. American College of Sports Medicine, "Updated Physical Activity Guidelines." www.acsm .org (accessed August 1, 2007).

11. United States Department of Health and Human Services, Office of the Surgeon General, "Public Health Priorities," www.surgeon- general.gov/publichealthpriorities .html#disease (accessed October 29, 2007).

12. National Coalition on Health Care, "Health Insurance Cost," www .hchc.org (accessed August 7, 2007).

13. Ibid.

14. Ibid.

15. J. Prochaska, C. DiClemente, and J. Norcross, "In Search of How People Change: Application to Addictive Behaviors," *American Psychologist* 47, no. 9 (1983): 1102–14.

16. Achintya Dey and Jacqueline Lucas, "Physical and Mental Health Characteristics of U.S. Born and Foreign Born Adults, 1997–2002," Centers for Disease Control and Prevention, National Center for Health Statistics, www.cdc.gov (March 1, 2006).

17. United States Department of Agriculture, "Key Recommendations for the General Population," Dietary Guidelines for Americans, 2005, www.health.gov/ dietaryguidelines/dga2005/ recommendations.htm.

18. American College Health Association, "National College Health Assessment. Reference Group Executive Summary Fall 2006" (Baltimore: American College Health Association, 2007).

19. Masaru Yanai and others, "Smoking Incidence and the Effect of Smokefree Education Programs in Juveniles," *Chest,* American College of Chest Physicians (2005).

20. E. P. Sarafino, *Health Psychology* (New York: Wiley, 1990) 189–191.

21. American College Health Association, "National College Health Assessment. Reference Group Executive Summary Fall 2006" (Baltimore: American College Health Association, 2007).

22. University of Iowa Advising Center, "Motivation, Goal Setting, and Success," www.uiowa.edu/web/ advisingcenter/motivation.htm (accessed August 5, 2007).

Name: _____ Date: _____

Instructor: _____ Section: _____

Purpose: This lab will help you assess your current level of wellness in each of the six dimensions and identify which wellness areas to target for behavior change.

Directions: Complete sections I–VII. For each item, indicate how often you think the statements describe you. After each section, total your scores for that section and write your score in the space provided. After completing all sections, you will summarize and analyze your results.

SECTION I: PHYSICAL WELLNESS

	Never 1	Rarely 2	Sometimes 3	Often 4	Always 5
1. I listen to my body and make adjustments or seek professional help when something is wrong.					
2. I do moderate activity every day, such as taking the stairs instead of riding the elevator.					
3. I engage in vigorous exercise three to four times per week.					
4. I do exercise for muscular strength and endurance at least two times per week.					
5. I do stretching and limbering exercises at least five days per week.					
6. I do yoga, Pilates, tai chi, or other exercises for balance and core strength two or three times per week.					
7. I feel good about the condition of my body. I have lots of energy and can get through the day without being overly tired.					
8. I get adequate rest at night and wake on most mornings feeling ready for the day ahead.					
9. My immune system is strong, and my body heals quickly when I get sick or injured.					
10. I eat nutritious foods daily and avoid junk food.					

Total for Section I: Physical Wellness = _____

SECTION II: SOCIAL WELLNESS

	Never 1	Rarely 2	Sometimes 3	Often 4	Always 5
1. I am open, honest, and get along well with others.					
2. I participate in a wide variety of social activities and enjoy all kinds of people.					
3. I try to be a "better person" and work on behaviors that have caused friction in the past.					
4. I am open and accessible to a loving and responsible relationship.					
5. I have someone I can talk to about private feelings.					
6. When I meet people, I feel good about the impression they have of me.					
7. I get along well with members of my family.					
8. I consider the feelings of others and do not act in hurtful or selfish ways.					
9. I try to see the good in my friends and help them feel good about themselves.					
10. I am good at listening to friends and family who need to talk.					

Total for Section II: Social Wellness = _____

SECTION III: EMOTIONAL WELLNESS

	Never 1	Rarely 2	Sometimes 3	Often 4	Always 5
1. I find it easy to laugh, cry, and show emotions like love, fear, and anger and try to express them in positive ways.					
2. I avoid using alcohol or drugs as a means to forget my problems or relieve stress.					
3. My friends regard me as a stable, well-adjusted person who they trust and rely on for support.					
4. When I am angry, I try to resolve issues in nonhurtful ways rather than stewing about them.					
5. I try not to worry unnecessarily, and I try to talk about my feelings, fears, and concerns rather than letting them build up.					
6. I recognize when I'm stressed and take steps to relax through exercise, quiet time, or calming activities.					
7. I view challenging situations and problems as opportunities for growth.					
8. I feel good about myself and believe others like me for who I am.					
9. I try not to be too critical or judgmental of others.					
10. I am flexible and adapt to change in a positive way.					

Total for Section III: Emotional Wellness = _____

SECTION IV: INTELLECTUAL WELLNESS

	Never 1	Rarely 2	Sometimes 3	Often 4	Always 5
1. I carefully consider options and possible consequences as I make choices.					
2. I am alert and ready to respond to life's challenges in ways that reflect thought and sound judgment.					
3. I learn from my mistakes and try to act differently the next time.					
4. I actively learn all I can about products and services before buying them.					
5. I manage my time well rather than letting time manage me.					
6. I follow directions or recommended guidelines and act in ways likely to keep myself and others safe.					
7. I consider myself to be a wise health consumer and check for reliable sources of information before making decisions.					
8. I have at least one personal-growth hobby that I make time for every week.					
9. My credit card balances are low, and my finances are in good order.					
10. I examine my own perceptions and then check evidence to see if I was correct or not.					

Total for Section IV: Intellectual Wellness = _____

SECTION V: ENVIRONMENTAL WELLNESS

	Never 1	Rarely 2	Sometimes 3	Often 4	Always 5
1. I am concerned about environmental pollution and actively try to preserve and protect natural resources.					
2. I buy recycled paper and purchase biodegradable products whenever possible.					
3. I recycle my garbage, reuse containers, and try to minimize the amount of paper and plastics that I use.					
4. I try to wear my clothes for longer periods of time between washings to save on water and reduce detergent in our water sources.					
5. My workplace is safe from toxic exposures and other hazards.					
6. I write my elected leaders about environmental concerns.					
7. I turn down the heat and wear warmer clothes at home in the winter and use the air conditioner only when really necessary.					
8. I am aware of potential hazards in my area and try to reduce my exposure whenever possible.					
9. I use both sides of the paper when taking notes and doing assignments.					
10. I try not to leave the water running too long when I shower, shave, or brush my teeth.					

Total for Section V: Environmental Wellness = _____

SECTION VI: SPIRITUAL WELLNESS

	Never 1	Rarely 2	Sometimes 3	Often 4	Always 5
1. I take time alone to think about life's meaning and where I fit in to the greater whole.					
2. I believe life is a gift we should cherish.					
3. I look forward to each day as an opportunity for further growth.					
4. I experience life to the fullest.					
5. I take time to enjoy nature and the beauty around me.					
6. I have faith in a greater power, nature, or the connectedness of all living things.					
7. I engage in acts of care and goodwill without expecting something in return.					
8. I look forward to each day as an opportunity to grow and be challenged in life.					
9. I work for peace in my interpersonal relationships, my community, and the world at large.					
10. I have a great love and respect for all living things and regard animals as important links in a vital living chain.					

Total for Section VI: Spiritual Wellness = _____

SECTION VII: REFLECTION—YOUR PERSONAL WELLNESS CONTINUUM

1. Write your totals for sections I–VI below:

Physical Wellness _____

Social Wellness _____

Emotional Wellness _____

Intellectual Wellness _____

Environmental Wellness _____

Spiritual Wellness _____

2. Understanding your scores:

Scores of 35–50: Outstanding! Your answers show that you are aware of the importance of these behaviors in your overall wellness. More important, you are putting your knowledge to work by practicing good habits that should reduce your overall risks. Although you received a very high score on this dimension of wellness, you may want to consider areas where your scores could be improved.

Scores of 30–34: Your wellness practices in these areas are very good, but there is room for improvement. Look again at the items on which you scored one or two points. What changes could you make to improve your score? Even a small change in behavior can help you achieve better wellness.

Scores of 20–29: Your wellness risks are showing. Find information about the risks you are facing and why it is important to change these behaviors. Perhaps you need help in deciding how to make the changes you desire. Assistance is available from this book, your instructor, and student health services at your school.

Scores below 20: You may be taking unnecessary risks. Perhaps you are not aware of the risks and what to do about them. Identify each risk area and make a mental note as you learn about that topic in this course. Whenever possible, seek additional resources, either on your campus or through your local community health resources. If any area is causing you to be less than functional in your class work or personal life, seek professional help and make a serious commitment to behavior change.

Name: _____   **Date:** _____

Instructor: _____   **Section:** _____

Purpose: To learn how to chart your current personal wellness balance and identify the wellness areas in which you would like to improve

Materials: Results from Lab 1.1

Directions: Follow the instructions below.

SECTION I: YOUR PERSONAL WELLNESS BALANCE

1. Create a personal wellness balance chart with your scores from sections I–VI of Lab 1.1. Allocate a larger "piece of the pie" for dimensions of wellness where your scores are higher and a smaller slice for dimensions with lower scores. Another option: allocate a larger slice for areas where you spend most of your time during a week.

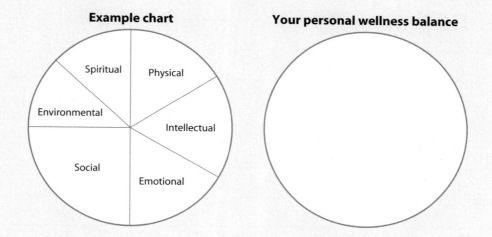

Example chart

Your personal wellness balance

2. Now create your **goal wellness balance chart.** Change your current balance chart to reflect your desired scores in each wellness dimension, or to reflect the optimal percentage of time you would like to allocate to each dimension.

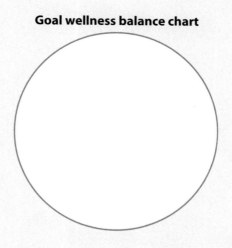

Goal wellness balance chart

SECTION II: YOUR PERSONAL WELLNESS CONTINUUM

1. Below is a figure showing the **wellness continuum.**

| Chronic illness | Irreversible damage | Signs of illness | Average wellness | Increased wellness | Optimum wellness |

a. Draw an arrow on the wellness continuum, indicating *where you currently are* on the continuum. Label the arrow "CURRENT."

b. Draw another arrow on the wellness continuum, indicating *where you would like to be* on the continuum. Label this arrow "GOAL."

SECTION III: REFLECTION

Reflect on your answers, your wellness balance charts, and your wellness continuum. What are your major areas of concern regarding your wellness? What two or three behaviors could you change easily to improve your wellness? Which one needs attention first?

_____

_____

_____

_____

_____

_____

_____

_____

_____

_____

LAB1.3

Name: _____ **Date:** _____

Instructor: _____ **Section:** _____

Purpose: To introduce students to the process of writing a behavior change contract and planning for new lifestyle behaviors. This introduction will serve as a model for other behavior change plans in subsequent chapters.

Directions: Complete the following sections.

SECTION I: PERSONAL WELLNESS REVIEW

1. Review your answers from Lab 1.1 and Lab 1.2.

2. Consider the stages of change (precontemplation, contemplation, preparation, action, maintenance) and evaluate your readiness to make a behavior change.

3. Choose a target behavior to change. For this behavior, you should be in the contemplation or preparation stages. Write the behavior below.

My behavior to change is _____

SECTION II: SHORT- AND LONG-TERM GOALS

1. **Long-Term Goal:** Long-term goals are those set for over 6 months to a year or more. These goals should be achievable and may take many steps and an extended time to reach. Be sure to use SMART (specific, measurable, action-oriented, realistic, time-oriented) goal-setting guidelines when creating your long-term goal. After writing out your long-term goal, choose an appropriate target date and a reward for completing your goal.

    a. Long-Term Goal: _____

    b. Target Date: _____

    c. Reward: _____

2. **Short-Term Goals:** Short-term goals are those you want to achieve in less than 6 months. These goals will often help you reach your long-term goal. They may also be part of your long-term goal. Again, use SMART goal-setting guidelines when setting short-term goals. After writing out your short-term goals, choose appropriate target dates and rewards.

    a. Short-Term Goal #1: _____

    b. Target Date: _____

    c. Reward: _____

    a. Short-Term Goal #2: _____

    b. Target Date: _____

    c. Reward: _____

SECTION III: BEHAVIOR CHANGE OBSTACLES AND STRATEGIES

1. These are **three of my obstacles** to changing this behavior (things I am currently doing or situations that contribute to this behavior or make it harder to change):

a. _____

b. _____

c. _____

2. Here are **three strategies** I will use to overcome these obstacles:

a. _____

b. _____

c. _____

SECTION IV: GETTING SUPPORT

1. Resources I will use to help me change this behavior include

a friend/partner/relative: _____

a school-based resource: _____

a community-based resource: _____

a book or reputable website: _____

2. How will you use these supportive resources to help you with your goals?

_____

_____

SECTION V: CONTRACT, TRACKING, AND FOLLOW-UP

1. Contract: I intend to make the behavior change described above. I will use the strategies and rewards to achieve the goals that will contribute to a healthy behavior change.

Signed _____ Date _____

Witness _____ Date _____

2. Tracking: Tracking your progress toward your goals is very important to ensure successful behavior change. As you move through this course, you will be asked to monitor your progress on several of your health, wellness, and fitness goals. Accurate and regular record-keeping is important.

3. Follow-up: When reaching your target date, it is important to follow up and reassess your program. During this course, you will be answering questions such as, Did you accomplish your goal? Do you need to set a new and more challenging goal? Do you need to alter your goals or program to make it more realistic? This section in your labs is important to modify your goals and your program, and to set future goals.

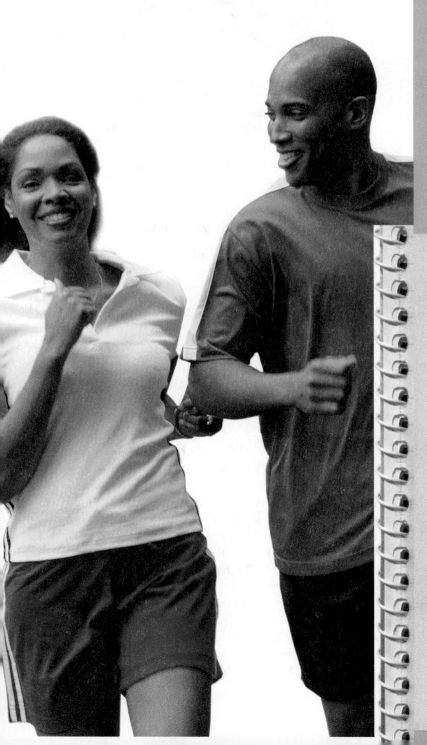

CHAPTER 2

Understanding Fitness Principles

OBJECTIVES

Identify the three primary levels of physical activity and describe the benefits of each.

Describe the five health-related components of fitness.

Identify the six skill-related components of fitness.

Explain the principles of overload, progression, specificity, reversibility, individuality, and recovery.

Describe how much physical activity is recommended for optimal health and wellness.

Describe general strategies for exercising safely.

Identify individual attributes that should be taken into account before beginning a fitness program.

Discuss strategies for beginning to design your own individualized fitness program.

CASE STUDY

Lily

"Hi, I'm Lily. I just started my junior year, and after a summer of lazing around, I want to get back into shape. I'm ready to put some serious time and energy into it, but the last time I started exercising, I tried to do too much and ended up getting injured. How do I keep from doing the same thing this time? How much exercise do I really need? And what does it actually mean to be fit, anyway—does it just mean being able to run a certain distance, or is there more to it than that?"

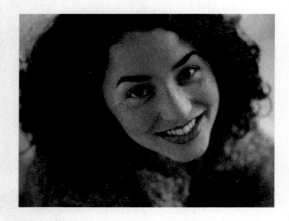

As we learned in Chapter 1, fitness is a critical component of overall wellness. The benefits of physical fitness are almost too numerous to list. Being physically fit can improve your mood, give you more energy for daily activities, help you maintain a healthy weight, and lessen your risk of developing chronic diseases. All of these benefits can, in turn, help you live a longer, healthier life.

In this chapter, we will cover the basic principles of fitness, address the question of how much exercise you need, introduce general guidelines for exercising safely, and discuss individual factors that should be taken into account when you design a personal fitness program. In Chapter 3, we will present several strategies to help you commit to fitness. Finally, in Chapters 4–6, we will turn to specific fitness goals—such as improving cardiorespiratory endurance, building muscular strength and endurance, and developing flexibility—and discuss how to design individual programs to achieve your goals in each of these key areas.

WHAT ARE THE THREE PRIMARY LEVELS OF PHYSICAL ACTIVITY?

Physical fitness is the ability to perform moderate to vigorous levels of physical activity without undue fatigue. Note that *physical activity* and *exercise* are not the same thing: **physical activity** technically means any bodily movement produced by skeletal muscles that results in an expenditure of energy, whereas **exercise** specifically refers to planned or structured physical activity done to achieve and maintain fitness.

Physical activity is often measured in metabolic equivalents, or **MET** levels. A MET level of 1 is equivalent to the energy you use at rest or while sitting quietly. A MET level of 2 equals two times the energy used at a MET level of 1, while a MET level of 3 equals three times the energy used at a MET level of 1, and so forth. Levels of physical activity can be grouped into three primary categories: (1) *lifestyle/light physical activities* (< 3 METS), (2) *moderate physical activities* (3 to 6 METS), and (3) *vigorous physical activities* (6+ METS). Figure 2.1 illustrates examples of each of these levels of physical activity, as well as the benefits that are associated with them.

physical fitness A set of attributes that relate to one's ability to perform moderate to vigorous levels of physical activity without undue fatigue

physical activity Any bodily movement produced by skeletal muscles that results in an expenditure of energy

exercise Physical activity that is planned or structured and involves repetitive bodily movement, done to improve or maintain one or more of the components of fitness

MET The standard metabolic equivalent used to estimate the amount of energy (oxygen) used by the body during physical activity; 1 MET = resting or sitting quietly

Lifestyle/ Light Physical Activities (< 3 METS)	Examples:	Benefits:
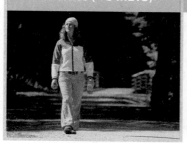	Light yard work and housework, leisurely walking, self-care and bathing, light stretching, light occupational activity	A moderate increase in health and wellness in those who are completely sedentary; reduced risk of some chronic diseases
Moderate Physical Activities (3–6 METS)	Examples:	Benefits:
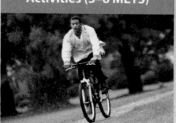	Walking 3–4.5 mph on a level surface, weight training, hiking, climbing stairs, bicycling 5–9 mph on a level surface, dancing, softball, recreational swimming, moderate yard work and housework	Increased cardiorespiratory endurance, lower body fat levels, improved blood cholesterol and pressure, better blood glucose management, decreased risk of disease, increased overall physical fitness
Vigorous Physical Activities (6+ METS)	Examples:	Benefits:
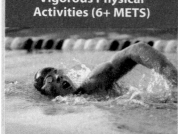	Jogging, running, circuit training, backpacking, aerobic classes, competitive sports, swimming laps, heavy yard work or housework, hard physical labor/ construction, bicycling over 10 mph up steep terrain	Increased overall physical fitness, decreased risk of disease, further improvements in overall strength and endurance

FIGURE 2.1

Examples and benefits of lifestyle/light physical activity, moderate physical activity, and vigorous physical activity.

WHAT ARE THE HEALTH-RELATED COMPONENTS OF PHYSICAL FITNESS?

The five **health-related components of physical fitness** are *cardiorespiratory endurance, muscular strength, muscular endurance, flexibility,* and *body composition.* Minimal competence in each of these areas is necessary for you to carry out daily activities, lower your risk of developing chronic diseases, and optimize your health and well-being.

CARDIORESPIRATORY ENDURANCE

Cardiorespiratory endurance (also called *cardiovascular fitness/endurance, aerobic fitness,* and *cardiorespiratory fitness*) is the ability of the cardiovascular and respiratory systems to provide oxygen to working muscles during sustained exercise.

health-related components of physical fitness Components of physical fitness that have a relationship with good health

Achieving adequate cardiorespiratory endurance decreases your risk of diabetes, heart disease, obesity, and other chronic diseases.[1] Increased cardiorespiratory endurance also improves your ability to enjoy recreational activities, such as bicycling and hiking, and to participate in them for extended periods of time. Your cardiorespiratory endurance level is determined by measuring your oxygen consumption during exercise, your heart rate response to exercise, and your rate of recovery after exercise. Chapter 4 will cover the various aspects of testing and training your cardiorespiratory system.

MUSCULAR STRENGTH

Muscular strength is the ability of your muscles to exert force. You may think of it as your ability to lift a heavy weight. Improved muscular strength decreases your risk of low bone density and musculoskeletal injuries.[2] In order to improve muscular strength, you need to tax your muscles in a controlled setting. This typically involves a weight room, as well as supervision to avoid injury. Chapter 5 will provide step-by-step instructions for testing your muscular strength and for designing a program to improve it.

MUSCULAR ENDURANCE

Muscular endurance is the ability of your muscles to contract repeatedly over time. Along with cardiorespiratory endurance, muscular endurance allows you to participate in recreational sports without undue fatigue. For example, in order to play a continuous game of basketball, you need to have good cardiorespiratory endurance to move up and down the court for the entire 90 minutes—and you need to have good lower-body muscular endurance to keep guarding, blocking, and shooting the ball effectively. You can improve your muscular endurance with resistance exercises or by participating in certain sports and activities. Chapter 5 will provide assessments for testing your muscular endurance and strategies for improvement.

skill-related components of fitness Components of physical fitness that have a relationship with enhanced motor skills and performance in sports

FLEXIBILITY

Flexibility is the ability to move your joints in a full range of motion. This component of fitness is often overlooked but is crucial for successful exercise and sports performance. A minimal level of flexibility in your working muscles helps prevent injuries. Maintaining that minimal level also increases your ability to train and work toward specific fitness goals. Having adequate flexibility can be especially important to prevent lower back pain and the decreased range of motion that often occurs with aging.[3] Chapter 6 will provide labs for assessing your flexibility and will offer sample flexibility and back-health exercises and programs.

BODY COMPOSITION

Body composition refers to the relative amounts of fat and lean tissue in your body. Lean tissue consists of muscle, bone, organs, and fluids. A healthy body composition has adequate muscle tissue with moderate to low amounts of fat tissue. The recommendations for fat percentages will vary based upon your gender and age. Increased levels of fat will put you at risk for diabetes, heart disease, and certain cancers. Working toward (and maintaining) a healthy body composition should be one of the cornerstones of all health, fitness, and diet programs.

WHAT ARE THE SKILL-RELATED COMPONENTS OF PHYSICAL FITNESS?

In addition to the five health-related components of fitness, physical fitness also involves attributes that improve your ability to perform athletic and exercise tasks. These attributes are called the **skill-related components of fitness.** Often termed *sport skills,* these are qualities that athletes aim to improve in order to gain a competitive edge. Recreational athletes and general exercisers can also benefit from improving these skills, because doing so can improve their enjoyment of their chosen sports. The six skill-related components of fitness are:

- Agility: The ability to rapidly change the position of your body with speed and accuracy
- Balance: The maintenance of equilibrium while you are stationary or moving
- Coordination: The ability to use both your senses and your body to perform motor tasks smoothly and accurately

- Power: The ability to perform work or contract muscles with high force quickly
- Speed: The ability to perform a movement in a short period of time
- Reaction time: The time between a stimulus and the initiation of your physical reaction to that stimulus

Although skill-related fitness is largely determined by heredity,[4] regular training can result in significant improvements. In order to improve skill-related components of fitness, athletes and exercisers first need to target the skills that will be important to their specific sport or exercise. For instance, a runner can benefit from increasing power for hill running and speed for winning races, whereas a tennis player can benefit from increased agility and reaction time.

Improving your sport skills can be as easy as simply participating regularly in any sport or activity. Playing football will increase reaction time and power, while dancing will increase balance, agility, and coordination. Another way to increase sport skills is to perform drills that mimic a sport-specific skill, or work specifically on any of the skill-related components of fitness. You can practice drills in group exercise classes that incorporate sport skills, or you can work with a personal trainer. Specialized equipment is often used in such drills: for example, exercises utilizing obstacles such as ladders, hurdles, and cones can help you improve your speed, agility, and coordination, while working on balance boards or with exercise balls can help you improve your balance.

WHAT ARE THE PRINCIPLES OF FITNESS?

In order to design an effective fitness program, you need to take into account the basic **principles of fitness** (also called *principles of exercise training*). These guiding principles explain how the body responds or adapts to exercise training and inform the best methods of training to reach your fitness goals.

OVERLOAD

The principle of **overload** states that in order to see improvements in your physical fitness, the amount or dose of training you undertake must be more than your body or specific body system is used to. This applies to any of the components of physical fitness (health- or skill-related) discussed earlier. For example, in order to increase your flexibility, you must stretch a little farther than you are used to. If

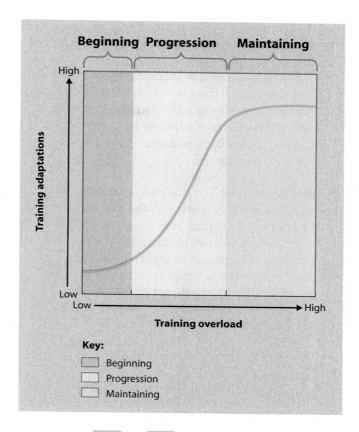

FIGURE 2.2

After adjusting to new training overloads at the beginning of your exercise program, you will see larger adaptations and improvements during the progression phase. As you approach your goal or genetic limits, your increases in overload will not result in further adaptations. This is a sign that you have reached a plateau and should maintain (if satisfied) or adjust your program for further improvement.

you have had the same fitness routine for years, you are *maintaining* your current level of fitness but are probably no longer seeing any improvements. To improve your current level of fitness, you must increase the frequency or intensity of your exercise.

Training Effects Consistent overloads or stresses on a body system will cause an **adaptation** to occur (Figure 2.2). An adaptation is a change in the body as a result of an overload. In exercise training this is

principles of fitness General principles of exercise adaptation that guide fitness programming

overload Subjecting the body or body system to more physical activity than it is used to

adaptation A change in a body system as a result of physical training

called a **training effect.** For example, if you normally run two laps around a track each day but gradually increase this to four laps each day, the overload to your cardiorespiratory and muscular systems will cause adaptations in those systems. While you may feel tired and out of breath the first time you run four laps, after a few weeks of running those four laps the adaptations in your body will allow you to cover that distance with greater ease.

Dose-Response The amount of adaptation you can expect is directly related to the amount of overload or training dose that you complete. This is called the *dose-response relationship.* An increase in your "dose," or amount of training, will result in increased responses or adaptations to that training. How much response or adaptation you can expect is dependent upon the body system trained, the health or fitness outcome measured, and your individual physical and genetic characteristics.

Diminished Returns The principle of *diminished returns* (also called the *initial values principle*) states that the rate of fitness improvement diminishes over time as fitness levels approach genetic limits. Initial fitness levels determine the amount of improvement that you can achieve from exercise training overloads. If you are sedentary and far from your genetic limits, you might experience large increases in fitness levels from moderate amounts of training. If you are active and closer to your genetic limits already, you may gain only small increases in fitness from larger amounts of training.

Diminished returns in overall health may occur from excessively high levels of physical activity. It is possible to be very fit while not being very healthy! Increasing physical activity only results in greater health gains to a certain point or *threshold.* After that threshold, extremely high levels of activity may actually start to harm you (see Figure 2.3). So, the goal is to design a fitness program that is vigorous enough to result in health benefits—but not one that is so hard on your body that you end up injuring yourself.

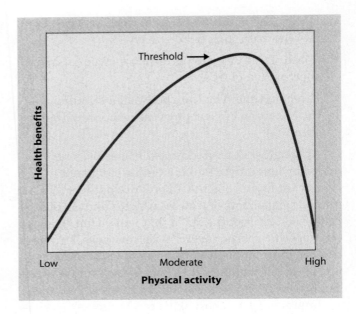

FIGURE 2.3

Increases in physical activity will result in greater health benefits until a threshold is reached; afterward, higher levels of physical activity will result in fewer overall health benefits.

PROGRESSION

The principle of **progression** states that in order to effectively and safely increase fitness, you need to apply an optimal level of overload to the body within a certain time period. Simply stated, you need to increase your workout levels enough to see results, but not so much that you increase your risk of injury. Your body will then progressively adapt to the overloads presented to it. To make sure that you are not progressing too quickly, follow the "10 percent rule": increase your program frequency, intensity, or duration by no more than 10 percent per week.

SPECIFICITY

The principle of **specificity** states that improvements in a body system will occur only if that specific body system is stressed or progressively overloaded by the physical activity. To follow this principle, make sure that you are training targeted muscle groups specific to your sport or that your program is specifically designed to meet your goals. For instance, if you are planning to walk a marathon, you should primarily *walk* during your training. If, instead, you decide to do lap swimming as your training, you may increase your cardiorespiratory fitness levels, but you will not be specifically training your lower body muscles to walk 26 miles.

training effect An increase in physical fitness as a result of overload adaptations in body systems

progression A gradual increase in a training program's intensity, frequency, and/or time

specificity The concept that only the body systems worked during training will show adaptations

REVERSIBILITY

All fitness gains are reversible, according to the principle of **reversibility.** This is the "use it or lose it" principle. If you do not maintain a minimal level of physical activity and exercise, your fitness levels will slip. Unfortunately, you cannot accumulate fitness or workout sessions in a "bank" for later. Doing a great deal of exercise during one week will not compensate for a subsequent month of doing no exercise. Whenever you stop exercising, it only takes about half the time that you spent exercising to lose any fitness gains you may have made while training.[5] For example, if you spent 4 months running 4 miles three times a week, you could lose any fitness gains from those 4 months within 2 months of *no* training.

INDIVIDUALITY

The principle of **individuality** states that adaptations to a training overload may vary greatly from person to person. Two people participate in the same training program but have very different responses. A person who responds well to a training program is considered a *responder.* One who does not respond well is considered a *nonresponder.* Of those individuals who show improvements, some may respond better to increases in total amount of physical activity, while others may show more improvement with increases in exercise intensity.

Genetics greatly influence all individual differences in training adaptations. While you cannot control your genetic makeup, understanding how

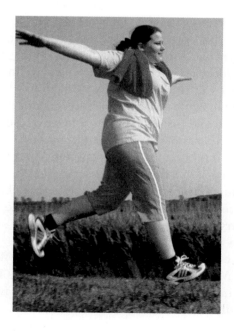

you respond to exercise is important in designing your personal fitness plan. In most cases, figuring out your individual response to certain exercise programs is a trial-and-error process. By completing regular fitness or performance assessments (and keeping a training log), you can track your individual response and adjust your program accordingly to meet your goals.

REST AND RECOVERY

The principle of rest and recovery (also called the *principle of recuperation*) is critical to ensuring continued progress toward your fitness goals. As you will recall, the overload principle states that you must subject your body to more exercise than it is used to doing. However, your body also needs time to recover from the increased physiological and structural training stresses that you place

reversibility The concept that training adaptations will revert toward initial levels when training is stopped

individuality Refers to the variable nature of physical activity dose-response or adaptations in different persons

SIX EASY WAYS TO GET MORE ACTIVE

You can improve your fitness level simply by adding more physical activity to your daily life. Below are a few ways you can incorporate more physical activity into your daily life:

- Instead of driving your car to campus, ride your bike or walk.
- If you must drive to campus, park your car farther from your destination than usual.
- If you have a dog, walk it daily. If you already do that, add a second daily walk—your dog will love you for it!
- While grocery shopping, carry a handbasket instead of pushing a cart (assuming your grocery list is not very long).
- If you have children, actively play with them.
- If you have a desk job, get up, stretch, and walk around often.

Source: U.S. Department of Health and Human Services, "Choices." Small Step Program. www.smallstep.gov/ga/choices.html.

on it. In resistance training (also called *weight training*) in particular, most of the training adaptations actually take place during the rest periods between workouts.

Constant training day after day with insufficient rest periods can result in reduced health benefits and can eventually lead to **overtraining.** If you are exercising consistently and start feeling more fatigue and muscle soreness than usual during and after exercise, you could be doing too much. Reduce the duration or intensity of your exercise and rest for a day or two. To prevent overtraining and to gain optimal benefits from your training program, schedule regular rest days (1 to 3 per week) in any cardiorespiratory endurance program and every other day for any strength-training program. Another important tip to avoid overtraining and injury is to alternate hard workout days with easier workout days during your weekly plan.

overtraining Excessive volume and intensity of physical training leading to diminished health, fitness, and performance

HOW MUCH EXERCISE IS ENOUGH?

How much exercise or physical activity do you really need? The answers will vary, depending on which sources you turn to and on your individual fitness goals.

VARIOUS ORGANIZATIONS RECOMMEND MINIMAL ACTIVITY LEVELS

The best sources of information rely on credible scientific research in developing their recommendations. These sources can be *government agencies* (such as the President's Council on Physical Fitness and Sports), *professional organizations* (such as the American College of Sports Medicine), or *private organizations* (such as the American Heart Association). Table 2.1 on pp. 38–39 compares the major physical activity guidelines from various organizations. Notice that, for adults, most organizations recommend at least 30 minutes of moderate exercise per day, for most days of the week.

THE PHYSICAL ACTIVITY PYRAMID SUMMARIZES GENERAL GUIDELINES

The Physical Activity Pyramid (Figure 2.4) visually summarizes minimal physical activity and exercise guidelines. Similar in concept to the USDA's Food Guide Pyramid, the Physical Activity Pyramid presents recommended levels of activity for optimal health and wellness. The pyramid's bottom layer represents light recreational "lifestyle" activities that you should strive to incorporate into your everyday life, especially walking. The next layer of the pyramid represents moderate-to-vigorous aerobic and/or sports activities (such as bicycling or jogging) that you should try to do three to five times per week in order to build cardiorespiratory endurance and fitness. The third layer of the pyramid represents strength-training and flexibility-building exercises that you should try to incorporate 2 to 3 days per week. The top layer of the pyramid represents the activities that should ideally receive the least amount of your time— sedentary activities such as watching TV or surfing the Web—in favor of more active pursuits.

The box **Tools for Change: Six Easy Ways to Get More Active** provides suggestions for how to incorporate more physical activity into your daily life.

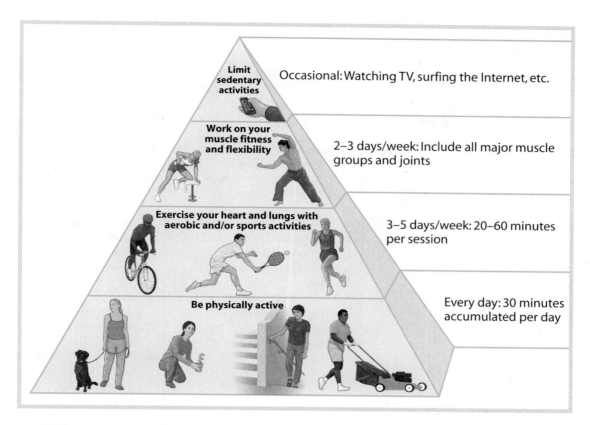

The Physical Activity Pyramid presents recommended levels of activity for optimal health and wellness.
Adapted from The Activity Pyramid. Pyramids of Health, Park Nicollet Health Source.

Try it NOW! Examine the Physical Activity Pyramid. • How does your weekly physical activity match up to its recommendations? • In which areas of the pyramid should you try to improve?

THE FITT FORMULA CAN HELP YOU PLAN YOUR PROGRAM

The **FITT formula** stands for *frequency, intensity, time,* and *type*. These are all factors that you should consider when planning your personal exercise program.

- *Frequency* is the number of times per week that you will perform an exercise.

- *Intensity* refers to how "hard" you will exercise. For aerobic activities, intensity is often measured in terms of how much the given activity increases the heart rate. For resistance activities, intensity is represented in the amount of resistance or weight lifted and the number of repetitions.

- *Time* is the amount of time that you will devote to a given exercise. It can be the total amount of time you spend on an aerobic or sport activity or the amount of time you spend holding a stretch for a flexibility exercise.

- *Type* refers to the kind of exercise you will do. Within each of the exercise components of fitness (cardiorespiratory endurance, muscular

FITT formula A formula for designing a safe and effective exercise program that specifies frequency, intensity, time, and type

TABLE **2.1**

General Exercise and Physical Activity Recommendations

Title & Organization(s)	Youth (< 18 Years)	Adults (18–65 Years)	Seniors (> 65 Years)
American College of Sports Medicine[1,2] and American Heart Association[1,2]	60 minutes or more of moderate to vigorous physical activity.	1. Moderate-intensity aerobic activity a minimum of 30 min., 5 days per week or vigorous-intensity aerobic activity a minimum of 20 min., 3 days per week or a combination of each. 2. Moderate and vigorous activities *in addition* to light activities of daily living. 3. Muscular strength and endurance exercises of major muscle groups two times per week or more, 8–12 repetitions.	1. Moderate-intensity aerobic activity a minimum of 30 min., 5 days per week or vigorous-intensity aerobic activity a minimum of 20 min., 3 days per week or a combination of each. 2. Moderate and vigorous activities are *in addition* to light activities of daily living. 3. Muscular strength and endurance of major muscle groups two times per week or more, 10–15 repetitions. 4. Flexibility exercises two days a week or more for at least 10 min. per day. 5. Balance exercises to reduce the risk of injury from falls.
U. S. Department of Agriculture[3] and U. S. Department of Health[3] and Human Services	At least 60 min. of physical activity on most, preferably all, days of the week.	1. *Reduce chronic disease*— At least 30 min. of moderate-intensity activity, above usual activity, on most days of the week. 2. *Prevent weight gain*—60 min. of moderate- to vigorous-intensity activity on most days of the week while not exceeding caloric intake. 3. *Sustain weight loss*— 60–90 min. of moderate-intensity physical activity while not exceeding caloric intake.	Participate in regular physical activity to reduce functional declines associated with aging and to achieve the other benefits of physical activity identified for all adults.
World Health Organization[4]	N/A	At least 30 min. of regular, moderate-intensity physical activity on most days reduces the risk of cardiovascular disease and diabetes, colon cancer, and breast cancer. More activity may be required for weight control.	Muscle strengthening and balance training can reduce falls and increase functional status among older adults.

strength and endurance, and flexibility), there are many types of exercises that will increase fitness levels. Your type, or **mode,** of exercise will be determined by your preferences, physical abilities, environment, and personal goals.

If you are beginning a fitness program for the first time, you may want to start with the Physical Activity Pyramid recommendations, and then customize your program using the FITT formula concepts to suit your personal goals.

mode The specific type of exercise performed

TABLE 2.1 *continued*

Title & Organization(s)	Youth (< 18 Years)	Adults (18–65 Years)	Seniors (> 65 Years)
Institute of Medicine[5]	An average of 60 min. of daily moderate physical activity.	An average of 60 min. of daily moderate physical activity (e.g., walking/jogging at 3–4 miles/hr) or shorter periods of more vigorous exertion (e.g., jogging for 30 min. at 5.5 miles/hr)	N/A
Office of the Surgeon General[6] and U. S. Department of Health[6] and Human Services	1. Parents can help their children maintain a physically active lifestyle by providing encouragement and opportunities for physical activity. Family events can include opportunities for everyone in the family to be active. 2. Teenagers—regular physical activity improves strength, builds lean muscle, and decreases body fat. It can build stronger bones to last a lifetime.	Minimum of 30 min. of moderate physical activity (150 calories) on most, if not all, days of the week.	Muscle-strengthening exercises can reduce the risk of falling and fracturing bones and can improve the ability to live independently.

Sources:

1. Haskell, W.L. et.al. "Physical Activity and Public Health: Updated Recommendation for Adults from the American College of Sports Medicine and the American Heart Association." *Medicine & Science in Sports and Exercise,* 2007; *39*(8): 1423–34. www.acsm-msse.org
2. Nelson, M.E. et.al. "Physical Activity and Public Health in Older Adults: Recommendation from the American College of Sports Medicine and the American Heart Association." *Medicine & Science in Sports and Exercise,* 2007; *39*(8): 1435–45. www.acsm-msse.org
3. U.S. Department of Health and Human Services and U.S. Department of Agriculture. *Dietary Guidelines for Americans,* 2005. 6th Edition, Washington, DC: U.S. Government Printing Office, January 2005.
4. World Health Organization. *Global Strategy on Diet, Physical Activity and Health.* Geneva, Switzerland: Marketing and Dissemination, World Health Organization, 2004.
5. Institute of Medicine of the National Academies. *Dietary Reference Intakes for Energy, Carbohydrate, Fiber, Fat, Fatty Acids, Cholesterol, Protein, and Amino Acids.* Food and Nutrition Board, Washington, DC: The National Academies Press, September 2002.
6. U.S. Department of Health and Human Services. *Physical Activity and Health: A Report of the Surgeon General.* Atlanta. U.S. Department of Health and Human Services, Centers for Disease Control and Prevention, National Center for Chronic Disease Prevention and Health Promotion, 1996.

WHAT DOES IT TAKE TO EXERCISE SAFELY?

Exercise-related injuries have risen in recent decades. Over 7 million Americans receive medical attention for sports-related injuries each year, with the greatest numbers of injuries affecting 5- to 24-year-olds.[6] To reduce your risk of exercise injury, follow the guidelines below.

WARM UP PROPERLY BEFORE YOUR WORKOUT

A proper warm-up consists of two phases: a general warm-up and a specific warm-up. In a *general warm-up,* your goal is to warm up the body by doing 3 to 10 minutes of light physical activity similar to the activities you will be performing during exercise. During this period of time (called the *rest-to-exercise*

FACTS AND FALLACIES

SHOULD YOU STRETCH WHILE WARMING UP?

Many people incorrectly think that a good warm-up consists primarily of stretching. While stretching can be a component of an effective warm-up, it is not the most important. In fact, in power athletes, too much stretching can actually decrease muscle power output during an athletic event.[1] If you enjoy stretching during your warm-up, limit it to 10-to-15-second stretches of the major muscle groups used during the activity, and stretch during the end of your specific warm-up.

Source: Young W. B., and Behm D. G. "Effects of Running, Static Stretching and Practice Jumps on Explosive Force Production and Jumping Performance," *The Journal of Sports Medicine and Physical Fitness* 2003; *43*(1): 21–7.

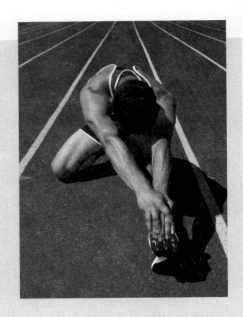

transition), you are preparing your body to withstand the more vigorous exercise to come. Your core body temperature should rise a few degrees, and you should break a slight sweat. This movement and temperature rise will increase your overall blood flow, ready the joint fluid and structures, and improve muscle elasticity.

During a *specific warm-up,* your goal is to focus on the particular muscle groups and joints that you will be using during the activity set. This part of the warm-up should consist of 3 to 5 minutes of **range-of-motion** movements. You should move the joints involved in your exercise through the range of motion that they will experience during the activity. Move joints through a full range of motion in a relaxed and controlled manner. If you want to add light stretching to your warm-up, do so at the end of your specific warm-up. The box **Facts and Fallacies: Should You Stretch While Warming Up?** addresses the misconceptions about stretching before a workout.

COOL DOWN PROPERLY AFTER YOUR WORKOUT

After you finish your workout, cool down in a manner that is appropriate to the activity that you performed. This *exercise-to-rest transition*

should last anywhere from 5 to 15 minutes. If your heart rate and temperature rose during your workout, you should perform a *general cool-down* in which your goal is to bring your heart rate, breathing rate, and temperature closer to resting levels. This cool-down is usually a less vigorous version of the activity you just performed. For example, if you jogged for 25 minutes, your general cool-down may consist of 10 minutes of walking.

If you have just finished a resistance-training program and your heart rate is not elevated, you should perform a *specific cool-down* for the joints and muscles you have exercised. A specific cool-down can be performed after a general cool-down for aerobic activities and right after exercise for resistance-training activities. During a specific cool-down, you should stretch the muscle groups worked during the activity. See Chapter 6 for more specifics on stretching during the cool-down process.

TAKE THE TIME TO PROPERLY LEARN THE SKILLS FOR YOUR CHOSEN ACTIVITY

There are hundreds of different activities that you can do to increase your health and fitness, each with a specific set of physical skills required for participation. You might choose simple activities like walking or jogging, which require little skill and have short learning curves, or you might focus on activities that require more complex skills, such as fencing or hockey. Whatever you choose, *properly learn the*

range of motion The movement limits that limbs have around a specific joint

physical skills required for the activity to enhance your enjoyment and to avoid injury. If you are just beginning a sport for the first time—for example, skiing—do not immediately approach the sport the way a more experienced athlete would. Take lessons, start on the beginner slopes, and give yourself time to safely perform your chosen activity.

CONSUME ENOUGH ENERGY AND WATER FOR EXERCISE

Deciding how much to eat and drink prior to exercise can be tricky. You need enough energy to work out, but you should not exercise on a full stomach. Eating a small meal 1 1/2 to 2 hours before exercise is a good way to make sure that you have energy (but not an upset stomach) during the workout. A *light* snack 30 to 60 minutes before your workout is acceptable as well.

Dehydration is more likely than food intake to affect your exercise performance. During the hours before your workout, be sure to drink enough water so that you do not feel thirsty as you go into your exercise session. Guidelines for drinking before, during, and after exercising should be tailored to the individual and the exercise session.[7] General guidelines are 17 to 20 oz. of fluid 2 to 3 hours before exercise and 7 to 10 oz. 10 to 20 minutes prior to exercise.[8] During your workout, hydrate when you feel thirsty, and increase the amount of water you consume as you start to sweat more profusely.

SELECT APPROPRIATE FOOTWEAR AND CLOTHING

Consider this: Your feet will typically strike the ground 1,000 times during 1 mile of running. Over weeks of training, that translates to a great deal of wear and tear on your feet and lower body. Needless to say, proper footwear is critical to a safe and successful training program—regardless of the activity you choose.

While some sports require specialized footwear, most beginning exercisers just need one pair of good, all-around cross-trainers or running shoes. The most important aspect of footwear is proper fit and cushioning. Always try on shoes before purchasing them, and if possible, spend a few minutes mimicking the activity you will be doing in them. The best shoes are not always the most expensive ones, but you should aim to purchase the highest quality footwear you can afford. Ask for assistance from a knowledgeable salesperson—let him or her know what activities you are planning to pursue, and ask which shoes would be most appropriate for your plans.

Clothing for exercise can be very simple (e.g., shorts and a T-shirt) or very technical (e.g., clothing with wicking fibers or special treatments for protection against harsh weather). The most important thing is to *dress appropriately for your chosen activity.* Make sure that your clothing is comfortable and does not restrict your range of motion. Women may wish to wear supportive athletic bras, and men may want to consider wearing supportive compression shorts or undergarments. If you are planning to exercise outdoors, take temperature into consideration and dress accordingly. The longer you plan to exercise, the more carefully you should think about what kind of attire will be most conducive to a successful workout.

WHAT INDIVIDUAL FACTORS SHOULD YOU CONSIDER WHEN DESIGNING A FITNESS PROGRAM?

There is no such thing as a "one-size-fits-all" physical fitness program. Different individuals have different needs, and general recommendations often need to be adapted to fit those individual needs. Your age, weight, current fitness level, and any disabilities and special health concerns are all factors that should be considered in order to design a safe and effective exercise routine.

AGE

Older adults may require additional precautions in order to prevent injury while exercising. Men over age 45 and women over age 55 should obtain medical clearance before beginning an exercise program.[9] Moderate aerobic activity, muscle-strengthening exercises, and flexibility work are all recommended activities for older adults. In addition, balance exercises should be included to help prevent the risk of falls and injury.

WEIGHT

Overweight individuals are at higher risk of musculoskeletal injuries due to increased stress on their muscles and joints, and they should take precautions to ensure safe workouts. If you are overweight,

UNDERSTANDING DIVERSITY

GETTING ACTIVE DESPITE DISABILITY

In the documentary film *Murderball,* muscular, aggressive rugby players compete in fierce, international competitions alongside other world-class athletes—all of them in wheelchairs. Their stories are an inspiration to disabled and nondisabled people alike, and demonstrate that while disability does pose undeniable obstacles, it does not have to hinder the achievement of even the highest levels of physical fitness.

With personal motivation, support from friends and family, and assistance from medical and fitness professionals, persons with disability can make exercise part of their daily routine and live physically active lives. For example, most strength-training machines are used from a seated position and can be operated by people in wheelchairs. Rubber exercise bands, meanwhile, can serve as alternative strength-building aids.[1] Many companies also offer modified sports equipment for people with disabilities: Handcycles allow people to ride bikes using arm power, and wakeboards and flotation devices enable waterskiing and swimming activities. Several kinds of seated skis make downhill skiing accessible to those with physical handicaps.

And disabled people can play a long list of sports—with modified rules and equipment—including volleyball, tennis, golf, soccer, basketball, bowling, bocci, archery, tai chi, and karate.

If you have a physical disability, consult with your doctor or physical therapist about what kinds of activities will best meet your goals and needs.

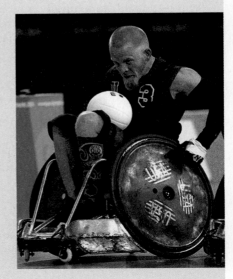

Source: Mayo Clinic, "Exercise and Disability: Physical Activity Is Within Your Reach." Mayo Clinic, June 22, 2006, www.mayoclinic.com/health/exercise/SM00042.

---

consider a cross-training routine with a mix of moderate weight-bearing (e.g., walking, stair-climbing) and non-weight-bearing (e.g., bicycling, water exercise) activities. If you feel pain in your lower-body joints during exercise, shift to more non-weight-bearing activities during your workout.

Underweight individuals, on the other hand, should perform more strength-training and weight-bearing activities to ensure proper muscle and bone maintenance.

CURRENT FITNESS LEVEL

Design a program that is appropriate to your current fitness level. If you already exercise regularly, consider gradually increasing the frequency or intensity of your workouts to realize more fitness gains. If you are currently sedentary and are just beginning to think about starting an exercise routine, do not just suddenly attempt to participate in a triathlon! Pick an activity that you find enjoyable, start at a level that is comfortable for you, and proceed from there.

DISABILITIES

If you have mobility restrictions, poor balance, dizziness, or other conditions that are physically limiting, you can still incorporate fitness into your daily life with alternative or adaptive exercises. Many colleges, community centers, parks and recreation facilities, and fitness centers offer adaptive courses, equipment, and instructors who are specially trained to help you meet your fitness goals. After obtaining medical clearance, seek out such facilities; your physician or a physical therapist may have good recommendations. The box **Understanding Diversity: Getting Active Despite Disability** provides additional suggestions.

SPECIAL HEALTH CONCERNS

Certain medical conditions may require you to exercise under medical supervision. Individuals with asthma, heart disease, hypertension, and diabetes all need medical clearance prior to beginning exercise and may need to be monitored by medical personnel during exercise. If you have special health concerns, seek out the advice of a qualified medical professional on how to exercise safely.

Individuals with significant bone or joint problems can benefit from selecting lower-impact activities such as swimming, water exercise, bicycling, walking, or low-impact aerobics. They can also benefit from resistance-training exercises that can strengthen

SPOTLIGHT

CAN YOU EXERCISE WHILE PREGNANT?

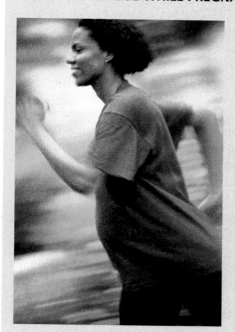

Although pregnancy is not the time to start an intense fitness or weight-loss program, most pregnant women can maintain pre-pregnancy activities with just a few modifications. The American College of Obstetrics and Gynecology recommends the following guidelines:

- First, be sure to get medical clearance for the particular exercise that you intend to do. Your physician may have some specific recommendations for your fitness program.

- If you are relatively new to exercising, seek out a pregnancy fitness exercise program where qualified instructors lead safe exercise sessions. These programs can also provide a good social support network for mothers-to-be.

- Choose fitness activities that do not increase risk of injury to you or the fetus. Avoid high-intensity sports, activities with the potential for falls or abdominal injury, and environmental extremes (such as temperature or barometric pressure—no scuba diving, in particular). Pay attention to your body temperature and avoid getting too hot during exercise, especially during the first trimester. Choose low-impact activities like swimming, water exercise, indoor cycling, yoga, and walking.

- In the absence of medical complications, perform 30 minutes or more of moderate exercise on most, if not all, days of the week.

- Monitor your exercise intensity levels by determining how you feel during exercise.

- In the third trimester, avoid supine exercises (i.e., exercises that require you to lie on your back), because these may restrict blood flow to the fetus. Also, exercise moderately and avoid higher-intensity workouts during this time.

- Add pelvic floor exercises to your fitness routine. These exercises, called *kegels,* involve tightening the pelvic floor muscles for 5 to15 seconds at a time and will help with pregnancy-induced incontinence and delivery recovery. Add three to five sets of 10 to your daily routine.

Pregnancy can be both a wonder-filled and scary time. Maintaining a minimum level of fitness can help you cope with the stresses coming your way. Consult your physician and other pregnancy fitness resources to get started.

Source: American College of Obstetrics and Gynecology, "Exercise During Pregnancy and the Postpartum Period." *Obstetrics & Gynecology* 2002; *99*(1): 171–173.

CASE STUDY

Lily

"I've started jogging again! I'm back to jogging 30 minutes twice a week and thinking of bumping things up to three times a week. I'm hoping to eventually work my way up to jogging for 45 minutes straight, each time I go out. I'm not tempted to run a 10k again any time soon, but if I can keep this new routine going, maybe I will be ready for a 5k—without hurting my knees this time."

1. Describe Lily's exercise routine, using the FITT formula.

2. What kinds of things would you advise Lily to do, in order to reduce her chances of injury?

3. Think back to Lily's question at the beginning of the chapter about what it means to be fit. Given what you have learned in this chapter, how would you answer that question?

muscles and joint structures, and contribute to bone-density maintenance and improvement (if their joint limitations will allow it).

If you are taking any prescription medications, ask your doctor if there are side effects that you should consider before exercising. In addition, beware of over-the-counter medications and other products that may cause drowsiness (such as antihistamines, certain cough/cold medicines, and alcohol), as this will decrease your reaction time, coordination, and balance during exercise.

If you are pregnant, read the box **Spotlight: Can You Exercise While Pregnant?** for advice on exercising safely while expecting.

HOW CAN YOU GET STARTED?

Preparing to exercise for the first time (or after a long sedentary period) can be daunting. Most people are unsure how to start, what to do, and how much to exercise. This often leads people to just jump right in, do something their friends are doing, or try something they saw on TV or in a magazine. This haphazard, impulsive approach often leads to disappointment and frustration—not to mention muscle soreness and even injury.

A better approach is to think carefully about your exercise motivations, goals, and needs, select activities that will meet those needs (and that you enjoy!), apply the FITT formula to each of those activities, and then make a conscious long-term commitment to your exercise program. We designed this textbook to help you along this process! To begin, fill out *Lab2.1* to assess your current readiness for physical activity and to determine if you need medical clearance to begin an exercise program. Next, read Chapter 3 for strategies to help you commit to a fitness program, including understanding your motivations, overcoming common obstacles to sticking with an exercise program, and selecting activities that are best suited to you. Then read Chapters 4–6 on cardiorespiratory endurance, strength training, and flexibility. Each of these chapters provides guidelines for beginning programs designed to help you meet your individual fitness goals in each of these health-related components of fitness.

To further assist you on your road to fitness, *Lab2.2* will teach you a basic skill—how to use a pedometer—and *Lab2.3* will help you begin to plan ways to incorporate more physical activity into your daily life.

REVIEW QUESTIONS

1. Moderate physical activity is best defined as activity that is:
   a. Less than 3 METS
   b. 3–6 METS
   c. 7–9 METS
   d. Over 10 METS

2. Which health-related component of fitness involves moving your joints through a full range of motion?
   a. Cardiorespiratory fitness
   b. Muscular endurance
   c. Flexibility
   d. Body composition

3. Which skill-related component of fitness is most involved in braking quickly when a car in front of you stops suddenly?
   a. Agility
   b. Power
   c. Coordination
   d. Reaction time

4. Which principle of fitness relies on the idea that the rate of improvement in a fitness program depends upon your initial fitness level?
   a. Progression
   b. Overload
   c. Diminished returns
   d. Specificity

5. The principle of individuality states that:
   a. Adaptations to training overload may vary widely from person to person
   b. All individuals respond the same way to exercise
   c. Genetic makeup has nothing to do with individual responses to exercise
   d. *Nonresponders* are individuals who do not benefit from exercise

6. The Physical Activity Pyramid recommends which of the following?
   a. Two to 3 days/week of cardiorespiratory activity, 3 to 5 days/week of strength-training and flexibility activities
   b. Two to 3 days/week of strength-training and flexibility exercises, 3 to 5 days/week of cardiorespiratory activity
   c. Constant sedentary activity every day
   d. Limiting the amount of time you spend walking

7. The F in the FITT formula stands for what?
   a. Family
   b. Friends
   c. Frequency
   d. Fitness

8. A proper warm-up consists of how many phases?
   a. One
   b. Two
   c. Three
   d. Four

9. If you are learning a sport for the first time, you should:
   a. Challenge yourself by immediately attempting to perform the exercise the way an experienced athlete would
   b. Not care about clothing and footwear
   c. Do whatever your friends are doing
   d. Take the time to properly acquire the physical skills necessary for your chosen activity

10. When designing your own fitness program, it is important to consider all of the following factors EXCEPT:
    a. Your weight
    b. Your current fitness level
    c. Any special health concerns
    d. A one-size-fits-all approach

CRITICAL THINKING QUESTIONS

1. Give an example of how a training overload can lead to adaptations and training effects.

2. Describe the similarities and differences between the principle of diminished returns and the principle of progression.

3. Imagine you are about to begin a fitness program centered around bicycling. Apply the FITT formula to describe how you might set up your program.

ONLINE RESOURCES

1. **Centers for Disease Control and Prevention: Physical Activity for Everyone**
   www.cdc.gov/nccdphp/dnpa/physical/everyone.htm
   Information about the importance of physical activity, measuring physical activity, getting started, incorporating lifestyle physical activity, resources, and more.

2. **Medline Plus**
   www.medlineplus.gov
   Health information from the U.S. National Library of Medicine and the National Institute for Health.

3. **MyPyramid.gov**
   www.mypyramid.gov
   USDA site with personal planning and tracking programs for diet and physical activity.

4. **National Institutes of Health (NIH)**
   www.health.nih.gov/result.asp/245
   Health information about exercise and physical fitness from various member institutions.

   Web addresses are subject to change. Please visit this book's website at **www.aw-bc.com/hopson** for updates and additional Web resources.

REFERENCES

1. M.R. Carnethon and others. "Prevalence and Cardiovascular Disease Correlates of Low Cardio-respiratory Fitness in Adolescents and Adults." *The Journal of the American Medical Association.* 2005; 294(23): 2981–88.

2. H. Suominen, "Muscle Training for Bone Strength." *Aging, Clinical and Experimental Research.* 2006; 18(2): 85–93.

3. M.A. Jones and others. "Biological Risk Indicators for Recurrent Non-Specific Low Back Pain in Adolescents." *British Journal of Sports Medicine.* 2005; 39(3): 137–40.

4. T.D. Brutsaert and E.J. Parra. "What Makes a Champion? Explaining Variation in Human Athletic Performance." *Respiratory Physiology and Neurobiology.* 2006; 151: 109–23.

5. W.D. McArdle and others. *Exercise Physiology: Energy, Nutrition, and Human Performance.* 6th Edition. Lippincott Williams & Wilkins, Baltimore, MD, 2007.

6. J.M. Conn and others. "Sports and Recreation Related Injury Episodes in the U.S. Population, 1997–99." *Injury Prevention.* 2003; 9(2): 117–23.

7. M.N. Sawka and others. "American College of Sports Medicine Position Stand: Exercise and Fluid Replacement." *Medicine and Science in Sports and Exercise.* 2007; 39(2): 377–90.

8. F.H. Fink and others. *Practical Applications in Sports Nutrition.* Jones and Bartlett Publishers, Inc, Sudbury, MA, 2006.

9. American College of Sports Medicine. *ACSM's Guidelines for Exercise Testing and Prescription.* 7th Edition. Lippincott Williams & Wilkins, Baltimore, MD, 2006.

Name: _____   **Date:** _____

Instructor: _____   **Section:** _____

SECTION I: THE PHYSICAL ACTIVITY READINESS QUESTIONNAIRE

Physical Activity Readiness
Questionnaire - PAR-Q
(revised 2002)

PAR-Q & YOU

(A Questionnaire for People Aged 15 to 69)

Regular physical activity is fun and healthy, and increasingly more people are starting to become more active every day. Being more active is very safe for most people. However, some people should check with their doctor before they start becoming much more physically active.

If you are planning to become much more physically active than you are now, start by answering the seven questions in the box below. If you are between the ages of 15 and 69, the PAR-Q will tell you if you should check with your doctor before you start. If you are over 69 years of age, and you are not used to being very active, check with your doctor.

Common sense is your best guide when you answer these questions. Please read the questions carefully and answer each one honestly: check YES or NO.

YES	NO	
☐	☐	1. Has your doctor ever said that you have a heart condition <u>and</u> that you should only do physical activity recommended by a doctor?
☐	☐	2. Do you feel pain in your chest when you do physical activity?
☐	☐	3. In the past month, have you had chest pain when you were not doing physical activity?
☐	☐	4. Do you lose your balance because of dizziness or do you ever lose consciousness?
☐	☐	5. Do you have a bone or joint problem (for example, back, knee or hip) that could be made worse by a change in your physical activity?
☐	☐	6. Is your doctor currently prescribing drugs (for example, water pills) for your blood pressure or heart condition?
☐	☐	7. Do you know of <u>any other reason</u> why you should not do physical activity?

If   **you**   **answered**

YES to one or more questions

Talk with your doctor by phone or in person BEFORE you start becoming much more physically active or BEFORE you have a fitness appraisal. Tell your doctor about the PAR-Q and which questions you answered YES.

• You may be able to do any activity you want — as long as you start slowly and build up gradually. Or, you may need to restrict your activities to those which are safe for you. Talk with your doctor about the kinds of activities you wish to participate in and follow his/her advice.

• Find out which community programs are safe and helpful for you.

NO to all questions

If you answered NO honestly to <u>all</u> PAR-Q questions, you can be reasonably sure that you can:

• start becoming much more physically active – begin slowly and build up gradually. This is the safest and easiest way to go.

• take part in a fitness appraisal – this is an excellent way to determine your basic fitness so that you can plan the best way for you to live actively. It is also highly recommended that you have your blood pressure evaluated. If your reading is over 144/94, talk with your doctor before you start becoming much more physically active.

DELAY BECOMING MUCH MORE ACTIVE:

• if you are not feeling well because of a temporary illness such as a cold or a fever – wait until you feel better; or

• if you are or may be pregnant – talk to your doctor before you start becoming more active.

PLEASE NOTE: If your health changes so that you then answer YES to any of the above questions, tell your fitness or health professional. Ask whether you should change your physical activity plan.

<u>Informed Use of the PAR-Q:</u> The Canadian Society for Exercise Physiology, Health Canada, and their agents assume no liability for persons who undertake physical activity, and if in doubt after completing this questionnaire, consult your doctor prior to physical activity.

No changes permitted. You are encouraged to photocopy the PAR-Q but only if you use the entire form.

NOTE: If the PAR-Q is being given to a person before he or she participates in a physical activity program or a fitness appraisal, this section may be used for legal or administrative purposes.
"I have read, understood and completed this questionnaire. Any questions I had were answered to my full satisfaction."

NAME _____

SIGNATURE _____   DATE_____

SIGNATURE OF PARENT _____   WITNESS _____
or GUARDIAN (for participants under the age of majority)

Note: This physical activity clearance is valid for a maximum of 12 months from the date it is completed and becomes invalid if your condition changes so that you would answer YES to any of the seven questions.

 © Canadian Society for Exercise Physiology   Supported by: 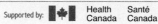 Health Canada   Santé Canada

Physical Activity Readiness Questionnaire (PAR-Q) © 2002. Used with permission from the Canadian Society for Exercise Physiology. www.csep.ca.

SECTION II: HEALTH/FITNESS PRE-PARTICIPATION SCREENING QUESTIONNAIRE

Assess your health status by marking all TRUE statements:

History—You have had:

_____ a heart attack

_____ heart surgery

_____ cardiac catheterization

_____ coronary angioplasty

_____ pacemaker/implantable cardiac defibrillator

_____ heart rhythm disturbance

_____ heart valve disease

_____ heart failure

_____ heart transplantation

_____ congenital heart disease

Symptoms:

_____ You experience chest discomfort with exertion.

_____ You experience unreasonable breathlessness.

_____ You experience dizziness, fainting, or blackouts.

_____ You take heart medications.

Other Health Issues:

_____ You have diabetes.

_____ You have asthma or other lung disease.

_____ You have burning or cramping sensations in your lower legs when walking short distances.

_____ You have musculoskeletal problems that limit your physical activity.

_____ You have concerns about the safety of exercise.

_____ You take prescription medication(s).

_____ You are pregnant.

If you marked any of the statements above, consult your physician or other appropriate health care provider before engaging in exercise. You may need to use a facility with a medically qualified staff.

Cardiovascular Risk Factors:

_____ You are a man older than 45 years old.

_____ You are a woman older than 55 years, have had a hysterectomy, or are postmenopausal.

_____ You smoke, or quit smoking, within the previous 6 months.

_____ Your blood pressure is > 140/90 mmHg.

_____ You do not know your blood pressure.

_____ You take blood pressure medication.

_____ Your blood cholesterol level is > 200 mg/dL.

_____ You do not know your cholesterol level.

_____ You have a close blood relative who had a heart attack or heart surgery before age 55 (father or brother) or age 65 (mother or sister).

_____ You are physically inactive (i.e., you get < 30 min of physical activity on at least 3 days/week).

_____ You are > 20 pounds overweight.

If you marked two or more of the statements in this section, you should consult your physician or other appropriate health care provider before engaging in exercise. You might benefit from using a facility with a professionally qualified exercise staff to guide your exercise program.

If you did not mark any of the above statements, you should not need medical clearance to exercise safely in a properly designed self-guided exercise program.

Source: American College of Sports Medicine, *ACSM's Guidelines for Exercise Testing and Prescription,* 7th ed. Lippincott Williams & Wilkins, Baltimore, MD, 2006. Modified from: American College of Sports Medicine and American Heart Association, "ACSM/AHA Joint Position Statement: Recommendations for Screening, Staffing, and Emergency Policies at Health/Fitness Facilities," *Medicine and Science in Sports and Exercise* (1998): 1810.

Name: _____ **Date:** _____

Instructor: _____ **Section:** _____

Purpose: Using a pedometer, learn how many steps you walk each day.

Directions:

1. Borrow or buy an inexpensive pedometer, a portable device that counts the number of steps you take in a day.

2. Wear the pedometer every day for a week and fill out Worksheet A.

WORKSHEET A

	Monday	Tuesday	Wednesday	Thursday	Friday	Saturday	Sunday
Steps/Day							

Average/day (total divided by 7) = _____

3. The U.S. Surgeon General recommends walking at least 10,000 steps each day. How many steps each day do you currently walk (typically)? _____

Here are a few tips for pedometer walking:

- You can get an accurate pedometer at a sporting goods store or over the Internet. Brands like Digiwalker and Sportline have a good basic model for about $10.

- Tie on your pedometer, or get one with a key chain or belt clip so you don't lose it, since you'll be wearing it all of your waking hours (except while you are showering or swimming).

- If you want to know the total distance you've been walking each day, you can buy a more sophisticated pedometer and calibrate it to your stride length (see manufacturer's directions). Some pedometers also tell you how many calories you've burned.

- Look for ways to increase your steps each day by, for example, walking up stairways, parking farther from buildings, and walking during lunch hour.

Name: _____ **Date:** _____

Instructor: _____ **Section:** _____

Purpose: To create a plan for reducing your sedentary time and replacing it with active time.

Directions:

1. On Worksheet A, list your typical activity for each hour of your day in the column labeled "Activity."

2. Now examine your list. What are your major sedentary activities? Highlight or circle them on Worksheet A.

3. List three physical activities that you would like to do but typically don't have time to do:

_____

_____

_____

4. Go back to Worksheet A and examine the sedentary activities you highlighted or circled in #2. Can you replace some of these sedentary activities with any of the physical activities you listed in #3? If so, write in the revised activity (in the "Revised Activity" column) next to the sedentary activity it is replacing.

5. If the physical activities you'd like to add to your schedule won't work in the time slots you have allotted for sedentary activity (for example, it may not be possible or safe to go out running at 11:30 PM), what are alternative physical activities you can safely pursue? Write them in.

WORKSHEET A

Time of Day	Activity	Revised Activity
6:00 AM		
7:00 AM		
8:00 AM		
9:00 AM		
10:00 AM		
11:00 AM		
12:00 PM		
1:00 PM		
2:00 PM		
3:00 PM		
4:00 PM		
5:00 PM		
6:00 PM		
7:00 PM		
8:00 PM		
9:00 PM		
10:00 PM		
11:00 PM		

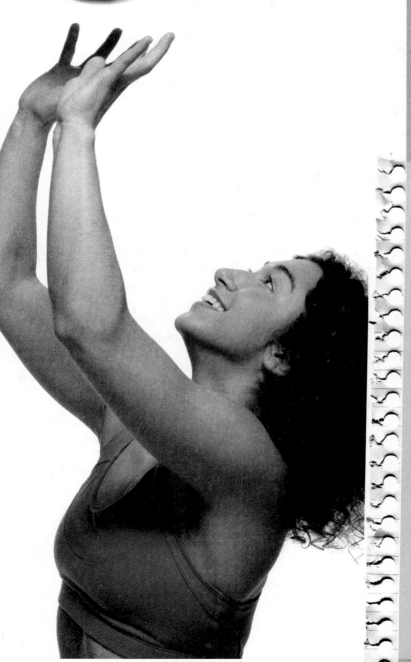

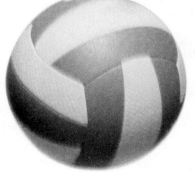

CHAPTER 3

Committing
to Fitness

OBJECTIVES

Commit to fitness behavior changes by assessing your motivations, setting appropriate goals, and creating a personal behavior change contract.

Identify common barriers and obstacles to exercise and develop rewards for overcoming them.

Discuss how your fitness needs may change over the life span.

CASE STUDY

Adam

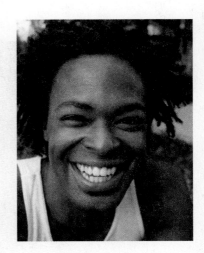

"Hi, I'm Adam. I'd like to be in better shape, but it seems like every time I try to get an exercise routine going, life gets in the way. I work 20 hours a week at a coffee shop, and I'm taking a full course load, so right off the bat, it's hard to find the time. I have a friend, Eric, who I used to play basketball with, but we have different schedules this semester, so that's stopped. I've been thinking about taking an indoor rock-climbing class but haven't actually gotten around to doing it. There always seems to be an errand to run or something else more important to do. Am I hopeless?"

Knowing that exercise is good for you is one thing. Starting a fitness program and sticking with it over the long-term is, too often, another thing altogether. According to a recent national survey, only 31 percent of adults in the United States participate in regular leisure-time physical activity. College-aged adults (18 to 24 years) fared slightly better, with 38 percent reporting regular physical activity patterns. The percentages drop as people age: Fewer than 27 percent of people 65 years and older reported regular leisure-time physical activity.[1]

Despite the statistics, making fitness part of your daily life is within your reach—and can be tremendously fun and rewarding. In this chapter, we will focus on various strategies to help you commit to fitness. We will ask you to assess your motivations for beginning an exercise program, suggest ways for you to set reasonable fitness goals, and present strategies for overcoming common obstacles to success. At the end of the chapter, we will discuss how fitness needs may change over the life span and will introduce ideas for how to successfully make regular physical activity a lifelong habit.

HOW CAN YOU PLAN A SUCCESSFUL FITNESS PROGRAM?

As you begin to plan your fitness program, think about the following:

- What motivates you?
- Where are you in the stages of behavior change (introduced in Chapter 1)?

- What are reasonable fitness goals you can set for yourself?
- Are you prepared to commit to a fitness program?

Answering each of these questions honestly is a good first step to a successful plan of action.

UNDERSTAND YOUR MOTIVATIONS FOR BEGINNING A FITNESS PROGRAM

People have many reasons for participating in sports, exercise, or other physical activities. Some people think of exercise as a chore—something they do more for health benefits than for fun. Some people like the thrill of participating in competitive sports. And some people exercise mainly for pleasure: They love the feeling they get from running outdoors, swimming laps in a pool, biking around a lake, or finishing a challenging hike.

Understanding your motivations for participating in a fitness program can help you plan activities in a way that make you more likely to stick with the program in the long run. Below are some of the most common reasons people decide to exercise, along with tips for how to maximize your chances of long-term fitness success.

- *I want to gain health benefits.* Many people want to exercise to maintain or improve their overall health. If this is your main motivation, try to design a program centered around physical activities that you find *enjoyable* and *easy to incorporate* in your day-to-day life. If you don't like gyms, don't sign up for one! Instead, select an activity in which you genuinely take pleasure such as walking the dog or jogging on a cross-country trail. Better yet, pick an activity that involves your friends and/or family. Having a partner can help keep both of you motivated to stay with the program.

- *I want to have fun.* If your main motivation is fun and recreation, consider taking lessons in a specific sport/activity that interests you, joining an intramural sports team on campus, or going on regular outdoor trips with friends. Seek out activities that, first and foremost, you know you will enjoy—for instance, a day hike in a beautiful spot—and that have the beneficial "side effect" of fitness.

- *I want to meet new people or exercise with friends.* Participating in a fitness program can be a great way to socialize and meet new people. Even if you do not consider this one of your main reasons to start exercising, social motivations can often keep you coming back. Look for activity classes that you can take with friends or where you can meet new people with similar interests. Consider joining a gym, club, or group (such as a running club or a soccer team) that meets regularly for group workout sessions or games.

- *I like the challenge of setting goals and doing well in competition.* Some people are highly motivated by personal challenges or competition. If this sounds like you, regardless of what activity you choose, be sure to set realistic, attainable goals. You may find a clearly defined target—such as an upcoming 5K race—to be just what you need to get started. Find a fun, competitive, active event happening in your area, and sign up!

- *I really want to lose some weight.* Losing weight is one of the most common reasons people exercise. If weight loss is your main motivation, you will need to consider your nutrition and diet plan along with your fitness plan. Choose activities that burn plenty of calories and that you genuinely enjoy. Chapter 9 on weight management offers more guidance for designing a weight-loss program.

- *I would like to have a stronger, more toned body.* If this is your primary reason for exercise, you have plenty of options. Select your favorite

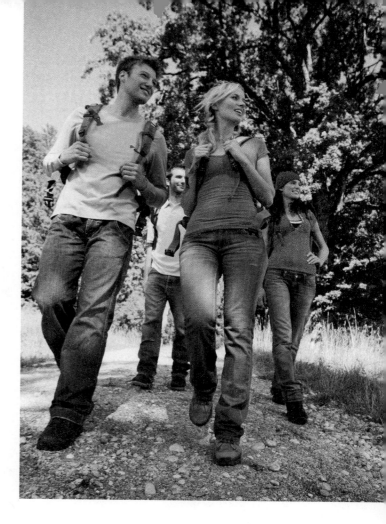

aerobic activity, begin strength training, or take a sport-specific class regularly. Chapter 5 provides a wide variety of options for strength training, regardless of your level of experience.

Lab3.1 will help you assess your motivations for beginning a fitness program. If you are not currently physically active, spend some time thinking about why that is. Are you too busy? Do you simply dislike exercise? Maximize your focus on the pleasurable aspects of being active and try to minimize the negatives. Be open to the possibility that your thinking may change—especially once you experience the benefits of a physically active life.

KNOW WHERE YOU ARE IN THE STAGES OF BEHAVIOR CHANGE

The *transtheoretical model of behavior change* outlines six stages of behavior change: precontemplation, contemplation, preparation, action, maintenance, and termination (see Chapter 1). When it comes to physical activity, where are you within this model? Recall that you can be in different stages of behavior change for different behaviors. For example, as you adopt daily lifestyle physical activities (action), you may be preparing to add some weekly jogging (preparation) to your routine and thinking about hitting the weight room sometime soon (contemplation). *Lab3.2* will help you start planning for physical activity behavior changes by determining where you currently are in the stages of behavior change.

SET REASONABLE GOALS
FOR INCREASED FITNESS

Setting appropriate, realistic goals can mean the difference between success and failure in fitness programming. As outlined in Chapter 1, goals need to be SMART—*specific, measurable, action-oriented, realistic,* and *time-oriented.* If you are new to exercise, your knowledge about what is "reasonable" may be limited. People will often start a fitness program and think they can lose 10 pounds in 2 weeks or train to run a 10K in 3 weeks. These goals are unrealistic and unreasonable for the beginning exerciser.

Remember the fitness principles covered in Chapter 2. A fitness program needs to be *progressive* in order for you to achieve results and avoid injury. As you begin a fitness program, your progress may initially be slow, while your body adjusts to the new activity. Eventually, consistent exercise will result in noticeable improvement. Setting reasonable goals includes considering everything that you have assessed about yourself: your fitness level when you begin, your reasons for exercise, and your motivations and attitudes about physical activity. Keep your physical limitations in mind, as well as constraints that other aspects of your life may impose—for instance, how much activity you can honestly fit into your schedule right now.

---

barriers to physical activity Personal or environmental issues that hinder your participation in regular physical activity

---

MAKE A PERSONAL COMMITMENT
TO REGULAR EXERCISE

How many times have you made a New Year's resolution, only to have it fall by the wayside a mere month later? Deciding that you are going to lead a more physically active lifestyle is the first step to changing your exercise behaviors. The harder step is to *commit* to that decision. Examine what a more active lifestyle would mean to you and write out your *personal commitment statement:* a list of reasons to commit to fitness. Review this list regularly until your new behaviors become routine.

Remember that committing to a new behavior takes perseverance. Whenever you feel your commitment flagging, reread your personal commitment statement and remind yourself of the reasons you began your program in the first place.

HOW CAN YOU OVERCOME
OBSTACLES TO EXERCISE?

You can probably immediately identify several things that keep you from being as active as you want to be. Obstacles, or **barriers to physical activity,** can be categorized as either environmental or personal. *Environmental* barriers include both external/physical factors and social/interpersonal factors that may make it harder or easier for you to exercise. Do you feel safe exercising on the streets around your campus? Is the weather conducive to exercising? Are facilities open during the hours that you need them? Do you have friends who exercise and who might be interested in exercising with you? Where you live, the facilities that are available to you, and the social support that you have to help keep you motivated are all environmental factors that can affect your exercise habits.

Likewise, *personal barriers* can play a role in whether you are successful in sticking to an exercise plan or if you give up after a minimal effort. Typical personal barriers include such things as lack of time, lack of self-motivation, injury, starting fitness levels and weight, disability, relationship difficulties, or psychological problems such as depression or anxiety. Older-than-average students, students with children, and those who must work long hours while attending school often face unique challenges as they work to improve their fitness levels.

Lab3.3 will help you identify the obstacles to physical activity in your life. Meanwhile, the following section provides suggestions for how to overcome some common obstacles to maintaining a regular fitness routine. The box **Tools for Change: Overcoming Common Obstacles to Exercise** on page 56 provides additional suggestions.

MAKE TIME FOR EXERCISE

Making time for exercise means making it a priority in your life and rearranging your schedule accordingly. People often state that they don't exercise because they don't have enough time. That might be the case—or they may simply be assigning exercise a lesser priority in their life than other activities, such as watching TV or text-messaging friends. While socializing and scheduling downtime in a busy life *are* important, consider how much time you spend in your life on sedentary activities like surfing the Internet. Then consider the benefits to your health and sense of well-being that would result if you replaced some of that sedentary time with physical activity.

To successfully stick with a fitness program, you need to prioritize exercise the same way that you prioritize your classes, homework, job, and social life. Schedule your exercise sessions into your calendar/appointment book the same way you schedule time for, say, a chemistry class or seeing a movie with friends. Prove to yourself that you are serious about getting fit by *making* the time for exercise.

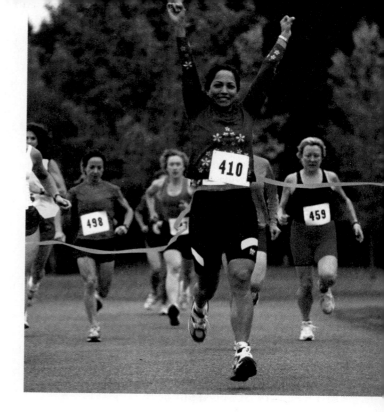

SET UP A REWARD STRUCTURE

If you find yourself unmotivated to get active, try coming up with personal rewards to motivate yourself. Rewards can be highly individual; after all, different things motivate different people. The key is to come up with rewards that reinforce your new, more active lifestyle. A common reward for people trying to lose weight, for example, is to shop for new clothes. But rewards do not necessarily have to be material. If competition or personal challenge motivate you, for example, you may find the exhilaration of finishing a half-marathon or completing a race in the top 10 percent of contenders to be considerable reward of its own.

Rewards can be internal or external. **Internal exercise rewards** commonly involve feeling better about yourself, feeling healthier, and having better life satisfaction from exercising. Long-term exercisers often report that internal exercise rewards are their primary motivation. New exercisers, however,

internal exercise rewards Rewards for exercise that are based upon how one is feeling physically and mentally (sense of accomplishment, relaxation, increased self-esteem)

TOOLS FOR CHANGE

OVERCOMING COMMON OBSTACLES TO EXERCISE

Below are lists of strategies for overcoming common obstacles to exercise.

Obstacle: Lack of Time

- Identify available time slots. Monitor your daily activities for 1 week. Identify at least three 30-minute time slots you could use for physical activity. Make physical activity a priority.
- Add physical activity to your daily routine. For example, walk or ride your bike to work or shopping, organize school activities around physical activity, walk the dog, exercise while you watch TV, park farther away from your destination, and so on.
- Make time for physical activity. For example, walk, jog, or swim during your lunch hour, or take fitness breaks instead of coffee breaks.
- Select activities requiring minimal time, such as walking, jogging, or stair-climbing.

Obstacle: Lack of Social Support

- Explain your interest in physical activity to friends and family. Ask them to support your efforts.
- Invite friends and family members to exercise with you. Plan social activities involving exercise.
- Develop new friendships with physically active people. Join a group, such as the YMCA or a hiking club.

Obstacle: Lack of Energy

- Schedule physical activity for times in the day or week when you feel energetic.
- Convince yourself that if you give it a chance, physical activity will increase your energy level; then try it.

Obstacle: Lack of Willpower

- Plan ahead. Make physical activity a regular part of your daily or weekly schedule and write it on your calendar.
- Invite a friend to exercise with you on a regular basis and write it on both your calendars.
- Join an exercise group or class.

Obstacle: Fear of Injury

- Learn how to warm up and cool down to prevent injury.
- Learn how to exercise appropriately considering your age, fitness level, skill level, and health status.
- Choose activities involving minimum risk.

Obstacle: Lack of Skill

- Select activities requiring no new skills, such as walking, climbing stairs, or jogging.
- Exercise with friends who are at the same skill level as you are.

- Find a friend who is willing to teach you some new skills.
- Take a class to develop new skills.

Obstacle: Lack of Resources

- Select activities that require minimal facilities or equipment, such as walking, jogging, jumping rope, or calisthenics.
- Identify inexpensive, convenient resources available in your community (community education programs, park and recreation programs, worksite programs, etc.).

Obstacle: Weather Conditions

- Develop a set of regular activities that are always available regardless of weather (indoor cycling, aerobic dance, indoor swimming, calisthenics, stair-climbing, rope-skipping, mall-walking, dancing, gymnasium games, etc.).
- Look at outdoor activities that depend on weather conditions (cross-country skiing, outdoor swimming, outdoor tennis, etc.) as "bonuses"—extra activities possible when weather and circumstances permit.

Obstacle: Travel

- Put a jump rope in your suitcase and jump rope.
- Walk the halls and climb the stairs in hotels.
- Stay in places with swimming pools or exercise facilities.
- Join the YMCA or YWCA.
- Visit the local shopping mall and walk for half an hour or more.
- Pack your favorite aerobic exercise tape.

Obstacle: Family Obligations

- Trade babysitting time with a friend, neighbor, or family member who also has small children.
- Exercise with the kids—go for a walk together, play tag or other running games, get an aerobic dance or exercise tape for kids (there are several on the market) and exercise together. You can spend time together and still get your exercise.
- Hire a babysitter and look at the cost as a worthwhile investment in your physical and mental health.
- Jump rope, do calisthenics, ride a stationary bicycle, or use other home gymnasium equipment while the kids are busy playing or sleeping.
- Try to exercise when the kids are not around (e.g., during school hours or their nap time).

Source: Adapted from U.S. Dept. of Health and Human Services, Public Health Service, Centers for Disease Control and Prevention, National Center for Chronic Disease Prevention and Health Promotion, Division of Nutrition, Physical Activity and Obesity. *Promoting Physical Activity: A Guide for Community Action* (Champaign, IL: Human Kinetics, 1999).

often rely on **external exercise rewards**—at least initially. External exercise rewards can be anything from a new workout wardrobe to a celebratory dinner to the admiration and praise of your peers or fitness instructor.

As you incorporate regular physical activity and exercise into your lifestyle, you may find that just having fun and feeling good while exercising is reward enough. If this switch to an internal reward motivation does not happen right away, keep setting external rewards to keep yourself motivated until it does. Don't be surprised if the switch happens faster than you think. Studies have shown that exercise releases endorphins in your body that can fill you with a sense of well-being.[2] For many long-term exercisers, the physical activity itself is truly its own reward.

SELECT FUN AND CONVENIENT ACTIVITIES

Even if you have committed to set aside time to exercise, you may not always *want* to. If you are used to a sedentary lifestyle, it can be difficult to tear yourself away from the computer or to get off the couch. One way to counter a lack of motivation is to *choose activities that you really enjoy*. We have mentioned this a few times already, but it bears repeating: If you dread your workout activity, you are not likely to stick with it for long. On the other hand, if your workout is a form of play, you will look forward to it time and time again. If you have not found a physical activity that you like yet, keep trying new things!

Choosing the best type of exercise is often also about convenience. Ask yourself: How close is the fitness club or walking path to my home? What classes can I take during my free times during the day? How much money do I need to spend in order to get started? How much time will this activity take? Despite your good intentions and high level of motivation when starting a new activity, if it's not convenient for your existing lifestyle and commitments, you will have a hard time sticking with it. Look for activities, facilities, and workout times that make sense for your schedule. If that is not possible, rearrange your current schedule to make a permanent place in your daily and weekly schedule for exercise.

Table 3.1 lists various activities along with the training effects of each on the key health-related aspects of fitness. Examine the table and consider which activities you find most appealing. Select those that seem most enjoyable and that meet your fitness-training goals. The table includes three categories: lifestyle physical activities, exercise

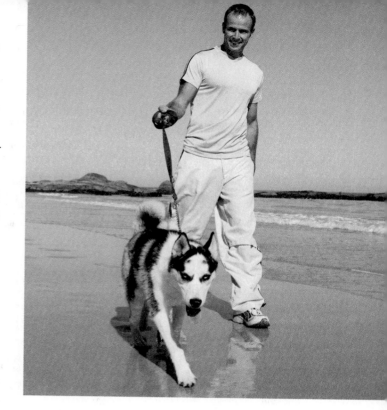

training options, and sports and recreational activities. Let's look at each of these in more detail.

Lifestyle Physical Activities
Lifestyle physical activities are those that you perform during daily life. If you are just starting your fitness program, increasing your lifestyle physical activity is a great place to start. These activities can be light, moderate, or vigorous, depending on what the task is and how long it takes you. For instance, watering your garden for 15 minutes may be a light activity, but doing yard work for 4 hours can be vigorous. Lifestyle physical activities include things like walking the dog, shopping, housework, gardening, bicycling to work, and so on.

Exercise Training Options
Most people think of typical exercise options when asked how they are going to increase their fitness. These include aerobics classes, jogging or running, weight training, indoor cardio workouts, yoga, tai chi, lap swimming, and water aerobics. These activities are great for specifically increasing your fitness. However, consider including a variety of activities to counter the boredom that may come from doing the same

external exercise rewards Rewards for exercise that come from outside of a person (trophy, compliment, day at the spa)

TABLE **3.1**

Training Effects of Various Physical Activities on Cardiorespiratory Endurance, Muscular Strength, Muscular Endurance, and Flexibility

Activity Type	Activity	Cardiorespiratory Endurance	Muscular Strength	Muscular Endurance	Flexibility
Lifestyle Physical Activities	Walking	**	—	**	*
	Bicycling	***	**	***	*
	Yard work	*	*	**	**
	Climbing stairs	***	**	***	*
	Housework	*	—	*	**
Exercise Training	Dance/step aerobics	***	*	**	*
	Resistance training	—	***	***	*
	Jogging/running	***	*	**	—
	Swimming	***	**	***	**
	Yoga	*	**	***	***
	Tai chi	*	*	**	**
Sports and Recreation Activities	Tennis	**	*	**	*
	Basketball	**	*	**	*
	Soccer	***	*	***	*
	Rock climbing	—	***	***	**
	Squash & racquetball	**	*	**	*
	Martial arts	**	**	***	***
	Snowboarding	**	*	***	**
	Golf	*	*	**	**
	In-line skating	***	*	***	—
	Canoeing	**	**	**	*

Legend: — = *negligible training effect,* * = *small training effect,* ** = *moderate training effect,* *** = *strong training effect*
Source: Adapted from R. Chevalier, K. Olijemark, and C. Cook, *Fitness Now!* Toronto, Ontario Canada: Pearson Prentice Hall, 2006.

exercise week after week. Add a few sports and recreational activities every now and then to keep yourself motivated and your body challenged.

Sports and Recreational Activities

Traditional team sports offer a great deal of fun, motivation, and fitness. Most cities have sports leagues for adult soccer, softball, basketball, ultimate Frisbee, and other team sports. If you like the camaraderie of working with a team and enjoy the challenge of team sports, strongly consider this option. You may be able to find team sports classes on campus, at community centers, and in sports clubs.

Other sports activities can offer great fitness benefits as well. Court sports like tennis, squash,

and racquetball will increase your cardiorespiratory fitness and muscle endurance and will improve your agility, coordination, and reaction time. Many sports are recreational for some people but a competitive pastime for others.

If you are going to rely on a sport or recreational activity for your regular fitness routine, just make sure that it really is regular. For instance, skiing and snowboarding are great activities but do not constitute a good fitness program if you only get to the mountain a couple of times a month four months of the year. Golf, mountain biking, in-line skating, hiking, ice skating, kayaking, and rock climbing are additional examples of recreational and competitive sports that can maintain or increase fitness if done regularly.

Less vigorous, more time

- Washing and waxing a car for 40–60 minutes
- Washing the windows or floors for 45–60 minutes
- Playing volleyball for 45 minutes
- Playing touch football for 30–45 minutes
- Gardening for 30–45 minutes
- Wheeling self in wheelchair for 30–40 minutes
- Walking 1¾ miles in 35 minutes (20 min/mile)
- Basketball (shooting baskets) for 30 minutes
- Bicycling 5 miles in 30 minutes
- Fast social dancing for 30 minutes
- Pushing a stroller 1½ miles in 3 minutes
- Raking leaves for 30 minutes
- Walking 2 miles in 30 minutes (15 min/mile)
- Water aerobics for 30 minutes
- Swimming laps for 20 minutes
- Wheelchair basketball for 20 minutes
- Basketball (playing a game) for 15–20 minutes
- Bicycling 4 miles in 15 minutes
- Jumping rope for 15 minutes
- Running 1½ miles in 15 minutes (10 min/mile)
- Shoveling snow for 15 minutes
- Stairwalking for 15 minutes

More vigorous, less time

FIGURE 3.1
Examples of moderate to vigorous physical activities.

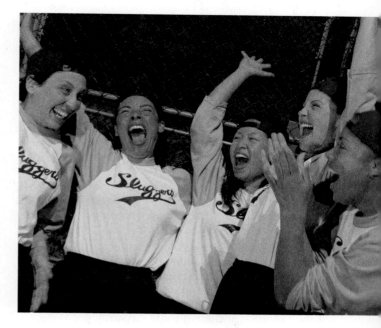

Figure 3.1 illustrates examples of moderate to vigorous lifestyle, exercise, and sports activities that can help you raise your fitness level.

CHOOSE ENVIRONMENTS
CONDUCIVE TO REGULAR EXERCISE

A major obstacle to exercise for many people is having a suitable, convenient place to work out. The following are some factors to consider when deciding where to exercise.

Exercise Facility Options
Exercise facilities are often located in colleges, community centers, health and fitness clubs, athletic and tennis clubs, parks and recreation facilities, YMCAs, corporate fitness centers, and schools. Choosing a facility based upon its location is a good idea because the farther away a facility is from your home, the less likely you are to use it.[3] Other things to consider when choosing a basic exercise facility are ease of parking (if you drive), variety of classes, quality of cardio and weight equipment, and hours that are compatible with your schedule. Additionally, you may be interested in facilities with a swimming pool, basketball and racquetball courts, locker rooms, showers, and spa.

Cost can be a big factor. Larger facilities with more offerings will likely be more expensive per month than a basic fitness center. Community centers and parks facilities often offer reasonable day use or multiday use fees. Almost all facilities offer day use passes for a fee, or even one-time free passes to check out the facility. Be sure to try the facility for several days to see if you like the atmosphere, the equipment, and the instructors.

If you have not taken advantage of your college facilities yet, you may be missing out on the best deal in town. As a student, you can typically get access to classes, courts, leagues, equipment, and even personal trainers. College is the perfect time to try out new sports and activities that you have always been curious about.

Neighborhood
Where you live can help or hinder your goal of regular physical activity. When people live in safe neighborhoods where it is easy to walk or bike to the store, they are more likely to be active.[4] This is becoming a bigger issue as growing cities and suburbs lead to a dramatic increase in urban sprawl. Some even suggest that urban sprawl is partially to blame for the rise in obesity

TOOLS FOR CHANGE

ADJUSTING TO YOUR ENVIRONMENT

In order to maintain a regular exercise routine, you need to feel safe and comfortable in your surroundings. Below are some suggestions for exercising safely in different environments:

- If your neighborhood is not safe, consider exercising with a friend or training group, or consider driving to a different nearby neighborhood to exercise.

- If you are exercising where there are many cars around, wear bright clothing and face traffic when walking or running. Seek out areas that are less busy and where speed limits are lower.

- If you are heading into a wilderness area for a hike, trail run, or mountain-bike ride, plan your outing with a friend, or at least let someone know specifically where you are going and when you will return. Know your route and carry a map, a cell phone, and basic safety supplies, including food and water for at least a day, a flashlight or headlamp, first-aid supplies, a pocketknife, and a space or emergency blanket.

- Exercise facilities are typically safe places to work out. If you have any concerns for your safety in the locker room, workout areas, parking areas, or anywhere around the building, talk to the manager and get an escort to your car at night.

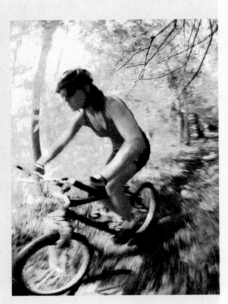

in the United States in recent years. For example, researchers in New Jersey found that residents of sprawling counties were less likely to walk during leisure time, weighed more, and had high blood pressure more often than residents living in compact urban areas.[5] Living near streets that are conducive to physical activity (with sidewalks, bike lanes, street lights, slower traffic) and parks with bike and walking paths might make the difference between whether you stay regularly active or not.

Weather If you are an outside exerciser, the weather can create obstacles to regular physical activity. The impact of weather will, of course, depend on where you live and the time of year. If you are prepared, you can exercise in most weather conditions. Pay attention to your body. If you feel too hot when exercising outside, slow down, move into the shade, and consider suspending your workout for the day. Limit your exercise time in the rain if you are getting too wet and cold. Exercising in the heat and the cold is covered further in Chapter 4.

Safety Do you feel safe walking to the local gym to exercise? Do you feel comfortable jogging around your neighborhood? These are important questions, and your answers can affect your exercise participation. The box **Tools for Change: Adjusting to Your Environment** presents tips for exercising safely in different environments.

CASE STUDY

Adam

"I took an honest look at where all my time goes, and I admit, I do spend a few hours goofing off each day. I spend a lot of that time online, checking e-mail and downloading music. I don't want to give that up, but I can see cutting back on it a little to make time for this rock-climbing class. My first class is tomorrow. If I can make it through the beginner series, I'm going to plan a trip out of town to take an outdoor climbing class."

1. Give three examples of things Adam is doing to increase his chances of sticking to his new exercise plans.

2. What are three things you can do to make exercise a regular part of your life?

HOW CAN YOU MAKE A LIFELONG COMMITMENT TO FITNESS?

Ideally, once you start a regular exercise program, you will be having so much fun and feeling so good that you will not want to stop. The reality for most of us, however, is that we will have some good days and some bad days when it comes to exercising consistently. How can you keep yourself committed to fitness once you have started?

MODIFY YOUR BEHAVIOR TO ESTABLISH NEW HABITS

Establishing new habits (and getting rid of old ones) can be one of the hardest things for people to do. It seems that you should be able to just stop an unhealthy behavior and replace it with a healthy one at any time. However, life is not that simple, because behavior patterns can be ingrained for years, and motivations for unhealthy behaviors can be very complicated. In Chapter 1, you learned about the essential steps and skills for behavior change. Recall the following steps for preparing to change a behavior:

- Examine your current habits and behavior.
- Assess your current beliefs and attitudes.
- Assess your motivation for change.
- Anticipate and overcome barriers to change.
- Make a commitment to change.
- Target a specific behavior to change.

> **Try it NOW!** Apply the steps for preparing to change a behavior to your plans to start a fitness program. • What are your main motivations to exercise? • What are obstacles that you can anticipate, and how might you work around them?

RECORD AND TRACK YOUR PROGRESS OVER TIME

One of the best ways to make sure that you stay on track with your fitness program is to record your activity and track your progress over time. The box **Spotlight: Tracking Your Fitness Progress Online** lists a variety of free, convenient online logs and self-assessments. Regularly record your progress—your successes as well as your setbacks. This will allow you to examine your program carefully on a regular basis, as well as provide motivation to keep up a consistent program. It can also help you determine if your goals or your program need to be adjusted over time. Set yourself up for success by setting short-term, achievable goals specifically designed for you and your needs.

RECOGNIZE THAT YOUR FITNESS NEEDS MAY CHANGE OVER TIME

Your body and lifestyle will change as you age, and over time, you may need to adjust your fitness program accordingly.

Children and Adolescents Keeping active during the day helps children maintain a healthy body weight, gain developmental motor skills, increase and maintain self-esteem, connect socially with peers and adults, and keep typically "adult" diseases (like type 2 diabetes) from afflicting them in their youth. Children should try to accumulate at least 60 minutes per day of moderate to vigorous physical activity.

Young and Midlife Adults As college or work demands increase, many people find that regular sports, recreation, and exercise get put on the back burner. The challenge for young and midlife adults is to make exercise a priority while balancing all of life's other demands. Remember that your overall health and wellness is one of the most important things to attend to. This is too often forgotten until something goes wrong—you start feeling sick, have signs of a chronic disease, or have a doctor advising you to lose weight. The best time to start being active is before any of these things happen.

Older Adults and Seniors Older adults are one of the fastest growing groups of exercisers.

TRACKING YOUR FITNESS PROGRESS ONLINE

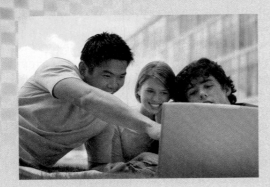

There are several Web resources that allow you to keep a log of your physical activity online, track your progress, and access information about recommended guidelines for physical activity. Below are just a few:

AllSport GPS
www.allsportgps.com

This site allows exercisers to map and save their walking, running, or bicycling routes using GPS or basic online mapping tools.

MyPyramid Tracker
www.mypyramidtracker.gov

MyPyramid Tracker is a free online assessment tool that lets you track your diet and physical activity, as well as assess how your habits compare to USDA and USDHHS (U.S. Dept. of Health and Human Services) nutrition and physical activity standards. You can enter data daily and record your results for up to a year.

Nike+
http://nikeplus.nike.com

This site offers the ability for runners to track their distance, pace, calories, and time.

President's Challenge
www.presidentschallenge.org

The President's Challenge is a program for those wanting to get active or are already active. Their website offers an online Activity Log that allows you to enter your activity data, track your progress, and earn rewards.

Many retirees are now turning to active pursuits rather than inactive hobbies to fill their leisure time. Seniors are forming cycling groups, hiking the Grand Canyon, joining health clubs, running or walking marathons, and taking active vacations. In general, older adults can participate in the same activities as younger adults and have similar physical activity guidelines (see Chapter 2), though they should seek medical clearance before beginning an exercise program if they have any preexisting health concerns.

Aging adults may experience loss of coordination, balance, muscle strength, and bone density, all of which increase the risk of fall-related fractures. Regular physical activity can actually reduce the chances of falling in the first place and reduce the risk of fracture if a fall occurs.[6] Thus, in addition to the general adult activity guidelines, seniors should engage in strength training and balance exercises to help prevent fall-related fractures. With an active lifestyle throughout adulthood, older adults can experience a similarly active and rewarding life in their later years.

REVIEW QUESTIONS

1. What percentage of American adults participate in regular leisure-time physical activity?
   a. 10%
   b. 25%
   c. 31%
   d. 50%

2. Which of the following is NOT one of the stages of behavior change?
   a. Precontemplation
   b. Action
   c. Maintenance
   d. Indecision

3. What does the "M" in SMART stand for?
   a. Motivation
   b. Measurable
   c. Muscle strength
   d. Mobility

4. Which of the following is an example of an environmental barrier to physical activity?
   a. Being injured
   b. Disliking exercise
   c. Not having anywhere safe to exercise
   d. Being unmotivated

5. Experiencing knee pain can be categorized as having a(n) _____ barrier to physical activity.
   a. personal
   b. scheduling
   c. social
   d. environmental

6. Which of the following is an example of an internal exercise reward?
   a. Buying new workout clothing
   b. Having fun while exercising
   c. Placing third in your age group at the local 5K
   d. Taking a celebratory trip after meeting an exercise goal

7. Which of the following is least likely to result in a successful long-term exercise routine?
   a. Making exercise a priority in your life
   b. Setting up a reward structure
   c. Selecting fun and convenient activities
   d. Forcing yourself to go to a gym even though you don't enjoy it

8. If one of your obstacles to exercise is fear of injury, all of the following can help, EXCEPT
   a. warming up and cooling down properly.
   b. exercising appropriately given your age, fitness level, skill level, and health status.
   c. choosing high-risk activities to "face down" your fear.
   d. choosing activities involving minimal risk.

9. If you are planning to exercise in the wilderness, all of the following is good advice EXCEPT
   a. let someone know where you are going and when you will return.
   b. be adventurous; don't worry about carrying a map or a cell phone.
   c. know your route.
   d. carry enough food and water for at least a day.

10. Which of the following groups has a specific exercise recommendation for strength and balance training?
    a. Children
    b. Adolescents
    c. Adults
    d. Older adults

CRITICAL THINKING QUESTIONS

1. Why is it important to understand your motivations for beginning a fitness program?

2. Explain the difference between internal and external exercise rewards.

ONLINE RESOURCES

See the Spotlight box on page 62. Also, please visit this book's website at **www.aw-bc.com/hopson** to access additional links related to topics in this chapter.

REFERENCES

1. P. Barnes and J. S. Schiller. "Early Release of Selected Estimates Based on Data from the 2006 National Health Interview Survey." National Center for Health Statistics. http://www.cdc.gov/nchs/nhis.htm (accessed July 19, 2007).

2. L. Carrasco, C. Villaverde, and C. M. Oltras. "Endorphin Responses to Stress Induced by Competitive Swimming Event." *The Journal of Sports Medicine and Physical Fitness* 47, no. 2 (2007): 239–245.

3. E. M. Berke, R. T. Ackermann, E. H. Lin, and others. "Distance as a Barrier to Using a Fitness-Program Benefit for Managed Medicare Enrollees." *Journal of Aging and Physical Activity* 14, no. 3 (2006): 313–324.

4. J. F. Sallis and K. Glanz. "The Role of Built Environments in Physical Activity, Eating, and Obesity in Childhood." *The Future of Children* 16, no. 1 (2006): 89–108.

5. R. Ewing, T. Schmid, R. Killingsworth, A. Zlot, and S. Raudenbush. "Relationship between Urban Sprawl and Physical Activity, Obesity, and Morbidity." *American Journal of Health Promotion* 18, no. 1 (2003): 47–57.

6. K. E. Ensrud, S. K. Ewing, B. C. Taylor, and others for the Study of Osteoporotic Fractures Research Group. "Frailty and Risk of Falls, Fracture, and Mortality in Older Women: The Study of Osteoporotic Fractures." *The Journals of Gerontology Series A, Biological Sciences and Medical Sciences* 62, no. 7 (2007): 744–751.

Name:_____ **Date:** _____

Instructor: _____ **Section:** _____

Purpose: To identify your motivations for starting a physical activity, exercise, or sport (or maintaining your current fitness routine).

SECTION I: WHAT MOTIVATES YOU?

Assign a rating of 1–7 for each of the motivations listed below, using the following scale: 1= not at all true, 7 = very true

I participate (or want to participate) in my physical activity or sport because:

____ 1. I want to be physically fit.

____ 2. It's fun.

____ 3. I like engaging in activities which physically challenge me.

____ 4. I want to obtain new skills.

____ 5. I want to maintain my weight and/or look better.

____ 6. I want to be with my friends.

____ 7. I like to do this activity.

____ 8. I want to improve existing skills.

____ 9. I like the challenge.

____ 10. I want to define my muscles so that I look better.

____ 11. It makes me happy.

____ 12. I want to keep up my current skill level.

____ 13. I want to have more energy.

____ 14. I like activities which are physically challenging.

____ 15. I like to be with others who are interested in this activity.

____ 16. I want to improve my cardiovascular fitness.

____ 17. I want to improve my appearance.

____ 18. I think it's interesting.

____ 19. I want to maintain my physical strength to live a healthy life.

____ 20. I want to be attractive to others.

____ 21. I want to meet new people.

____ 22. I enjoy this activity.

____ 23. I want to maintain my physical health and well-being.

____ 24. I want to improve my body shape.

____ 25. I want to get better at my activity.

____ 26. I find this activity stimulating.

____ 27. I will feel physically unattractive if I don't.

____ 28. My friends want me to.

____ 29. I like the excitement of participation.

____ 30. I enjoy spending time with others doing this activity.

SECTION II: SCORING

Fill in your scores for the questions above in the appropriate boxes (for example, in the box for "Q 2," enter the numerical value you wrote in for question #2). Then add the totals for each type of motivation. Your total scores reflect which category motivates you the most.

Motivation Type →	Interest/ Enjoyment	Competence	Appearance	Fitness	Social
	Q 2:	Q 3:	Q 5:	Q 1:	Q 6:
	Q 7:	Q 4:	Q 10:	Q 13:	Q 15:
	Q 11:	Q 8:	Q 17:	Q 16:	Q 21:
	Q 18:	Q 9:	Q 20:	Q 19:	Q 28:
	Q 22:	Q 12:	Q 24:	Q 23:	Q 30:
	Q 26:	Q 14:	Q 27:		
	Q 29:	Q 25:			
Totals:					

Source: R. M. Ryan, C. M. Frederick, D. Lepes, N. Rubio, and K. M. Sheldon, "Intrinsic Motivation and Exercise Adherence," *International Journal of Sport Psychology* 28 (1997): 335–354; C. M. Frederick and R. M. Ryan, "Differences in Motivation for Sport and Exercise and Their Relationships with Participation and Mental Health," *Journal of Sport Behavior* 16 (1993): 125–145.

SECTION III: REFLECTION

1. Do the results surprise you? Explain why or why not.

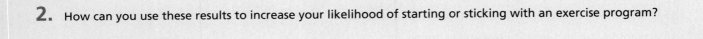

2. How can you use these results to increase your likelihood of starting or sticking with an exercise program?

Name: _____   Date: _____

Instructor: _____   Section: _____

Purpose: To identify your physical activity stage of change and complete a physical activity behavioral change contract.

SECTION I: PHYSICAL ACTIVITY STAGES OF CHANGE QUESTIONNAIRE

1. After carefully reading each of the following statements, please circle **YES** or **NO**.

(1) I am currently physically active.*	NO	YES
(2) I intend to become more physically active in the next 6 months.	NO	YES
(3) I currently engage in regular** physical activity.	NO	YES
(4) I have been regularly physically active for the past 6 months.	NO	YES

* Physical activity or exercise: Activities such as walking briskly, jogging, bicycling, swimming, or any other activity in which the exertion is at least as intense as these activities.

** Regular activity: Activity that adds up to a total of 30 minutes or more per day and is done at least 5 days per week.

2. Identify your physical activity stage of change (circle your stage):

→ If you answered NO to questions 1 and 2, you are in **PRECONTEMPLATION.**

(To move toward behavior change, it is important at this stage to start thinking about physical activity and its benefits.)

→ If you answered NO to question 1 and YES to question 2, you are in **CONTEMPLATION.**

(In order to move into preparation, you must gain information about how to get started moving toward your goal.)

→ If you answered YES to question 1 and NO to question 3, you are in **PREPARATION.**

(In this stage, it is important to remove barriers that are preventing regular physical activity.)

→ If you answered YES to questions 1 and 3, but NO to question 4, you are in **ACTION.**

(In order to maintain your new behavior, in this stage you need to track your progress, maintain your motivation, and head off potential relapses before they occur.)

→ If you answered YES to questions 1, 3, and 4, you are in **MAINTENANCE.**

(To keep your active lifestyle habits, try new activities and cross-training, make it fun, and strive to keep a consistent program despite life's obstacles.)

Sources: B. H. Marcus and B. A. Lewis, "Physical Activity and the Stages of Motivational Readiness for Change Model," *President's Council on Physical Fitness and Sports Research Digest* 4, no.1 (2003): 1–8; B. H. Marcus, S. W. Banspach, R. C. Lefebvre, J. S. Rossi, R. A. Carleton, and D. B. Abrams, "Using the Stages of Change Model to Increase the Adoption of Physical Activity Among Community Participants," *American Journal of Health Promotion* 6, no.6 (1992): 424–429; Canadian Fitness and Lifestyle Research Institute, "Stages of Change in Exercise," *Progress in Prevention* (1996): Bulletin 5.

SECTION II: SHORT- AND LONG-TERM GOALS

1. **Long-term physical activity goal:** Be sure to use SMART goal-setting guidelines (specific, measurable, action-oriented, realistic, time-oriented) when creating your goal for 6 months or longer.

Long-term physical activity goal: _____

_____

Target Date: _____

2. **Short-term physical activity goals:** Short-term goals are goals you can achieve in less than 6 months.

Short-term physical activity goal #1: _____

_____

Target Date: _____

Short-term physical activity goal #2: _____

_____

Target Date: _____

SECTION III: GETTING SUPPORT

1. Resources I will use to help me change this behavior include:

A friend/partner/relative: _____

A school-based resource: _____

A community-based resource: _____

A book or reputable website: _____

2. How will you use these supportive resources to help you with your goals?

_____

_____

SECTION IV: CONTRACT, TRACKING, AND FOLLOW-UP

1. **Contract:** I intend to make the behavior change described above.

Signed _____ Date _____

Witness _____ Date _____

2. **Tracking:** Keeping track of your progress toward your goals is very important to ensure successful behavior change. Consider keeping a physical activity log on paper, in a journal, on the computer, or on the Web.

3. **Follow-Up:** After reaching your target date, follow up and reassess your program and goals. Did you accomplish your goal? Do you need to set a new and more challenging goal? Do you need to alter your goals or program to make it more realistic?

Name: _____   **Date:** _____

Instructor: _____   **Section:** _____

Purpose: To identify your barriers to exercise and learn how to set up exercise-specific rewards to overcome those barriers.

SECTION I: WHAT KEEPS YOU FROM BEING ACTIVE?

Listed below are common reasons that people give to describe why they do not get as much physical activity as they would like. Read each statement and indicate how likely you are to state the same reason.

How likely are you to say:	Very likely	Somewhat likely	Somewhat unlikely	Very unlikely
1. My day is so busy now, I just don't think I can make the time to include physical activity in my regular schedule.	3	2	1	0
2. None of my family members or friends like to do anything active, so I don't have a chance to exercise.	3	2	1	0
3. I'm just too tired after work to get any exercise.	3	2	1	0
4. I've been thinking about getting more exercise, but I just can't seem to get started.	3	2	1	0
5. I'm getting older, so exercise can be risky.	3	2	1	0
6. I don't get enough exercise because I have never learned the skills for any sport.	3	2	1	0
7. I don't have access to jogging trails, swimming pools, bike paths, etc.	3	2	1	0
8. Physical activity takes too much time away from other commitments—work, family, etc.	3	2	1	0
9. I'm embarrassed about how I will look when I exercise with others.	3	2	1	0
10. I don't get enough sleep as it is. I just couldn't get up early or stay up late to get some exercise.	3	2	1	0
11. It's easier for me to find excuses not to exercise than to go out to do something.	3	2	1	0
12. I know of too many people who have hurt themselves by overdoing it with exercise.	3	2	1	0
13. I really can't see learning a new sport at my age.	3	2	1	0
14. It's just too expensive. You have to take a class or join a club or buy the right equipment.	3	2	1	0
15. My free periods during the day are too short to include exercise.	3	2	1	0
16. My usual social activities with family or friends do not include physical activity.	3	2	1	0
17. I'm too tired during the week, and I need the weekend to catch up on my rest.	3	2	1	0
18. I want to get more exercise, but I just can't seem to make myself stick to anything.	3	2	1	0
19. I'm afraid I might injure myself or have a heart attack.	3	2	1	0
20. I'm not good enough at any physical activity to make it fun.	3	2	1	0
21. If we had exercise facilities and showers at work, then I would be more likely to exercise.	3	2	1	0

Source: Centers for Disease Control and Prevention, "Overcoming Barriers to Physical Activity." Available at: www.cdc.gov/nccdphp/dnpa/physical/life/overcome.htm. Accessed August 22, 2007.

SECTION II: SCORING

Follow these instructions to score the results from your quiz in Section I:

- Enter the circled number in the spaces provided, putting together the number for statement 1 on line 1, statement 2 on line 2, and so on.

- Add the three scores on each line. Your barriers to physical activity fall into one or more of seven categories below. Circle any physical activity barrier category with a score of 5 or above, because this is an important barrier for you to overcome.

____ + ____ + ____ = _____
1   8   15   **Lack of time**

____ + ____ + ____ = _____
2   9   16   **Social influence**

____ + ____ + ____ = _____
3   10   17   **Lack of energy**

____ + ____ + ____ = _____
4   11   18   **Lack of willpower**

____ + ____ + ____ = _____
5   12   19   **Fear of injury**

____ + ____ + ____ = _____
6   13   20   **Lack of skill**

____ + ____ + ____ = _____
7   14   21   **Lack of resources**

SECTION III: OVERCOMING BARRIERS TO EXERCISE

See the Tools for Change box on page 56 for strategies to overcome your personal barriers to exercise.

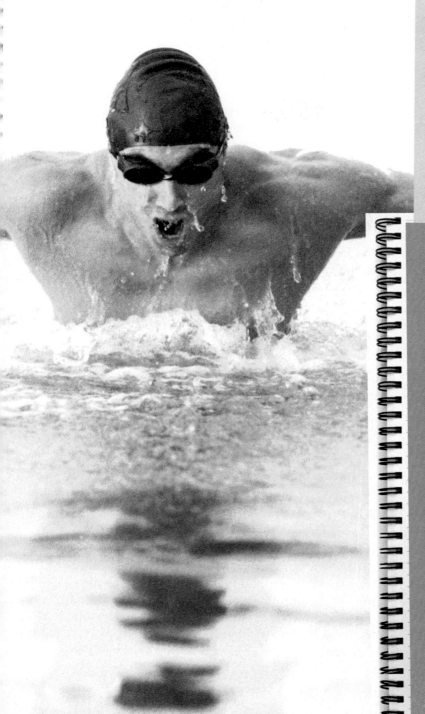

CHAPTER 4

Conditioning Your Cardiorespiratory System

OBJECTIVES

Define cardiorespiratory fitness.

Discuss the structures and functions of the cardiorespiratory system at rest and during exercise.

Describe how the three metabolic systems work during exercise.

Describe the benefits of cardiorespiratory training.

Assess your cardiorespiratory fitness level.

Set appropriate cardiorespiratory fitness goals.

Create a cardiorespiratory exercise plan compatible with your goals and lifestyle.

Describe how to prevent injuries during cardiorespiratory training.

CASE STUDY

Angela

"Hi, I'm Angela. In high school, I was on the varsity tennis team—I played #2 singles and was pretty competitive! After high school, I spent a few years working and saving up money for college, so I'm a little older than most of my classmates. Unfortunately, I got out of shape during that time, too. Our coach used to have us do all kinds of cardio and cross-training drills. I want to start playing tennis again, but without a coach or a team, I'm not sure how to go about getting in shape for it. Should I just find a partner and dive right back in?"

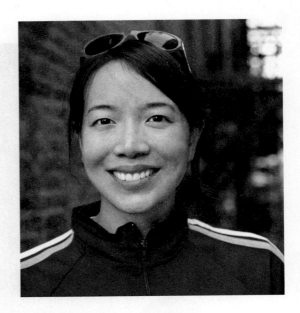

Cardiorespiratory fitness is the ability of your cardiovascular and respiratory systems to supply oxygen and nutrients to large muscle groups in order to sustain continuous activity. It is a key component of your overall fitness and wellness. A healthy cardiorespiratory system can be the difference between having adequate energy to sustain daily, recreational, and sports activities, and getting tired out by performing simple physical tasks.

When people decide to "get in shape," they often choose cardiorespiratory activities such as jogging or running. In fact, the number-one fitness activity in the United States is also the easiest and most convenient of cardiorespiratory activities: walking.[1] In this chapter, we will provide a brief overview of how the cardiorespiratory system works. We will discuss the benefits of regular cardiorespiratory training. We will then cover how to set goals for cardiorespiratory fitness and how to design a cardiorespiratory exercise program that is personalized for your needs.

HOW DOES THE CARDIO-RESPIRATORY SYSTEM WORK?

The cardiorespiratory system is made up of the cardiovascular system and the respiratory system. Together, these systems deliver essential oxygen and nutrients to your body's cells and tissues, while also removing carbon dioxide and wastes.

AN OVERVIEW OF THE CARDIORESPIRATORY SYSTEM

The **respiratory system** (also called the *pulmonary system*) consists of the air passageways and the lungs, while the **cardiovascular system** consists of the heart and blood vessels (see Figure 4.1).

Air Passageways Air enters your body via your nose and mouth. It then continues through your throat (*pharynx*), voice box (*larynx*), and windpipe (*trachea*) (see Figure 4.2). These upper respiratory passageways warm, humidify, and filter the air, promoting optimal gas exchange. Mucus and small, hairlike projections called *cilia* filter out unwanted particles in the air; you expel these particles through your nose or mouth, or you swallow them.

---

cardiorespiratory fitness The ability of your cardiovascular and respiratory systems to supply oxygen and nutrients to large muscle groups in order to sustain dynamic activity

respiratory system The body system responsible for the exchange of gases between the body and the air

cardiovascular system The body system responsible for the delivery of oxygen and nutrients to body tissues and the delivery of carbon dioxide and other wastes back to the heart and lungs

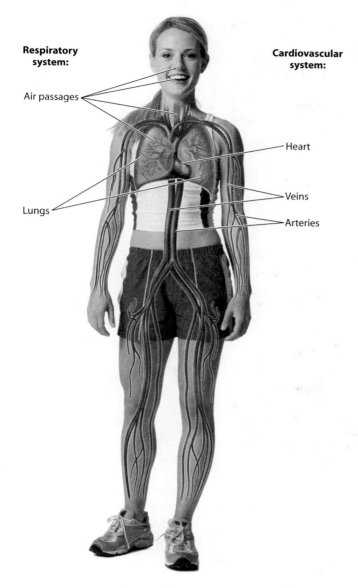

Respiratory system:
Air passages
Lungs

Cardiovascular system:
Heart
Veins
Arteries

FIGURE 4.1

The cardiorespiratory system consists of the cardiovascular and respiratory systems.

The inspired air travels down through the lower respiratory tract—the lower trachea, *bronchi,* and *bronchioles*—eventually reaching air sacs (*alveoli*) in the lungs, where gas exchange (i.e., the delivery of oxygen and the removal of carbon dioxide) occurs.

Lungs The air passageways in the lungs have extensive branching, similar to the branches on a large tree. At the very ends of the smallest branches (the bronchioles) are alveoli, which are surrounded by small blood vessels called *capillaries*. Because the walls of the alveoli and capillaries are very thin, oxygen moves easily from the alveolar sacs into the

capillary blood, where vessels then transport it to the heart and the rest of the body. Meanwhile, carbon dioxide moves from the capillaries into the alveoli and exits the body when you exhale. This exchange of oxygen and carbon dioxide is called **respiration.**

Heart The heart is a fist-sized pump consisting of four chambers: the *right atrium,* the *right ventricle,* the *left atrium,* and the *left ventricle* (Figure 4.3). Small *valves* regulate the steady, rhythmic flow of blood between chambers and prevent the blood from moving in the wrong direction. The two **atria** are collecting chambers that receive blood from the rest of the body. The two **ventricles** pump blood out again. The heart pumps blood through two different circulatory systems: in **pulmonary circulation,** blood circulates from the heart to the lungs and back; in **systemic circulation,** blood circulates from the heart to the rest of the body and back.

Blood returning to the heart enters the heart through the right atrium. When the atrium is full, it contracts, pumping blood into the right ventricle. The right ventricle fills and contracts, pumping blood through the **pulmonary artery** into the lungs. The ventricles are more muscular than the atria, because contraction of these chambers must be forceful enough to send blood out of the heart.

Blood returning from the lungs enters the heart through the left atrium. When the atrium is full, it contracts, pumping blood into the left ventricle. The left ventricle fills and contracts, pumping the blood out of the heart via the **aorta** and transporting it to the cells of the heart, brain, and body. The left

respiration The exchange of gases in the lungs or in the tissues

atria Upper chambers of the heart that collect blood from the rest of the body

ventricles Lower chambers of the heart that pump blood to the rest of the body

pulmonary circulation Blood circulation from the heart to the lungs and back

systemic circulation Blood circulation from the heart to the rest of the body and back

pulmonary artery The artery that carries blood from the right ventricle to the lungs

aorta The artery that carries blood from the left ventricle to the rest of the body

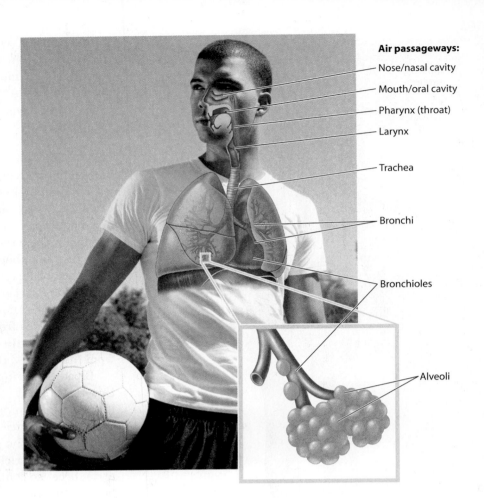

Air passageways:
- Nose/nasal cavity
- Mouth/oral cavity
- Pharynx (throat)
- Larynx
- Trachea
- Bronchi
- Bronchioles
- Alveoli

FIGURE 4.2
The respiratory system consists of the air passageways and the lungs.

ventricle is the most muscular chamber, because it must contract forcefully enough to send blood to the rest of the body.

The heart cycle consists of two phases: systole and diastole. During **systole,** the ventricles contract and blood is pumped out of the heart. During **diastole,** the ventricles relax and fill back up with blood from the right and left atria. Specialized heart tissue involuntarily and automatically starts the heart cycle. This tissue, located in the right atrium, is called the *pacemaker,* because it

determines how fast your heart beats. One "beat" of your heart consists of a full heart cycle. Through a stethoscope, you can hear your heartbeat as a "lub dub." The "lub" signals the end of the diastole phase (ventricular relaxation), and the "dub" signals the end of the systole phase (vertricular contraction). The number of times your heart beats in one minute is your **heart rate.**

Blood Vessels Blood vessels transport blood throughout your body. There are two types of blood vessels: **arteries,** which carry blood away from the heart, and **veins,** which carry blood back toward the heart. As arteries branch off from the heart, they divide into smaller blood vessels called *arterioles,* and then into even smaller blood vessels known as *capillaries.* As mentioned earlier, capillaries have thin walls that permit the exchange of oxygen, carbon dioxide, nutrients, and waste products with body cells. The carbon dioxide and waste products are transported to the lungs and kidneys through veins and *venules* (small veins.)

The pressure that blood exerts on the walls of your vessels is called **blood pressure.** The blood

systole The contraction phase of the heart cycle

diastole The relaxation phase of the heart cycle

heart rate The number of beats of the heart in 1 minute

arteries High-pressure blood vessels that carry blood away from the heart to the lungs or cells

veins Low-pressure blood vessels that carry blood from the cells or lungs back to the heart

blood pressure The pressure that blood in the arteries exerts on the arterial walls

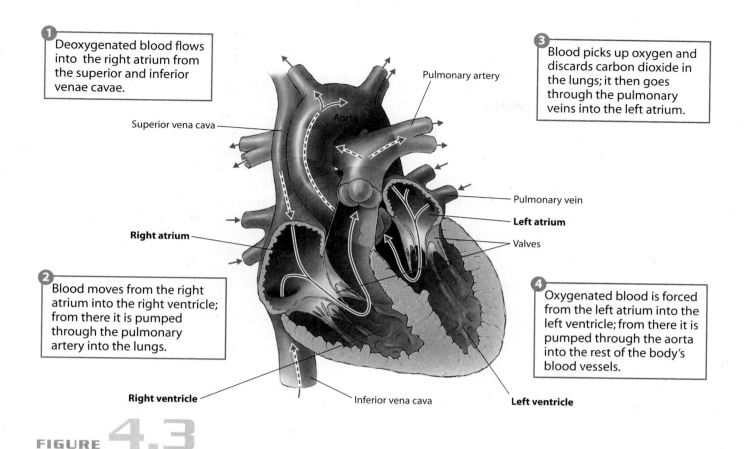

1 Deoxygenated blood flows into the right atrium from the superior and inferior venae cavae.

3 Blood picks up oxygen and discards carbon dioxide in the lungs; it then goes through the pulmonary veins into the left atrium.

Pulmonary artery

Aorta

Superior vena cava

Pulmonary vein

Left atrium

Right atrium

Valves

2 Blood moves from the right atrium into the right ventricle; from there it is pumped through the pulmonary artery into the lungs.

4 Oxygenated blood is forced from the left atrium into the left ventricle; from there it is pumped through the aorta into the rest of the body's blood vessels.

Right ventricle

Inferior vena cava

Left ventricle

FIGURE 4.3

The heart is a four-chambered pump. The right atrium and left atrium collect blood from the rest of the body. The right and left ventricles pump blood back out. In pulmonary circulation, blood circulates from the heart to the lungs and back. In systemic circulation, blood circulates from the heart to the rest of the body and back.

pressure in arteries must be high in order to drive the flow of blood to all your cells. (In veins, blood pressure is close to zero.) Due to the strength of the heart contraction, pressure in the arteries is higher during systole. The pressure measured in the arteries during this phase is called **systolic blood pressure.** When the heart is relaxed, pressure in the arteries drops; this pressure is called **diastolic blood pressure.**

THREE METABOLIC SYSTEMS
DELIVER ESSENTIAL ENERGY

All of the cells in your body need energy to function. The cellular form of energy is called *adenosine triphosphate,* or **ATP.** ATP must be constantly regenerated from energy stored in your body and from food. The energy stores in your body consist of fat from adipose tissues and muscles, glucose from muscles and the liver, and protein and **creatine phosphate** from muscles. The energy in food comes from fat, carbohydrates, and protein. Your body breaks down stored and consumed nutrients to ATP

via three metabolic energy systems: the *immediate, nonoxidative* (anaerobic), and *oxidative* (aerobic) systems. To varying extents, your body draws upon all three systems while you are active, depending on the duration of the activity. Let's examine each of these systems in detail.

The Immediate Energy System When it needs quick, immediate access to energy, your body first draws upon the ATP stored in your muscles. "Explosive" activities like a basketball jump shot, a 50-meter sprint, or a dive off a diving board are all

systolic blood pressure Blood pressure during the systole phase of the heart cycle

diastolic blood pressure Blood pressure during the diastole phase of the heart cycle

ATP Adenosine triphosphate; the cellular form of energy

creatine phosphate A molecule that is stored in muscle cells and used in the immediate energy system to donate a phosphate to make ATP

examples of actions fueled by this immediate energy system. However, your body depletes energy stored in your muscles within a matter of seconds: ATP in muscle cells is typically used up in less than 10 seconds, and creatine phosphate (which is used to make more ATP) is typically gone within 30 seconds. As a result, your body must rely on other energy systems in order to sustain longer activities.

The Nonoxidative (Anaerobic) Energy System
As soon as you start moving, the nonoxidative energy system begins breaking down glucose for energy. This system breaks down glucose quickly and *anaerobically* (without oxygen) in order to produce ATP. Although this system is active immediately, it does not supply the majority of your needed ATP until about 30 seconds into an activity. Examples of nonoxidative, **anaerobic** activities include a sprint down a soccer field, running up a steep hill, and swimming a 100-meter sprint in the pool.

You may experience muscular fatigue with the nonoxidative energy system, because your body has a limited glucose supply and because the process of breaking down glucose can produce high levels of **lactic acid.** Lactic acid accumulation in the muscles and blood can produce a burning sensation in the muscles during intense activity. While annoying, an increase in lactic acid is temporary. Contrary to popular belief, your body clears lactic acid from muscles within minutes or hours of exercise. Lactic acid does *not* cause the muscle soreness you may feel a day or two after an exercise session. In fact, during and after exercise, lactic acid cleared from the muscles and blood is reused for energy.

The nonoxidative energy system supplies your body with most of its needed ATP until about 3 minutes into an activity. At that point, the oxidative energy system becomes the primary provider of ATP.

The Oxidative (Aerobic) Energy System
During the first 3 minutes of activity (when the immediate and nonoxidative systems are supplying most of the ATP you need), your body is also gradually increasing its *oxidative* production of ATP by utilizing oxygen in the **mitochondria** of your cells. The oxidative energy system is also called the *aerobic* energy system (*aerobic* means "with oxygen"). Mitochondria are often referred to as the "powerhouses of the cell," because most of your energy production occurs in these structures. The *complete* breakdown of fat, glucose, and protein occurs only in the mitochondria; thus, the oxidative energy system yields more ATP from each energy source than any other system.

Aerobic *activities* are low- to moderate-intensity activities that are usually sustained for 20 minutes or longer. Examples of aerobic activities include cycling, treadmill walking, jogging, and water aerobics.

Figure 4.4 illustrates how the proportion of each energy system's contribution of ATP changes, depending on the duration of a given activity.

THE CARDIORESPIRATORY
SYSTEM AT REST AND DURING EXERCISE

Your cardiorespiratory system must adapt in order to meet your body's needs during exercise.

Resting Conditions
At rest, your body works to maintain **homeostasis,** a stable, constant internal environment. If healthy, your resting heart rate is between 50 to 90 beats per minute, your breathing rate is around 12 to 20 breaths per minute, and your resting blood pressure is below 120 systolic and below 80 diastolic. During homeostasis, your oxygen and nutrient delivery matches the needs of your cells. Your body breaks down fat via the oxidative energy system in order to supply ATP to the body. Although you "burn" fat for energy, your total energy expenditure is low.

Response to Exercise
Physical activity disrupts your body's homeostasis. During exercise, your body must increase blood flow to working muscles in order to maintain adequate oxygen and nutrient delivery. Your heart rate increases, and stronger heart contractions result in an increase in **cardiac output**—the amount of blood exiting your heart in 1 minute. Your breathing rate also increases to

---

anaerobic Without oxygen (nonoxidative)

lactic acid An end-product of the nonoxidative breakdown of glucose that can increase acidity in muscles and the blood and cause muscular fatigue

mitochondria Cellular structures where oxidative energy production takes place

aerobic Dependent on oxygen (oxidative)

homeostasis A stable, constant internal environment

cardiac output The volume of blood ejected from the heart in 1 minute; expressed in liters or milliliters per minute

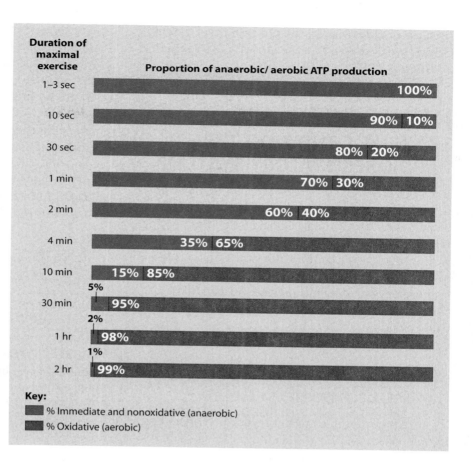

Duration of maximal exercise | **Proportion of anaerobic/ aerobic ATP production**

Duration	Anaerobic	Aerobic
1–3 sec	100%	
10 sec	90%	10%
30 sec	80%	20%
1 min	70%	30%
2 min	60%	40%
4 min	35%	65%
10 min	15%	85%
30 min	5%	95%
1 hr	2%	98%
2 hr	1%	99%

Key:
▬ % Immediate and nonoxidative (anaerobic)
▬ % Oxidative (aerobic)

FIGURE 4.4

In the first 2 minutes of exercise, your body primarily uses ATP generated by the two anaerobic energy systems. After about 3 minutes into the exercise, your body begins to primarily use ATP generated by the oxidative (aerobic) energy system.

ensure that enough oxygen is transported into the blood.

The increased volume of blood moving from your heart into your blood vessels results in an increase in systolic blood pressure. The body directs this increased blood flow to active tissues during exercise. Arteries leading to contracting muscles will *dilate* (open up wider) to accommodate the increased blood flow. This arterial dilation allows diastolic blood pressure to stay the same or even decrease during aerobic exercise. In addition, capillaries that were not open at rest will open up to allow for oxygen and nutrient exchange with muscles.

When you begin to exercise, it takes a few minutes for your body to increase blood flow and to fully engage the oxidative energy system. This is why your body must rely on the faster immediate and nonoxidative energy systems in the first few minutes of exercise. The slower ATP production of the oxidative system also means that during your exercise session, you may have to draw upon the nonoxidative energy system more than once. For example, if you are jogging and suddenly sprint to the end of the street, your oxidative energy system may not be able to supply ATP quickly enough. Your body will

CASE STUDY

Angela

"I thought I would kick-start my plan to get back into shape by doing one of the workouts my tennis coach had us do in high school. I jogged for a mile, did some calisthenics on the court, and then played two sets of tennis with a friend. That was a mistake. My friend has a killer serve—it's like a bullet coming at you. She won every point she served, because I couldn't move fast enough to return the ball. Also, I was surprised at how much that jog tired me out. I used to run a mile with no problem at all! By the end of the first set, I was completely exhausted. My friend won 6-1, 6-1."

1. Which energy system do you think Angela's friend relied on most while hitting her explosive serves?

2. Assume that Angela jogged for 12 minutes during her warm-up. Describe how each of the three energy systems played a part in fueling her jog.

then need to draw upon the nonoxidative system (which breaks down glucose quickly) to supply the additional ATP you need.

HOW DOES AEROBIC TRAINING CONDITION THE CARDIORESPIRATORY SYSTEM?

Recall that aerobic activities are low- to moderate-intensity activities performed for an extended period of time (i.e., 20 minutes or longer). Regular aerobic training conditions your cardiorespiratory system by improving your body's ability to (1) deliver large amounts of oxygen to working muscles, (2) transfer and use oxygen efficiently in the muscles, and (3) utilize energy sources for sustained muscular contractions.

AEROBIC TRAINING INCREASES OXYGEN DELIVERY TO MUSCLES

With regular aerobic training, your body gets better at delivering oxygen to working muscles. Your respiratory muscles become more efficient and you experience less fatigue in an extended workout.

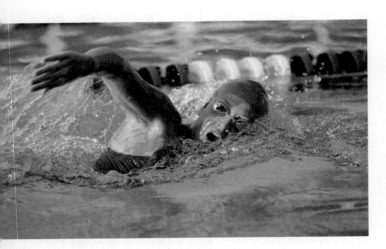

hemoglobin A four-part globular, iron-containing protein that carries oxygen in red blood cells

plasma The yellow-colored fluid portion of blood that contains water, proteins, hormones, ions, energy sources, and blood gases

stroke volume The volume of blood ejected from the heart in one heartbeat; expressed in liters or milliliters per beat

You can carry more oxygen in your blood, due to an increase in **hemoglobin,** the oxygen-carrying protein. Since the fluid portion of your blood, the **plasma,** also increases with aerobic training, you will see an increase in your total blood volume. Your heart will adapt to this greater volume by increasing the blood-holding capacity of your left ventricle. The ventricle will not only hold more blood, but (with training) it will also have stronger contractions. All of this will allow you to pump more blood out of your heart with every heartbeat, thus increasing your heart's **stroke volume.**

AEROBIC TRAINING IMPROVES THE TRANSFER AND USE OF OXYGEN

Delivering oxygen to working muscles is only part of the picture. Your body also needs to transfer oxygen into the muscles and use it efficiently. With consistent aerobic training, your body will increase the number of capillaries in the muscles that you train. This will enable increased blood flow to these muscles and improve oxygen transfer from the blood into the muscles. Once inside the muscle cells, the oxygen will be transported to mitochondria for use in the oxidative energy system. Mitochondria numbers will increase within each muscle cell, improving oxygen utilization by muscles and subsequently improving oxidative production of ATP as well.

AEROBIC TRAINING IMPROVES YOUR BODY'S ABILITY TO USE ENERGY EFFICIENTLY

Regular aerobic training will enhance your ability to store glycogen within muscles. When needed, glycogen can be broken down into glucose and used for energy during exercise. In fact, a minimal amount of glucose is needed during exercise to keep the oxidative energy system running efficiently.

Since fat breakdown for energy is accomplished within the mitochondria, an increase in the number of mitochondria will improve your body's ability to utilize fat for energy, sparing glucose and glycogen stores. Improving your body's ability to burn fat may allow you to have some glucose "left over" for that last-minute sprint to the finish! Less utilization of glucose and the nonoxidative energy system also means less lactic acid production during exercise and a delaying of fatigue.

Table 4.1 summarizes these and other adaptations that occur over time with aerobic training.

TABLE 4.1

Cardiorespiratory Training Adaptations

Cardiorespiratory Training Increases:	Cardiorespiratory Training Decreases:
VO$_2$max	Resting heart rate
Maximal cardiac output	Fatigue in respiratory muscles
Maximal stroke volume	Lactic acid produced in submaximal exercise
Heart contraction strength	Glucose use for energy in exercise
Left ventricle volume	Percentage of body fat (with calorie restriction)
Total blood volume	Blood pressure
Plasma volume	LDL cholesterol
Red blood cell mass/hemoglobin	Blood triglycerides
Mitochondria density	
Capillary density	
Fat use for energy in exercise	
Muscle endurance	
Muscle glycogen stores	
Muscle blood flow	
HDL cholesterol	

WHAT ARE THE BENEFITS OF CARDIORESPIRATORY FITNESS?

There are many reasons to improve your cardiorespiratory fitness.

CARDIORESPIRATORY FITNESS DECREASES YOUR RISK OF DISEASE

Having a low fitness level can put you at higher risk for disease and early death. The good news is that you don't need to increase your fitness to extremely high levels in order to see risk-reducing health benefits. Results of a multi-year federally funded trial indicate that just increasing your fitness to a moderate level can significantly reduce your risk of early mortality from several chronic diseases.[2] In particular, regular aerobic exercise helps protect you against the number-one killer in the world: cardiovascular disease. An increase in cardiorespiratory fitness can decrease your resting heart rate, decrease your blood levels of "bad" (LDL) cholesterol, and help prevent blood clots—all of which can lower your risk of heart attack and stroke. And it is never too early to start improving your fitness: in a study of children just 9 to 11 years old, higher cardiorespiratory fitness levels were associated with healthier arteries.[3] If children learn to be active and sustain an active lifestyle, they can avoid the stiffer, less healthy arteries that tend to accompany a sedentary lifestyle in later years.[4]

Cardiorespiratory fitness can also help you manage your weight and blood pressure, thus reducing your chances of developing conditions like **metabolic syndrome** (a group of obesity-related risk factors associated with cardiovascular disease and type 2 diabetes).[5] It can also help lessen your

metabolic syndrome A clustering of three or more heart disease and diabetes risk factors in one person (high blood pressure, impaired glucose tolerance, insulin resistance, decreased HDL cholesterol, elevated triglycerides, overweight with fat mostly around the waist)

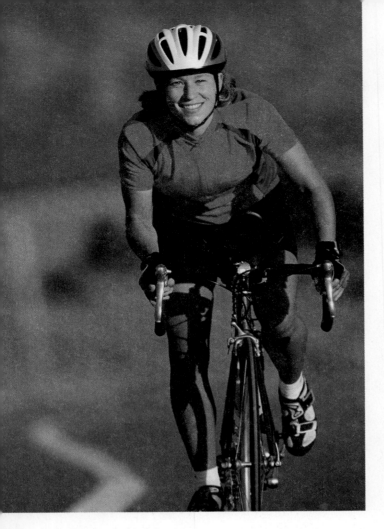

the exercise session—and long afterward. You can also burn many calories with light-to-moderate aerobic exercise by performing the activity for an extended period of time.

CARDIORESPIRATORY FITNESS
IMPROVES SELF-ESTEEM, MOOD, AND SENSE OF WELL-BEING

Exercise makes you feel good! A single aerobic exercise session can improve mood and reduce tension and anxiety as a result of chemical changes in the brain and nervous system.[9] Long-term changes are even more dramatic. One study has shown that over the course of a 12-week aerobic fitness program, men and women reported improved self-concept, anxiety, mood, and depression scores, compared to a control group, and maintained their improved psychological health for a year.[10] Numerous studies point to the importance of exercise in reducing symptoms of depression.[11]

CARDIORESPIRATORY FITNESS
IMPROVES IMMUNE FUNCTION

Light to moderate exercise can boost your immune system.[12] Regular, moderate aerobic exercise can reduce stress and improve the quality of your sleep (stress and sleep are both tied to immune system health). Research has also shown that regularly participating in aerobic exercise can slow the reduction in immune system function that tends to occur as you get older.[13]

CARDIORESPIRATORY FITNESS
IMPROVES LONG-TERM QUALITY OF LIFE

Cardiorespiratory fitness has a protective effect against age-related cognitive declines.[14] One study even suggests that aerobic exercise training can increase brain volume and thus *improve* cognitive function as you age.[15]

Increased cardiorespiratory fitness can also improve the quality of life for individuals with chronic diseases or other medical conditions. Research has shown that after a 6-month exercise program, men living with HIV improved their scores in cardiorespiratory fitness and in cognitive function and overall health.[16] Cardiorespiratory fitness has also been linked to better quality of life for survivors of breast cancer[17] and heart attacks.[18] Of course, the

risk of developing diabetes, since the regular rhythmic muscular contractions that occur in aerobic exercise improve your body's ability to utilize insulin and glucose.[6]

Regular physical activity stimulates hormones, anti-inflammatory agents, and immune responses that help protect against many forms of cancer. Studies have shown that regular physical activity and increased cardiorespiratory fitness can lower your risk of some of the most common cancers, including lung, colon, breast, and prostate.[7]

CARDIORESPIRATORY FITNESS
HELPS YOU CONTROL BODY WEIGHT AND BODY COMPOSITION

Cardiorespiratory training burns calories. By increasing your calorie expenditure through exercise, you can more effectively manage your body weight and keep your level of body fat low. A high-intensity aerobic exercise session can elevate your metabolic rate for hours,[8] burning calories during

best time to incorporate a cardiorespiratory program into your life is *before* you show signs of disease.

HOW CAN YOU ASSESS YOUR OWN CARDIORESPIRATORY FITNESS?

How fit is your cardiorespiratory system? Chances are, you already have a general idea. If you get easily winded after walking up a short flight of stairs or have trouble walking quickly for more than 10 minutes or so, you likely have a low cardiorespiratory fitness level.

Monitoring your **resting heart rate** is one way to keep track of general changes in your fitness level. Recall that your heart rate is the number of times your heart beats in 1 minute. Your resting heart rate decreases as your cardiorespiratory system becomes more conditioned. With an increase in stroke volume, your heart does not have to beat as many times per minute to deliver the same amount of blood to the body; at rest, your heart can slow down and still deliver adequate oxygen to all your cells.

When the heart contracts and pushes blood out, that wave of blood can be felt moving through the arteries. This is your **pulse.** To determine your heart rate, feel for your pulse at specific arteries around the body. The most common arteries to use for checking an exercise pulse are the *carotid* and the *radial* arteries (see Figure 4.5). Press your index and middle fingers gently against your skin and count the number of beats that you feel. Avoid using your thumb when taking your pulse, because the pulse in your thumb can interfere with your ability to count accurately. *Lab4.1* walks you through how to take an accurate heart rate reading at rest and during exercise.

UNDERSTAND MAXIMAL OXYGEN CONSUMPTION

Your body's maximal ability to utilize oxygen during exercise is called **maximal oxygen consumption** or **VO$_2$max.** Your VO$_2$max is determined by your body's ability to deliver oxygen to the muscles and the muscles' ability to consume or utilize the oxygen. VO$_2$max numbers range from 20 to 94 ml/kg·min, with male athletes typically ranging from 50 to 70 ml/kg·min and female athletes ranging from 40 to 60 ml/kg·min. Your maximal oxygen consumption is

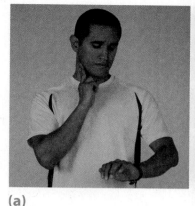 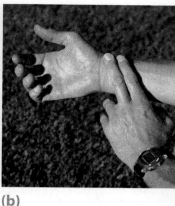

(a)   (b)

FIGURE 4.5

To determine your heart rate, feel for your pulse at either the (a) carotid artery, or (b) the radial artery.

largely determined by genetics and tends to decrease as you get older. That said, you can typically improve your VO$_2$max an average of 15 to 20 percent with training. The more deconditioned you are before beginning a training program, the more dramatic an improvement you can achieve with training.

The most accurate measurements of VO$_2$max are performed in a laboratory setting (see Figure 4.6). The test is usually completed on a treadmill or stationary bike and requires specialized equipment and technicians to ensure safety. The technicians measure the precise amount of oxygen that enters and exits the body during a maximal exercise session.

TEST SUBMAXIMAL HEART RATE RESPONSES

An alternative to testing your true maximal oxygen consumption is to perform a *submaximal* test. Submaximal tests do not test your body's maximal oxygen consumption but rather test for submaximal values that can be compared against norm charts or

resting heart rate The number of times your heart beats in a minute while the body is at rest; typically between 50 to 90 beats per minute

pulse The pressure wave felt in the arteries due to blood ejection with each heartbeat

maximal oxygen consumption (VO$_2$max) The highest rate of oxygen consumption your body is capable of during maximal exercise; expressed in either liters per minute (L/min) or milliliters per minute per kilogram of body weight (ml/kg·min)

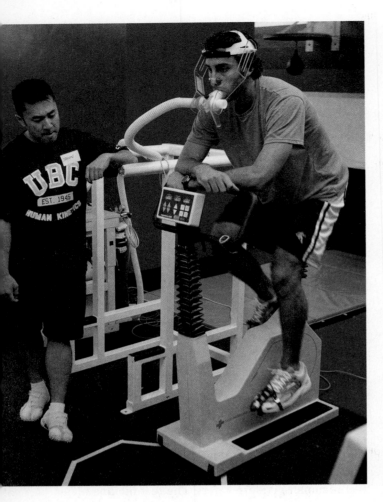

FIGURE 4.6
The most accurate measurements of VO₂max are performed in a laboratory setting.

used to predict maximal values. Submaximal tests are safer, require less equipment and expertise, and are performed in either a laboratory or field/classroom setting.

Submaximal tests in the laboratory are usually performed on a stationary bike or treadmill. These tests predict your maximal effort level and oxygen consumption by assessing your heart rate response. A higher heart rate means a higher oxygen consumption. By testing your heart rate response to different exercise intensities, an exercise technician can use your predicted **maximal heart rate (HRmax)** to

maximal heart rate (HRmax) The highest heart rate you can achieve during maximal exercise

estimate your maximal exercise intensity and oxygen consumption. Your maximal heart rate is the fastest your heart will beat in exhaustive exercise (a number that will decrease as you get older). One way to predict your HRmax is to subtract your age from the number 220. For example, if you are 18 years old, your predicted HRmax would be $220 - 18 = 202$ beats per minute. This formula is not as accurate as maximal laboratory tests, but it is used in many submaximal tests and heart rate training equations.

TEST CARDIORESPIRATORY
FITNESS IN THE FIELD/CLASSROOM

Most classes in health and fitness enroll too many students to perform laboratory testing. More appropriate for these classes are classroom or field tests of cardiorespiratory fitness. Like laboratory tests, these tests either predict your maximal oxygen consumption from submaximal test results or allow you to compare your results with norm tables. Typical tests include submaximal stepping, walking, and running assessments. In *Lab4.2* you will perform three different assessments of cardiorespiratory fitness: the 3-minute step test, the 1-mile walking test, and the 1.5-mile running test.

Three-Minute Step Test In this test, you will step up and down on a 12-inch high step bench. At the end of 3 minutes, take your 1-minute recovery heart rate and compare this to norm charts for your age and sex. The faster your heart recovers from exercise, the better conditioned you are.

One-Mile Walking Test In this test, you will walk as fast as you can for 1 mile. Record your finish time and your heart rate at the end of the 1 mile. Use your results to calculate an estimated VO₂max and determine your fitness level for your age and sex. A faster time and lower heart rate indicate a higher level of fitness.

1.5-Mile Running Test In this test, you will run 1.5 miles as fast as you can. If you cannot run the entire course, you may take walking breaks. Use your finish time to calculate your estimated VO₂max and determine your fitness level for your age and sex. A faster time indicates a higher level of fitness.

HOW CAN YOU CREATE YOUR OWN CARDIORESPIRATORY FITNESS PROGRAM?

Having a plan is one of the most important things you can do before beginning a personalized cardiorespiratory fitness program. Careful planning will help you reach your goals, prevent injuries, and ensure that you have fun while exercising!

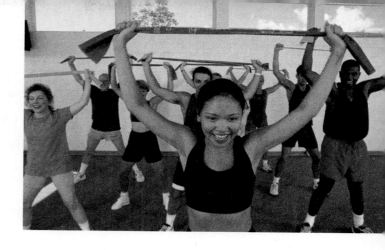

SET APPROPRIATE CARDIORESPIRATORY FITNESS GOALS

Goal-setting for cardiorespiratory fitness should follow the SMART goal-setting guidelines we first introduced in Chapter 1. Recall that SMART goals are *s*pecific, *m*easurable, *a*ction-oriented, *r*ealistic, and *t*ime-oriented. Setting a vague goal like "Build a stronger cardiorespiratory system" is not as useful as setting a specific goal that follows the SMART guidelines, such as "Improve my cardiorespiratory fitness from a 'fair' rating on my 3-minute step test to a 'good' rating, by exercising on the elliptical machine 3 days a week for 30 minutes for the next 2 months."

In *Lab4.3* you will set your own short- and long-term goals for cardiorespiratory fitness. Review the training adaptations and benefits of cardiorespiratory training discussed earlier in the chapter to guide your goal-setting. Try to set goals that are realistic and that involve an activity that you enjoy. If your goal is to run a marathon but you hate running, you will likely be setting yourself up for failure (unless your attitude toward running changes!). Choose goals that you can achieve, doing the types of activities that you enjoy most.

LEARN ABOUT CARDIORESPIRATORY TRAINING OPTIONS

There are a wide variety of cardiorespiratory training options available to you.

Classes If you enjoy the company of other people and like the motivating aspect of an instructor leading a workout, consider enrolling in a group exercise class. Classes that incorporate a continuous, rhythmic activity lasting more than 20 minutes will help you maintain or improve your cardiorespiratory fitness. Such classes can be found in colleges, recreational centers, and fitness centers in almost every community. Class formats and instructors can vary widely, so consider sampling a few different classes and instructors before deciding on a regular class. Choose classes where the instructors are not only motivating, but also experienced, certified, and have a realistic understanding of your current health/fitness levels.

Indoor Workouts If you are not sure about working out in a group or with an instructor, you can design your own cardiorespiratory workout using indoor cardio equipment. You can find cardio equipment at most gyms or fitness centers or purchase it for home use. Indoor cardio workout equipment includes stationary bicycles, treadmills, elliptical trainers, stair-climbing machines, recumbent bikes, arm cycle ergometers, rowing machines, and jump ropes. If you are using a machine in a fitness facility, get an introduction to the features, use, and safety from a facility employee. In addition, consider running

---

Try it NOW! **Sign up for a cardio class! Examples of cardio classes include aerobics, hi/lo aerobics, step aerobics, kickboxing, cardio conditioning, boot camp, hip-hop, dance aerobics, water aerobics, Jazzercise, power step, cardio funk, cycling, and spinning. • All of these are designed to increase your heart rate and get you moving in a fun, supportive environment.**

on an indoor track, swimming in a pool, deep-water jogging, or participating in a racquet sport.

Outdoor Workouts If you like to be outside, explore outdoor options for a cardiorespiratory workout. It is not uncommon to pursue a combination of indoor and outdoor exercise routines, depending on the weather and the facility options available to you. Exercising outdoors can be very rewarding if you live in an area with interesting sights, safe pathways, and beautiful trails. The options for outdoor cardio workouts are endless. Here are just a few ideas: walking, jogging, running, cycling, track workouts, trail running, hiking, tennis, cross-country skiing, open-water swimming, and inline skating.

Differing Workout Formats (Continuous, Interval, Circuit) Aerobic training is a type of *continuous* training—i.e., you perform a rhythmic activity and sustain it for a period of time (ideally 20 minutes or more). While aerobic training should be the cornerstone of your cardiorespiratory training program, other workout formats can add variety, intensity, and other fitness benefits.

An **interval workout** alternates periods of higher-intensity exercise with periods of lower-intensity exercise or rest. An interval workout method allows you to increase the intensity of your workout to a level that you might not otherwise be able to sustain for a long period of time. If done correctly, this type of workout can further develop your body's aerobic training adaptations.

A **circuit-training** workout involves moving from location to location in a circuit-training room, exercising for a certain amount of time (or number of repetitions) at each "station." You can enroll in a circuit-training class or circuit-train on your own. The circuit can contain alternating aerobic and weight-training activities, just weight stations, or just

aerobic stations. The best circuit for cardiorespiratory conditioning is one with all aerobic exercise stations.

APPLY FITT PRINCIPLES TO CARDIORESPIRATORY FITNESS

After setting goals and selecting the types of cardiorespiratory exercise that you want to do, you must decide how much, how hard, and how long to exercise. Recall the FITT principles introduced in Chapter 2: *f*requency, *i*ntensity, *t*ime, and *t*ype. Let's look at how each of these principles applies to a cardiorespiratory fitness program.

Frequency According to the American College of Sports Medicine, you should spend 3 to 5 days per week on cardiorespiratory conditioning. If you are exercising at higher intensity levels, you can improve or maintain your VO_2max by working out only 3 days per week. If you are exercising at lower intensity levels, you may need more than 3 days per week to improve cardiorespiratory fitness.

If your goals include weight loss or disease prevention, you will benefit from exercising more often but at a lower intensity in order to prevent injuries and overtraining.

Intensity Your workouts should be intense enough to tax your cardiorespiratory system, but not so difficult as to discourage you or increase your chances of injury. You can measure the intensity of your exercise by various methods, including determining your heart rate, assessing your **rating of perceived exertion (RPE),** and administering a **talk test.**

Determining Your Heart Rate. Your heart rate provides a good indication of how hard your cardiorespiratory system is working, since it is related to the amount of oxygen that your body is consuming. You can determine your heart rate by using a heart rate monitor or (as we discussed earlier) by counting your pulse.

Heart rate monitors can be found on cardio equipment and merely require you to place your hands on the receiving pads for a few seconds. Personal heart rate monitors, which consist of a chest strap transmitter and a wrist receiver, are also widely available but can be expensive.

Counting your pulse while exercising is an easy and low-cost way to measure your heart rate. Your heart rate decreases rapidly after stopping exercise, especially after 15 seconds; therefore, count your pulse for only 10 seconds, and try to keep moving as

interval workout A workout that alternates periods of higher-intensity exercise with periods of lower-intensity exercise or rest

circuit training A workout where exercisers move from one exercise station to another, after a certain number of repetitions or amount of time

rating of perceived exertion (RPE) A subjective scale of exercise intensity

talk test A method of measuring exercise intensity based on assessing your ability to speak during exercise

TABLE 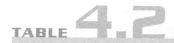 4.2

ACSM's Training Guidelines for Cardiorespiratory Fitness

Recommendations for the General Adult Population

Frequency (days/week)	3–5
Intensity (how hard)	64–90% of HRmax or 40–85% of HRR 12–16 RPE
Time (how long)	20–60 min
Type (exercises)	Large muscle group, dynamic activity

Source: American College of Sports Medicine, *ACSM's Guidelines for Exercise Testing and Prescription.* 7th ed. (Baltimore, MD: Lippincott Williams & Wilkins, 2006). Copyright © ACSM. Reprinted by permission of Wolters/Kluwer.

TABLE 4.3

Target Heart Rate Guidelines*

Age	Target HR Range (bpm)	10-Sec Count
18–24	139–179	23–30
25–29	135–174	22–29
30–34	132–169	22–28
35–39	129–165	21–28
40–44	125–160	21–27
45–49	122–156	20–26
50–54	118–151	20–25
55–59	114–147	19–25
60–64	110–142	18–24
65+	108–140	18–23

*Based upon the *HRmax method,* where 220 − age = HRmax and the training zone is 70 to 90% of HRmax. Individuals with low fitness levels should start below or at the low end of these ranges.

you count. Then multiply your 10-second count by 6 to convert to the number of beats per minute.

What **target heart rate** should you aim for in a workout? The answer depends on your goals and fitness level. As you can see in Table 4.2, the American College of Sports Medicine's recommendations for exercise intensity level cites a wide range of target heart rates: 64 to 90 percent of HRmax. Use the following guidelines to determine where within this range you should aim:

- If you are deconditioned or just starting out, you should aim for 64 to 70 percent of your HRmax.

- If you have a lower level of fitness but are regularly active, aim for 71 to 77 percent of HRmax.

- If you have a moderate level of fitness, try to reach 77 to 85 percent of your HRmax.

- Athletes or other highly conditioned individuals can regularly attain the highest levels during continuous or interval workouts (85% to 90% of HRmax).

Another method of determining your target heart rate is to measure your **heart rate reserve (HRR).** HRR is the difference between your resting heart rate and your maximum heart rate. Lab 4.1 will walk you through how to determine your HRR.

Table 4.3 also provides target heart rate guidelines for exercise, using the HRmax method based on your age.

Rating of Perceived Exertion. Another way to assess the intensity of your workout is by determining your *rating of perceived exertion (RPE)*. RPE is simply your perception of how hard you are working during exercise. Developed by Gunnar Borg in 1970, the RPE scale (Figure 4.7) is a subjective scale that can nonetheless be a very valuable tool when it is not easy or appropriate to use heart rate monitoring as an assessment for workout intensity. For example, if you participate in a water sport like swimming, heart rate

target heart rate The heart rate you are aiming for during an exercise session; often a range with high and low heart rates called your *training zone*

heart rate reserve (HRR) The number of beats per minute available or in reserve for exercise heart rate increases; maximal heart rate minus resting heart rate

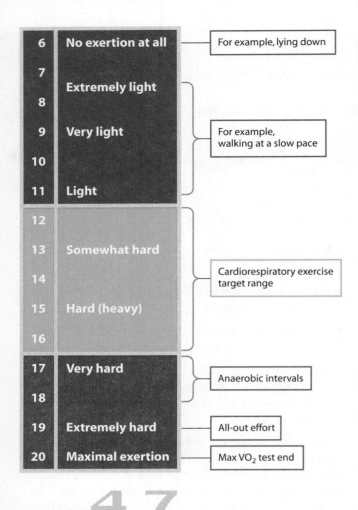

6	No exertion at all	For example, lying down
7		
8	Extremely light	
9	Very light	For example, walking at a slow pace
10		
11	Light	
12		
13	Somewhat hard	
14		Cardiorespiratory exercise target range
15	Hard (heavy)	
16		
17	Very hard	Anaerobic intervals
18		
19	Extremely hard	All-out effort
20	Maximal exertion	Max VO₂ test end

FIGURE 4.7

The rating of perceived exertion (RPE) scale is one way to estimate the intensity of your workout. A rating of 7 to 11 indicates light exertion. A rating of 12 to 16 indicates medium to heavy exertion and should be your target range in order to achieve cardiorespiratory improvements. A rating of 17 to 20 indicates extremely strenuous exertion, with a rating of 20 indicating the maximal exertion possible.

monitoring can be misleading, because heart rates tend to slow down while exercising in water, due to increased hydrostatic pressure and decreased temperature. For this reason, you may prefer to use RPE to determine your exercise intensity.

cross-training The practice of using different exercise modes or types in your cardiorespiratory training program

warm-up The initial 5-to-20-minute preparation phase of a workout

cool-down The ending phase of a workout where the body is brought gradually back to rest

To use the RPE scale, simply look at the scale, read the descriptions for each numerical rating, and assign a number corresponding to the description that best captures how you are feeling during your workout. If you choose a number between 12 to 16, you are most likely working in (or at least close to) your target heart rate training zone. As you become more experienced with a particular cardiorespiratory activity, your ability to use the scale accurately will improve, as you will become more attuned to how your body feels during exercise.

The Talk Test. The *talk test* method of measuring exercise intensity is based on assessing how easily you can talk during exercise. While exercising at a *light* intensity, you should be able to talk easily and continuously. If you are exercising at a *moderate* intensity, you should be able to talk easily, but not continuously, during the activity. If you are too out of breath to carry on a conversation, you are working at a high or *vigorous* intensity. To increase cardiorespiratory fitness, aim for at least a moderate intensity level for most of your workout. You can incorporate short periods of light and vigorous activity for workout variety or interval training.

Time For optimal cardiorespiratory conditioning, your exercise sessions should be between 20 to 60 minutes long. If you are just starting out, exercise continuously for as long as you can, and then work your way up to the minimum guideline of 20 minutes. The box **Facts and Fallacies: Can Shorter Workouts Benefit Health?** examines how workouts as short as 10 to 15 minutes can still benefit health.

Type For optimal motivation, training adaptation, and injury prevention, *choose activities that you enjoy.* Alternate your participation in these activities by the day or week for a **cross-training** effect. Cross-training can help you maintain muscle balance by working different muscle groups.

INCLUDE A WARM-UP AND COOL-DOWN PHASE IN YOUR WORKOUT SESSION

A cardiorespiratory workout session should consist of three components: the **warm-up** phase, the main cardiorespiratory endurance conditioning set, and the **cool-down** phase.

FACTS AND FALLACIES

CAN SHORTER WORKOUTS BENEFIT HEALTH?

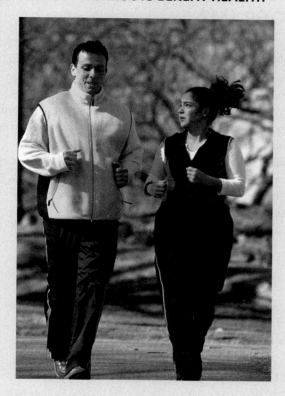

Experts used to believe that aerobic exercise must always be sustained for at least 30 minutes or more in order to result in health benefits. They felt that shorter workouts, or interrupted sessions where the heartbeat slows to resting rate, were less effective than longer workouts, where the heart rate stays continuously in the target training zone.

Recent research suggests otherwise. In one study, researchers instructed a group of obese women to walk briskly for 30 minutes three times per week, and another group to walk for two 15-minute sessions 5 days per week.[1] The intermittent walkers gained nearly as much aerobic capacity as the continuous walkers—and in both groups, blood fats and insulin measurements improved significantly. The continuous walkers lost weight, however, while the intermittent walkers did not.

In another study, young (around 25 years old) but sedentary people were instructed to eat a high-fat meal and then exercise.[2] Half of the eaters then ran for 30 minutes on a treadmill, while the other half ran for three 10-minute stretches separated by rest periods. Intermittent exercise proved to be *better* at lowering fats in the bloodstream than continuous exercise. The experimenters speculate that this may happen because each exercise session independently speeds the metabolic rate, adding up to a greater overall effect than longer, single sessions.[3]

The American College of Sports Medicine now endorses 30 minutes or more of accumulated short bouts of exercise for heart health. Knowing the value of these shorter sessions can encourage people with limited time to squeeze in 10 minutes of aerobic exercise whenever they can. Longer continuous bouts of moderate aerobic activity are excellent for burning excess body fat, so the ACSM also encourages those as well. Bottom line: Get moving, whether for short periods or long!

Sources:
1. J. E. Donnelly and others, "The Effects of 18 Months of Intermittent vs Continuous Exercise," *International Journal of Obesity,* May 2, no. 5 (2000).
2. T. S. Altena and others, "Single Sessions of Intermittent and Continuous Exercise and Postprandial Lipemia," *Medicine & Science in Sports & Exercise* 36, no. 8 1364–71.
3. American College of Sports Medicine, "Short Bouts of Exercise Reduce Fat in the Bloodstream After Meals," News release, August 5, 2004, www.acsm.org.

Figure 4.8 illustrates a sample workout for a moderately fit 20-year-old showing each of these components. Remember that your warm-up should ideally consist of light physical activity that mimics the movements of your main exercise set. For example, if your main exercise set is running, an ideal warm-up would be to jog. Likewise, your cool-down should ideally be a less-vigorous version of your main exercise set. Review Chapter 2 for more guidelines on warming up and cooling down. In addition, keep in mind that when you are starting an exercise program, you should generally perform longer warm-up (15 to 20 minutes) and cool-down (10 minutes or more) segments.

PLAN FOR PROPER PROGRESSION OF YOUR PROGRAM

When you are starting a new exercise program, it is easy to attempt to do too much too soon. In order to avoid injuring yourself, increase your workout by no more than 10 percent per week (the *10 percent rule*). That means that your weekly increases in frequency, intensity, and/or time

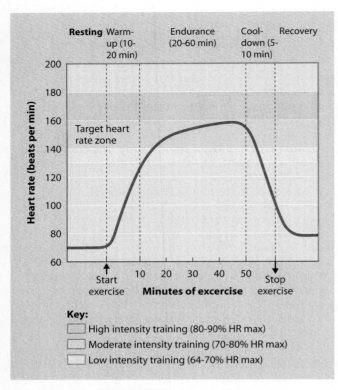

Resting | Warm-up (10-20 min) | Endurance (20-60 min) | Cool-down (5-10 min) | Recovery

Target heart rate zone

Start exercise — **Minutes of excercise** — Stop exercise

Key:
☐ High intensity training (80-90% HR max)
☐ Moderate intensity training (70-80% HR max)
☐ Low intensity training (64-70% HR max)

FIGURE 4.8

This graph charts the progression of a sample cardiorespiratory workout for a moderately fit 20-year-old. Note that it consists of a warm-up phase, an endurance phase, and a cooldown phase. Adapted from ACSM's Guidelines for Exercise Testing and Prescription. 7th ed. (Baltimore, MD: Lippincott Williams & Wilkins, 2006). Copyright © ACSM. Reprinted by permission of Wolters/Kluwer.

should not total more than 10 percent. For example, if you are jogging for 30 minutes per exercise session, next week you could safely increase each session to 33 minutes (10 percent increase in time).

Table 4.4 provides some sample cardiorespiratory programs.

HOW CAN YOU MAINTAIN YOUR CARDIORESPIRATORY PROGRAM?

How many times have you started a walking or jogging program only to quit after a few weeks? For many people, the biggest challenge to improving cardiorespiratory fitness is not beginning a program, but keeping it up. In Chapter 3, we covered several techniques for recognizing and overcoming common barriers to sustaining an exercise program. As we will discuss next, it also helps to keep in mind the stages of progression, to track your progress through journaling, and to periodically reassess your needs.

UNDERSTAND THE STAGES OF PROGRESSION

The stages of progression are simple: they consist of a start-up phase, an improvement phase, and a maintenance phase.

Start-up In the *start-up* phase of a cardiorespiratory program, you will be adjusting to the new activity in your weekly routine. During this stage, it is important to listen to your body carefully. Pay attention to how you feel during exercise so that you can make adjustments if necessary. Do you prefer exercising in the morning or in the evening? Is that aerobics class really right for you? In this first stage, your main concern should be fine-tuning your program until you settle on an activity and routine that is comfortable for you. Depending on your fitness level and exercise experience, this stage can last anywhere from 2 to 4 weeks.

CASE STUDY

Angela

"After practically killing myself on the tennis court last week, I did some research into exactly what it means to 'get in shape.' I was really interested to learn about things like target heart rates and the different ways to measure cardiorespiratory fitness. I took the 1.5-mile run test and found out that my current fitness rating is only 'fair.' So my plan is to design a cardio workout that will get my rating up to 'good' or 'excellent' before challenging my friend to another match!"

1. Pretend you are Angela's fitness trainer. Write a target goal for Angela that incorporates the SMART guidelines.

2. Consider your own cardiorespiratory fitness goals. Write a target goal for yourself that incorporates the SMART guidelines.

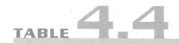

TABLE 4.4

Sample Cardiorespiratory Training Programs

	Beginning	Intermediate
Frequency	3 days/week	4–5 days/week
Intensity	64–75% of HRmax or 40–65% of HRR 12–14 RPE	70–85% of HRmax or 60–80% of HRR 13–16 RPE
Time	10–30 min	25–50 min

Sample Training Progression*

Program Stage	Week	Frequency (days/week)	Intensity (%HRmax)	Time (endurance min)
Initial Start-up	1	2–3	64–70	10–15
	2	2–3	64–70	15–20
	3	3–4	64–70	20–25
	4	3–4	68–72	20–25
Improvement	5–7	3–4	68–72	25–30
	8–10	3–4	70–75	25–30
	11–13	3–4	70–75	30–35
	14–16	3–5	74–80	30–35
	17–20	3–5	74–80	35–40
	21–24	3–5	78–85	35–40
Maintenance	24+	3–5	70–85	30–60

*This program is intended for someone starting a new program who has been medically cleared for moderate exercise levels.

Source: American College of Sports Medicine, *ACSM's Guidelines for Exercise Testing and Prescription.* 7th ed. (Baltimore, MD: Lippincott Williams & Wilkins, 2006). Copyright © ACSM. Reprinted by permission of Wolters/Kluwer.

Improvement Once you have the "kinks" worked out of your program, you are ready to move into the *improvement* phase. In this stage, your body starts adapting to the cardiorespiratory exercise. Some of these changes will be evident to you; some will not (see Table 4.2). You should, however, start feeling better during exercise, have more energy when *not* exercising, and feel like you can exercise for longer periods of time without fatigue. As in the initial stage, it is important to pay attention to your body so that you can make changes as needed. The improvement stage can last anywhere from 3 to 8 months, depending on your program and goals.

Maintenance After months of hard work, you are at the fitness level you desire, and you feel great! You have reached the *maintenance* stage. The key to this stage is to not interrupt your program. If you stop exercising, you can lose your newly achieved fitness level in only *half* the time it took you to acquire it. In fact, athletes can start losing cardiorespiratory fitness within just 2 weeks of inactivity. During the maintenance stage, it is important to keep your program consistent. If you really want to cut back, try cutting back on exercise time but not intensity level (it is easier to maintain cardiorespiratory fitness if you at least keep your workout intensity at an adequate level). The maintenance stage lasts for as long as you continue your program.

TRACK YOUR PROGRESS THROUGH JOURNALING

Do you remember how you felt during that spinning workout 3 weeks ago? How was the speed and incline of your treadmill workout last week? Keeping a workout journal or log will allow you to keep track of your progress and help you make changes for future workouts. Be sure to write down things like the FITT components of your workout, how you felt during the workout, the time of day, and any other information that may be relevant. Reviewing your journal entries can help you identify patterns or problems that you can address in future workouts. It can also provide positive reinforcement by reminding you of the progress you have made since beginning the program.

TROUBLESHOOT PROBLEMS
RIGHT AWAY

Everyone will experience some obstacles or problems when starting an exercise program. You may not have enough time in your day to work out, it may be difficult for you to physically get to your workout facility, you may be feeling pain in your knee, and so on. While these issues may set you back temporarily, they should not keep you from reaching your goals. Address the problems right away and brainstorm solutions to keep your fitness on track. Understand that you may have to reassess your program or target dates. Setbacks happen to everyone; the sooner you acknowledge a problem and address it, the sooner you can get back on track.

PERIODICALLY REASSESS YOUR
CARDIORESPIRATORY FITNESS LEVEL

The cardiorespiratory assessments introduced in Lab 4.2 can be completed any time throughout your program. Although you will certainly *feel* your progress by how your body responds to exercise, it is always nice to have quantitative measures of your progress as well. Complete the assessments in Lab 4.2 at least twice—once after 3 months of your new program and again at 6 months. Keep in mind that you will see the most improvements in assessments that are similar to your chosen workout activity (e.g., if you are doing step aerobics, you will probably see more improvement in the step test than in the 1.5-mile run test). Record your new results and check your level of improvement. If you have not improved, look at your program again and figure out if you need to redesign it.

REASSESS YOUR GOALS AND
PROGRAM AS NEEDED

Once a target date arrives, review your goals for that date. Did you achieve what you set out to do? If not, list the reasons why. Was there an issue with your program, motivation, or your life in general? Address these issues and then rewrite your goals, taking the issues into account. You may need to set more realistic goals with more realistic target dates, or select a different activity. If you need more motivation, consider finding a workout partner or working with a personal trainer.

HOW CAN YOU AVOID INJURY DURING CARDIORESPIRATORY EXERCISE?

The fastest way to disrupt a training program is to get injured. You can reduce your risks of injury by following a well-designed exercise program, wearing appropriate footwear and clothing, paying attention to your exercise environment, drinking enough water for your workout, and understanding how to prevent or treat common injuries.

DESIGN A PERSONALIZED, BALANCED
CARDIORESPIRATORY PROGRAM

The most common injuries from cardiorespiratory fitness programs are from overuse, such as strains and tendonitis, particularly in the lower body. If you attempt to do too much too soon, you put yourself at risk for such injuries. Make sure your exercise program considers your current level of fitness and make your FITT targets realistic and achievable. You may also want to consider incorporating cross-training into your program, since doing one activity exclusively can result in uneven muscle development, making you more vulnerable to injury.

WEAR APPROPRIATE FOOTWEAR
AND CLOTHING

Use common sense in wearing clothing and footwear that is appropriate to your chosen cardiorespiratory activity. If you are cycling, a helmet and bright clothing are essential. If you are running, walking, taking a group fitness class, or participating in a racquet sport, pay particularly close attention to your footwear. You might get away with running in your old gym shoes for a few short workouts, but you could quickly develop an injury if the shoes do not have enough support and cushioning. The box **Tools for Change: Selecting Proper Footwear** provides guidelines for finding the best shoes for your needs.

TOOLS FOR CHANGE

SELECTING PROPER FOOTWEAR

Below are some tips for how to select proper athletic shoes:
- Shop for shoes after a workout, preferably at the end of the day. This is when your feet will be at their biggest.
- When trying on shoes, wear the socks that you use when you exercise.

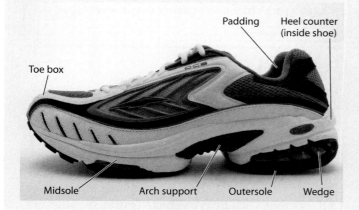

Padding
Heel counter (inside shoe)
Toe box
Midsole
Arch support
Outersole
Wedge

- When the shoe is on your foot, check to make sure you can freely wiggle all of your toes.
- The shoes should be comfortable as soon as you try them on.
- Walk or run a few steps in your shoes. They should feel comfortable.
- Always relace the shoes you are trying on. You should begin at the farthest eyelets and apply even pressure as you make a crisscross lacing pattern to the top of the shoe.
- There should be a firm grip of the shoe to your heel. Your heel should not slip as you walk or run.
- If you participate in a sport three or more times a week, you need a sports-specific shoe. Ask a knowledgeable salesperson for advice on purchasing sport-specific shoes.

Source: Modified with permission from Moseley CF (ed.), *Your Orthopaedic Connection,* Rosemont, IL, American Academy of Orthopaedic Surgeons. Available at http://orthoinfo.aaos.org.

PAY ATTENTION TO YOUR EXERCISE ENVIRONMENT

Extremes in hot and cold temperatures can affect your cardiorespiratory workout, as can air quality.

Prevent Heat-Related Illness When exercising indoors, be sure the exercise room is well-ventilated and cool enough to prevent your body from overheating. When exercising outdoors in hot weather, take precautions to avoid heat-related illnesses such as **heat cramps, heat exhaustion,** or **heat stroke.** Your risk of heat-related illness increases if you (1) exercise too hard for your fitness level, (2) exercise in high heat, humidity, and sunshine, (3) have a low fitness level overall, (4) are lacking in adequate sleep, (5) are not accustomed to the environment, (6) have an underlying infection, or (7) are overweight.[19] You can decrease your risk by being more fit, wearing light, sweat-wicking clothing, picking cooler times of the day to exercise, avoiding hazardous conditions, letting your body gradually become used to the environment, and increasing your workout slowly.

If you suspect you are developing a heat-related illness, act immediately. For heat cramps, cease activity, seek a cool environment, and restore your body's fluid and electrolyte balances by drinking water or

a sports drink. For heat exhaustion, rest in a cool environment, apply cold packs to your head and neck, drink water or a sports drink, and seek medical attention. If you suspect heatstroke, you will need medical attention immediately; ice-water immersion with IV fluids may be necessary. Because exercise increases your core body temperature, your risk of heat illness is greater when you are active, even in lower temperatures. Take extra precautions during difficult workouts to take breaks and drink fluids.

Prevent Cold-Related Illness Exercising in extreme cold also presents risks. If you like to cross-country ski, hike in the mountains, swim in cold

heat cramps Severe cramping in the large muscle groups and abdomen caused by high fluid and electrolyte loss in sustained exertion in the heat

heat exhaustion An elevated core body temperature, headache, fatigue, profuse sweating, nausea, and clammy skin brought on by sustained exertion in the heat with dehydration and electrolyte losses

heatstroke A core body temperature above 104 degrees, headache, nausea, vomiting, diarrhea, rapid pulse, cessation of sweating, and disorientation resulting from extreme exertion in very hot conditions

water, or just exercise in snowy, windy, rainy environments, you should take precautions to prevent **hypothermia,** a condition in which the body's internal temperature drops so low that it can no longer warm itself back up. If untreated, hypothermia leads to death. To avoid hypothermia, (1) minimize heat loss by wearing a warm hat and clothing, (2) keep yourself dry by wearing sweat-wicking clothing and changing out of any wet clothes as quickly as possible, (3) exercise with a workout partner who can help recognize early warning signs of cold-related illness, (4) avoid exercising in poor weather conditions, (5) warm up thoroughly, (6) drink fluids to stay hydrated, and (7) get out of the cold and warm up if you start shivering.

The early warning signs of hypothermia include shivering, goose bumps, and fast, shallow breathing. The next stage involves violent shivering, muscle incoordination, mild confusion, pale skin, and potentially blue lips, ears, fingers, and toes. In the most dangerous and potentially fatal stage of hypothermia, shivering will stop and the person will have trouble thinking, speaking, walking, and using his or her hands. If you suspect you are at risk of hypothermia, get dry and warm as soon as possible. If you are in an advanced stage of hypothermia, you will need medical attention immediately.

Be Aware of the Impact of Air Quality

Air pollution can irritate your air passageways and lungs, particularly if you have asthma, allergies, bronchitis, or other pulmonary disorders. If you experience a disruption in your breathing pattern, irritated eyes, or a headache, stop exercising and go indoors. Avoid exercising outdoors when the air quality is poor, particularly if you have a smog or air-quality alert in your city that day. If you must exercise outside on a regular basis, take measures to reduce your intake of air pollution. Exercise in wilderness areas, in parks, or on low-traffic streets. Try to exercise at times when the air quality is better, such as early in the morning and on weekends.

Watch for Hazards
Watch for hazards in your exercise environment that may cause you to trip

hypothermia A condition where the core temperature of the body drops below the level required for sustaining normal bodily functions

dehydration A process that leads to a lack of sufficient fluid in the body, affecting normal body functioning

Try it NOW! What hazards do you face in your exercise routine? • List three things about your workout routine, your clothing, or your environment that might put you at risk for injury or illness. • What can you do to minimize your risks?

and fall. When exercising indoors, seek out a space with a well-maintained floor and where you can work out without obstructions. When exercising outdoors, seek out lower-impact surfaces like a school track, running or bike path, or a dirt trail. Use your common sense: avoid slippery or muddy surfaces, as well as areas with heavy vehicle traffic. If you exercise outdoors at night, wear reflective clothing and clip a light somewhere on your body so that drivers can easily see you.

DRINK ENOUGH WATER

If you sweat profusely and do not replace the lost fluid, you will become dehydrated. Your body needs a certain amount of water in order to function. Loss of body water will decrease your blood volume and will subsequently decrease the blood flow to muscles, lowering exercise performance. **Dehydration** will also slow your sweat rate and significantly increase your susceptibility for heat-related illness.

According to the ACSM, you should lose no more than 2 percent of your body weight in fluid during an exercise session. A loss of fluid equivalent to 1 percent of your body weight will cause you to feel thirsty; losses over 3 percent may start to affect your exercise performance. Weigh yourself before and after exercise to determine how much water weight you have lost and adjust your fluid intake accordingly. Water loss is an individual issue. Everyone sweats at different rates in response to exercise. To decrease water loss, start ingesting additional fluid several hours before an exercise session and drink during exercise as well. If you are exercising for over an hour, you may benefit from drinking fluid with sugars and electrolytes (salts) in it, like a sports drink.

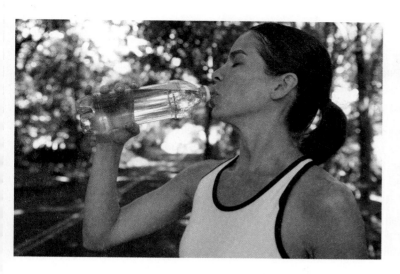

UNDERSTAND HOW TO PREVENT OR TREAT COMMON INJURIES

Below are some of the most common exercise injuries, as well as guidelines for how to prevent and treat them.

Delayed-Onset Muscle Soreness

Delayed-onset muscle soreness (DOMS) is the muscle tightness and tenderness you may feel a day or two after a hard workout session. This soreness is due to microscopic tears in your muscle fibers and connective tissues, and occurs when the body sustains excessive overloads. Most people experience DOMS at one point or another and typically recover quickly. DOMS is a sign that you did too much too soon. If you experience DOMS (especially common when starting an exercise program), examine your program design. Find ways to decrease the time, intensity, resistance, or repetitions of the exercise.

Muscle and Tendon Strains

A muscle or tendon strain is a soft-tissue injury that can be acute or chronic. An acute, sudden strain occurs due to a trauma or sudden movement/force that you are not accustomed to. A chronic, perpetual strain occurs from overstressed muscles that are worked in the same way over and over. Muscle strains involve damage to the muscle fibers, and tendon strains involve damage to the tissue that connects muscles to bones. The primary symptoms of a strain are muscle pain, spasms, and weakness. In addition, there may be swelling of the area, cramping, and difficulty moving the muscle involved. Commonly strained areas of the body are the lower back and the back of the thighs (hamstrings).

Ligament and Joint Sprains

A sudden movement or trauma can cause a sprain (damage to joint structures.) A *mild or first-degree sprain* involves overstretching or slight tearing of the ligament(s), resulting in some pain and swelling but little or no decrease in joint stability. In a *moderate or second-degree sprain,* ligaments are partially torn, and the area is painful, swollen, and bruised. In this level of sprain, mobility is limited and medical attention should be sought to determine the true severity of the injury. A *severe or third-degree sprain* involves a complete tearing or rupturing of the ligament or joint structures. Excessive pain, swelling, bruising, and an inability to move or put any weight on the joint are symptoms of a third-degree sprain. Immediate medical attention is necessary to determine if any bones were broken during the injury process. The most common sprains occur in the ankle while landing from a jump, the knee from a blow to the side or a fall, and the wrist during a fall.

Overuse Injuries

Overuse injuries are due to repetitive use. You are at an increased risk of an overuse injury if you are new to sports and exercise, if you dramatically change your exercise routine, or if you do the same type of activity day in and day out.

Tendonitis is a typical overuse injury that can result from overusing the lower- or upper-body muscles. The repetitive contractions of skeletal muscles can cause pain and swelling in the tendons near joints. Common tendonitis locations are the elbow, ankle, and shoulder and often result from tennis ("tennis elbow"), running, and weight-lifting, respectively.

A frequent overuse injury in runners and walkers is *plantar fasciitis,* or inflammation in the fascia on the underside of the foot. Pain in the arch and the heel of the foot, particularly when you are not warmed up (stepping out of bed in the morning), is the hallmark of this overuse injury.

Another injury common in runners is "runner's knee," or *patella-femoral pain syndrome.* Pain behind the kneecap or patella, inflammation, and tenderness can result from an imbalance in knee-stabilizing muscles that causes the patella to get "off track." If your patella is not tracking properly with your other knee joint structures and you contract it 1,000 times, you are bound to get irritation and pain. Women have more problems with this syndrome than men due to their wider hips contributing to knee alignment issues.

TABLE **4.5**

Common Exercise Injuries, Treatments, and Prevention

Injury	Description	Treatment and Prevention
DOMS	Muscle tenderness and stiffness 24–48 hours after strenuous exercise	*Treatment:* Reduce exercise to light activity until the pain stops, gently stretch the area; for some, heat and anti-inflammatory medications help as well *Prevention:* Follow proper exercise programming guidelines
Back Pain	Sharp or dull pain and stiffness in the mid to lower back	*Treatment:* Reduce exercise until the acute pain stops, gently stretch the area, ice, heat, anti-inflammatory medications *Prevention:* Strengthen abdominal and back muscles, stretch back and hip muscles, maintain a healthy body weight, have good posture and lifting techniques
Blisters	Red, fluid- or blood-filled pockets of skin, often on the feet after a long exercise session	*Treatment:* Change shoes that may have caused the blister, keep the area clean, and cover if needed; do not purposefully pop blisters *Prevention:* Use good-fitting, comfortable shoes and sweat-wicking socks (avoid all cotton socks)
Muscle Cramps	Muscle pain, tightness, and uncontrollable spasms	*Treatment:* Stop activity, massage and stretch the affected area until the cramp releases *Prevention:* Follow warm-up, cool-down, and general exercise guidelines, stay fully hydrated for exercise
Muscle Strain	Damage to the muscle or tendon fibers due to injury or overtraining resulting in pain, swelling, and decreased function; varying levels of severity	*Treatment:* Reduce painful activity, ice, heat after a few days, anti-inflammatory medications if desired, stretching *Prevention:* Follow warm-up, cool-down, and general exercise guidelines, reduce or stop activity if muscles feel overly weak and fatigued
Joint Sprain	Damage to ligaments or joint structures and a result of an acute injury resulting in pain, swelling, and loss of function; varying levels of severity	*Treatment:* Stop activity, ice, compression, elevation, seek medical attention *Prevention:* Avoid high joint stress activities, strengthen joint-supporting muscles, wear supportive bracing if necessary

Shin splints is the general term used to describe any pain that occurs in the front or sides of the lower legs. It is often tendonitis, a muscle strain, connective tissue inflammation, and sometimes a stress fracture. In response to repetitive stresses on hard surfaces, the muscles, tendons, and connective tissues of your lower-leg muscles get inflamed and become painful. Shin splints are common in runners and high-mileage walkers.

Over time, repeated stress to the lower leg can lead to a *stress fracture*. If you think you have shin splints but the pain won't go away with rest, ice, and therapy, you should get medical attention to rule out a stress fracture.

RICE Acronym for *rest, ice, compression,* and *elevation;* a method of treating common exercise injuries

Treating Injuries with RICE The **RICE** treatment for injuries involves <u>r</u>est, <u>i</u>ce, <u>c</u>ompression, and

TABLE 4.5   *continued*

Injury	Description	Treatment and Prevention
Dislocation	Separation of bones in a joint causing structural alterations and potential ligament and nerve damage	*Treatment:* Stop activity, ice, immobilization, seek medical treatment *Prevention:* Avoid high joint stress activities, strengthen joint-supporting muscles, wear supportive bracing if necessary
Tendonitis	Chronic pain and swelling in tendons as a result of overuse	*Treatment:* Reduce exercise to light activity until the pain stops, ice, gently stretch the area; antiinflammatory medications may help *Prevention:* Follow proper exercise programming guidelines, work for muscle balance in strength and flexibility
Plantar Fasciitis	Irritation, pain, and swelling of the fascia under the foot	*Treatment:* Reduce painful activities, gently stretch the area; for some people, ice, heat, and/or anti-inflammatory medications help as well *Prevention:* Wear good athletic shoes with adequate arch support and cushioning, warm up and stretch the plantar fascia prior to exercise
Runner's Knee	Patella-femoral pain syndrome where there is chronic pain behind or around the kneecap	*Treatment:* Reduce exercises that cause pain; use ice, anti-inflammatory medications if needed for pain and swelling *Prevention:* Work for balance in strength and flexibility in all of the knee-supporting muscles, good athletic shoes with support and foot control, exercise on softer surfaces, weight control
Shin Splints	Chronic pain in the front of the lower leg (the shins); can also occur as pain on the sides of the lower leg	*Treatment:* Reduce painful exercise, ice, gently stretch the area, switch to less weight-bearing activities *Prevention:* Work for balance in strength and flexibility in the lower-leg muscles, good athletic shoes with support and cushioning, exercise on softer surfaces
Stress Fracture	Small cracks or breaks in the bone in overused areas of the body causing chronic pain; must be medically diagnosed via X-ray	*Treatment:* Alter exercise to non-weight-bearing until the acute pain stops, seek medical attention, rest *Prevention:* Follow proper exercise programming guidelines to avoid overtraining, good athletic shoes with support and cushioning, exercise on softer surfaces

Source: Prentice, WE. *Arnheim's Principles of Athletic Training: A Competency-based Approach.* 12th ed. New York, NY: McGraw-Hill, 2006. Copyright © 2006 McGraw-Hill Companies, Inc. Used with permission.

*e*levation. After an injury, you need to *rest* or stop using that body part and allow for treatment and recovery. Most injuries will require *ice* immediately to reduce blood flow, acute inflammation, and pain. Apply ice or an ice pack for 10 to 30 minutes at a time, three to five times a day until symptoms lessen. *Compression* or applying pressure to the injury can be helpful for injuries that are bleeding or swelling. Using an elastic bandage around the injury will reduce swelling but still allow for adequate blood flow to the area. Tingling or discolored skin can be a sign that your wrapping is too tight. In order to promote blood flow back to the heart and lower the amount of swelling, *elevate* the injury above heart level. Following the RICE treatment is a good start for most exercise and sports-related injuries. Seek further medical attention if you are unsure how injured you are or if symptoms do not cease within a few hours. See Table 4.5 for a summary of common exercise injuries.

REVIEW QUESTIONS

1. Cardiorespiratory fitness is best improved by
   a. stretching your leg muscles every day.
   b. a 90-minute yoga class, three times per week.
   c. vigorously riding your bicycle every day for 30 minutes.
   d. walking to and from classes across campus.

2. Which of the following is NOT a benefit of cardiorespiratory fitness?
   a. Better sleep
   b. Increased muscle power
   c. Improved immune function
   d. Decreased risk of cancer

3. Which circulation delivers blood to the lungs and back?
   a. Pulmonary
   b. Systemic
   c. Hepatic
   d. Cardiac

4. Which energy system will provide most of the ATP during an hour-long bicycle ride?
   a. The immediate energy system
   b. The nonoxidative energy system
   c. The creatine phosphate energy system
   d. The oxidative energy system

5. Which of the following will decrease with regular, aerobic training?
   a. Muscle cell size
   b. Blood volume
   c. Resting heart rate
   d. Maximal cardiac output

6. Which test of the cardiorespiratory system requires specialized equipment and technicians?
   a. VO_2max test
   b. 3-minute step test
   c. 1-mile walk test
   d. 1.5-mile run test

7. The bulk of your cardiorespiratory training program should include
   a. interval training.
   b. circuit training.
   c. hill run training.
   d. continuous target heart rate training.

8. Which RPE value is associated with training in your target heart rate range?
   a. 8
   b. 11
   c. 14
   d. 18

9. Which of the following is the BEST way to plan for cardiorespiratory program progression?
   a. Follow the 10 percent rule
   b. Increase your exercise duration each time you work out
   c. Plan a race in 4 weeks to really get you going
   d. Follow the same program as your best friend

10. What is the most common type of injury or illness in cardiorespiratory exercisers?
    a. Heat illness
    b. Hypothermia
    c. Overuse injuries
    d. Head injuries

CRITICAL THINKING QUESTIONS

1. What adjustments does the body make during exercise to increase the delivery of oxygen to working muscles?

2. Describe two ways to determine your target heart rate during exercise.

ONLINE RESOURCES

1. **American Heart Association (AHA)**
   www.americanheart.org
   Information about cardiovascular disease prevention through nutrition and exercise.

2. **MyPyramid.gov**
   www.mypyramid.gov
   USDA site with personal planning and tracking programs for diet and physical activity.

3. **American Council on Exercise (ACE)**
www.acefitness.org
Health and fitness tips from a leading organization on fitness certification.

4. **America's Running Routes**
www.usatf.org/routes
USA Track and Field site for finding or mapping a walking or running route.

Website links are subject to change. Please visit this book's website at **www.aw-bc.com/hopson** for an updated list of links, as well as additional online resources.

REFERENCES

1. National Health Interview Survey (NHIS), U.S. Physical Activity Statistics: 1998 U.S. Physical Activity Statistics: Participation in Select Physical Activities. Available at www.cdc.gov/nccdphp/dnpa/physical/stats/pasports.htm. Accessed June 25, 2007.

2. J. L. Johnson and others. "Exercise Training Amount and Intensity Effects on Metabolic Syndrome," *American Journal of Cardiology* 100, no. 12 (2007): 1759–66.

3. K. E. Reed, D. E. Warburton, R. Z. Lewanczuk, and others, "Arterial Compliance in Young Children: The Role of Aerobic Fitness," *European Journal of Cardiovascular Prevention and Rehabilitation* 12, no. 5 (2005): 492–97.

4. J. M. McGavock, T. J. Anderson, and R. Z. Lewanczuk, "Sedentary Lifestyle and Antecedents of Cardiovascular Disease in Young Adults," *American Journal of Hypertension* 19, no. 7 (2006): 701–07.

5. C. E. Finley, M. J. LaMonte, C. I. Waslien, and others, "Cardiorespiratory Fitness, Macronutrient Intake, and the Metabolic Syndrome: The Aerobics Center Longitudinal Study," *Journal of the American Dietetic Association* 106, no. 5 (2006): 673–79.

6. C. R. Bruce, A. B. Thrush, V. A. Mertz, and others, "Endurance Training in Obese Humans Improves Glucose Tolerance and Mitochondrial Fatty Acid Oxidation and Alters Muscle Lipid Content," *American Journal of Physiology: Endocrinology and Metabolism* 291, no. 1 (2006): E99–E107.

7. S. A. Oliveria, H. W. Kohl, D. Trichopoulos, and S. N. Blair, "The Association between Cardiorespiratory Fitness and Prostate Cancer," *Medicine and Science in Sports and Exercise* 28, no. 1(1996): 97–104. Also C. M. Dallel and others. "Long Term Recreational Physical Activity and Risk of Invasive and in situ Breast Cancer: The California Teachers Study," *Archives of Internal Medicine* 167, no. 4 (2007): 408–15.

8. G. R. Hunter, N. M. Byrne, B. A. Gower, and others, "Increased Resting Energy Expenditure after 40 Minutes of Aerobic but Not Resistance Exercise," *Obesity (Silver Spring)* 14, no. 11 (2006): 2018–25.

9. D. L. Roth, "Acute Emotional and Psychological Effects of Aerobic Exercise," *Psychophysiology* 26, no. 5 (1989): 593–602.

10. T. M. DiLorenzo, E. P. Bargman, R. Stucky-Ropp, and others, "Long-Term Effects of Aerobic Exercise on Psychological Outcomes," *Preventative Medicine* 28, no. 1 (1999): 75–85.

11. E. W. Martensen and J. S. Raglin, "Themed Review: Anxiety/Depression," *American Journal of Lifestyle Medicine,* 1, no. 3 (2007): 159–166.

12. D. C. Nieman, "Current Perspective on Exercise Immunology," *Current Sports Medicine Reports* 2, no. 5 (2003): 239–42.

13. M. H. Arai, A. J. Duarte, and V. M. Natale, "The Effects of Long-Term Endurance Training on the Immune and Endocrine Systems of Elderly Men: The Role of Cytokines and Anabolic Steroid Hormones," *Immunity and Aging* 3(2006): 9.

14. R. S. Newson and E. B. Kemps, "Cardiorespiratory Fitness as a Predictor of Successful Cognitive Ageing," *Journal of Clinical and Experimental Neuropsychology* 28, no.6 (2006): 949–67.

15. S. J. Colcome, K. I. Erickson, P. E. Scalf, and others. "Aerobic Exercise Training Increases Brain Volume in Aging Humans," *Journal of Gerontology Series A: Biological Sciences and Medical Sciences* 61, no.11 (2006): 1166–70.

16. S. Fillipas, L. B. Oldmeadow, M. J. Bailey, and C. L. Cherry, "A Six-Month, Supervised, Aerobic and Resistance Exercise Program Improves Self-Efficacy in People with Human Immunodeficiency Virus: A Randomized Controlled Trial," *Australian Journal of Physiotherapy* 52, no. 3 (2006): 185–90.

17. M. McNeely and others, "Effects of Exercise on Breast Cancer Patients and Survivors," *Canadian Medical Association Journal* 175, no. 1 (2006): 34–41.

18. L. D. Dugmore, R. J. Tipson, M. H. Phillips, and others. "Changes in Cardiorespiratory Fitness, Psychological Wellbeing, Quality of Life, and Vocational Status Following a 12 Month Cardiac Exercise Rehabilitation Programme," *Heart* 81, no. 4 (1999): 359–66.

19. M. Rav-Acha, E. Hadad, Y. Epstein, and others, "Fatal Exertional Heat Stroke: A Case Series," *American Journal of the Medical Sciences* 328, no. 2 (2004): 84–87.

Name: _____   **Date:** _____

Instructor: _____   **Section:** _____

Materials: Calculator and a stopwatch

Purpose: (1) To measure your resting heart rate (RHR); (2) to calculate your personal target heart rate range for exercise; (3) to assess the intensity of your workout

SECTION I: DETERMINING YOUR RESTING HEART RATE

Practice Taking Your Pulse

Press your middle and index fingers *gently* on the side of your throat to take your *carotid pulse.* You can also take a *radial pulse* by placing your middle and index fingers at the thumbside of your wrist. Measure your resting heart rate (RHR) by counting your pulse for 60 seconds, then 30 seconds, then 10 seconds. Record your counts and complete the calculations below.

Pulse Rate #1 (1 min) _____ × 1 = _____ 1 full minute RHR

Pulse Rate #2 (30 sec) _____ × 2 = _____ 1 calculated minute RHR

Pulse Rate #3 (10 sec) _____ × 6 = _____ 1 calculated minute RHR

Determine Your True Resting Heart Rate

Take your pulse first thing in the morning on four different days. Record and average the results below. For an accurate resting heart rate, always count your pulse for a full minute. Ideally, you should take your pulse after waking up *without an alarm* and after a good night's rest.

	Resting Heart Rate (RHR)	Time of Day
Day 1		
Day 2		
Day 3		
Day 4		

Average RHR = _____

SECTION II: CALCULATE YOUR TARGET HEART RATE RANGE FOR EXERCISE

Calculate your personal target heart rate range for exercise using two methods: the maximum heart rate (HRmax) method and the heart rate reserve (HRR) method. Your target heart rate will provide a guideline for how many beats per minute your heart should be beating during exercise, in order to achieve improvements in cardiorespiratory fitness.

Note that you must count your pulse within 15 seconds of stopping exercise in order for your heart rate to reflect the exercise rate. Thus, if you take 5 seconds to find your pulse and start counting, that leaves you 10 seconds to take an exercise heart rate.

Method #1: Maximum Heart Rate (HRmax)

1. Find your predicted **HRmax** = 220 − _____ = _____
   $\qquad\qquad\qquad\qquad\qquad\qquad$ (age) $\qquad\qquad$ (predicted HRmax)

2. Find your low HR target = _____ × .70 = _____ bpm ÷ 6 = _____
   $\qquad\qquad\qquad\qquad\quad$ (predicted HRmax) $\qquad\quad$ *Low HR target* $\qquad\qquad$ *Low 10 sec target*

3. Find your high HR target = _____ × .90 = _____ bpm ÷ 6 = _____
   $\qquad\qquad\qquad\qquad\quad$ (predicted HRmax) $\qquad\quad$ *High HR target* $\qquad\qquad$ *High 10 sec target*

Method #2: Heart Rate Reserve (HRR)

1. Find your HRR = _____ − _____ = _____
   $\qquad\qquad\qquad$ (predicted HRmax) $\qquad\quad$ RHR $\qquad\qquad$ HRR
   $\qquad\qquad\qquad\qquad\qquad\qquad\qquad$ (from Section I)

2. Find 65% of HRR = (_____ × .65) + _____ = _____ bpm ÷ 6 = _____
   $\qquad\qquad\qquad\qquad$ HRR $\qquad\qquad\qquad\qquad$ RHR $\qquad\quad$ *Low HR target* $\qquad\qquad$ *Low 10 sec target*

3. Find 85% of HRR = (_____ × .85) + _____ = _____ bpm ÷ 6 = _____
   $\qquad\qquad\qquad\qquad$ HRR $\qquad\qquad\qquad\qquad$ RHR $\qquad\quad$ *High HR target* $\qquad\qquad$ *High 10 sec target*

SECTION III: MONITOR YOUR WORKOUT INTENSITY LEVEL

Practice monitoring your workout intensity during a 30-minute exercise session. You can choose any form of individual exercise that allows you to easily monitor your heart rate via a pulse check.

1. Calculate your estimated heart rate goal as a 10-second count for each time interval in the chart below.

2. Conduct your exercise session. Take your pulse and record your actual exercise heart rates.

3. In the last column of the chart, write your Rating of Perceived Exertion (RPE) scores 30 seconds before the end of the time period indicated on the workout schedule.

Time	Planned Intensity	Calculated HR 10 sec Count	Actual 10 sec HR	Rating of Perceived Exertion (RPE)
5 min warm-up	Slowly up to 55% HRmax	Predicted HRmax × .55 = _____ ÷ 6 = _____		
5 min	65% HRmax	Predicted HRmax × .65 = _____ ÷ 6 = _____		
4 min	75% HRmax	Predicted HRmax × .75 = _____ ÷ 6 = _____		
3 min	85% HRmax	Predicted HRmax × .85 = _____ ÷ 6 = _____		
4 min	75% HRmax	Predicted HRmax × .75 = _____ ÷ 6 = _____		
5 min	65% HRmax	Predicted HRmax × .65 = _____ ÷ 6 = _____		
4 min cool-down	55% HRmax	Predicted HRmax × .55 = _____ ÷ 6 = _____		

SECTION IV: REFLECTION

1. How close were your calculated and actual heart rates during your 30-minute exercise session?

2. Did the intensity levels feel higher or lower than you thought they would at each percentage of HRmax?

Name: _____   Date: _____

Instructor: _____   Section: _____

Materials: Calculator, 12-inch step, stopwatch, metronome

Purpose: To measure (1) recovery from physical activity, (2) walking speed, and (3) current level of cardiorespiratory fitness.

SECTION I: THE 3-MINUTE STEP TEST

For this test, you will be stepping on a 12-inch high step bench for 3 minutes and then measuring your recovery pulse for 1 full minute.

1. **Setup and preparation.** Set up a 12-inch-high step bench in a place that will be safe to perform the test. Set the metronome to a pace of 96 beats per minute, which means you will be doing 24 steps up and down in a minute. Listen to the metronome and do a couple of practice steps to ensure that you can step with the right cadence ("up, up, down, down"). One foot will be stepping up or down with each beat of the metronome. Have a stopwatch available to time your 3 minutes on the step and your 1 minute HR afterward.

2. **Step up and down for 3 minutes.** Start the metronome and march in place to the beat. Start stepping up on the bench and down to the floor after starting the stopwatch. Maintain this exact pace for the entire 3 minutes.

3. **Stop and count your pulse for 1 full minute.** At the end of 3 minutes, stop stepping, turn off the metronome, sit down on your bench, and find your carotid or radial pulse immediately. Within 5 seconds of stopping the exercise, start counting your recovery pulse and count for 1 full minute.

4. **Record your results and your fitness rating.** Record your recovery heart rate below in beats per minute (bpm). Locate your fitness rating on the chart below and record that as well.

The 3-Minute Step Test RESULTS

1-Minute Recovery HR: _____ **(bpm)**   **Fitness Rating:** _____

YMCA 3-Minute Step Test Ratings (bpm)							
Men	**Excellent**	**Good**	**Above Average**	**Average**	**Below Average**	**Poor**	**Very Poor**
18–25 yrs	<80	81–89	90–99	100–106	107–117	118–130	>131
26–35 yrs	<81	82–90	91–99	100–108	109–118	119–129	>130
36–45 yrs	<84	85–95	96–104	105–112	113–119	120–131	>132
46–55 yrs	<87	88–97	98–107	108–117	118–123	124–134	>135
56–65 yrs	<87	88–97	98–104	105–112	113–121	122–130	>131
66+ yrs	<87	88–97	98–103	104–113	114–121	122–132	>133

YMCA 3-Minute Step Test Ratings (bpm)							
Women	Excellent	Good	Above Average	Average	Below Average	Poor	Very Poor
18–25 yrs	<86	87–98	99–108	109–117	118–127	128–141	>142
26–35 yrs	<89	90–101	102–110	111–120	121–128	129–140	>141
36–45 yrs	<91	92–102	102–110	111–119	120–129	130–142	>143
46–55 yrs	<94	95–104	105–115	116–120	121–126	127–137	>138
56–65 yrs	<95	96–105	106–111	112–118	119–128	129–141	>142
66+ yrs	<91	92–103	104–115	116–122	123–128	129–134	>135

Source: Reprinted with permission from the *YMCA Fitness Testing and Assessment Manual,* Fourth Edition. © 2000 by YMCA of the USA, Chicago. All rights reserved.

SECTION II: THE 1-MILE WALK TEST

You will walk 1 mile and determine your heart rate response to the exercise immediately after. IMPORTANT REMINDERS: The accuracy of this test depends on three things: (1) Walk during this test. Do not run. (2) You must walk the mile as fast as you can. (3) You must keep a steady pace throughout the mile. Do not "sprint" at the end.

1. **Preparation and warm-up.** Make sure that you have an accurate 1-mile course to complete (four laps around a standard track) and a stopwatch. Warm up with 3 to 5 minutes of light walking and range-of-motion activities.

2. **Walk 1 full mile as fast as you can.** After completing the 1 mile, mark your finish time (from your watch, stopwatch, or someone calling out the time) below. Convert the time from minutes and seconds to minutes with a decimal fraction.

3. **Immediately take an exercise heart rate and cool-down.** Within 5 seconds of finishing the walk, find your carotid or radial pulse and count your pulse for 10 seconds. Multiply the number by 6 and record your HR below. After recording your finish time and your HR, cool down by walking slowly for another 5 minutes and doing some light stretching.

4. **Calculate your estimated maximal oxygen consumption (VO$_2$max).** Use the formula below to calculate your estimated VO$_2$max. This number will more accurately reflect your fitness level if you followed the test instructions carefully.

5. **Find the cardiorespiratory fitness level that corresponds to your predicted VO$_2$max.** Use the chart at the end of Section III to determine your cardiorespiratory fitness level, as determined by this 1-mile walking test.

The 1-Mile Walk Test RESULTS

1-Mile Walk Time: _____ (min:sec); divide sec by 60 = _____ (min w/ decimal)

Exercise HR: _____ (beats) × 6 = _____ (bpm)

(10 sec count)

Estimated VO$_2$max: Use the following equation to estimate VO$_2$max, where **gender = *0 for female*** and ***1 for male;*** time = walk time to the nearest hundredth of a minute; and HR = heart rate (bpm) at the end of the walking test. Plug in your weight and numbers from above and calculate the numbers in parentheses first. Complete the calculation to find your estimated VO$_2$max.

- VO$_2$max = 132.853 − [0.0769 × body weight (lb)] − [0.3877 × age (yr)] + [6.3150 × gender]
  − [3.2649 × time (min)] − [0.1565 × HR (bpm)]
- VO$_2$max = 132.853 − [0.0769 × _____ (lb)] − [0.3877 × _____ (yr)] + [6.3150 × _____ (gender)]
  − [3.2649 × ____ (min)] − [0.1565 × ____ (bpm)]
- VO$_2$max = 132.853 − _____ − _____ + _____ − _____ − _____
- VO$_2$max = _____ (ml/kg·min)

Walk Test VO$_2$max Fitness Rating: _____

SECTION III: 1.5-MILE RUN TEST

1. **Preparation and warm-up.** Make sure that you have an accurate 1.5-mile course to complete (six laps around a standard track) and a stopwatch. Warm up with 5 to 10 minutes of walking/jogging and range-of-motion activities.

2. **Run (with walk breaks if needed) 1.5 miles as fast as you can.** After reaching 1.5 miles, mark your finish time (from your watch, stopwatch, or someone calling out the time) below. You will be converting the time from minutes and seconds to minutes with a decimal fraction.

3. **Cool-down.** After recording your finish time, cool down by walking for 5 minutes and doing some light stretching.

4. **Calculate your estimated maximal oxygen consumption (VO$_2$max).** Use the formula below to calculate your estimated VO$_2$max.

5. **Find your cardiorespiratory fitness level that corresponds to your predicted VO$_2$max.** Use the chart at the end of this section to determine your cardiorespiratory fitness level, as determined by this 1.5-mile running test.

The 1.5-Mile Run Test RESULTS

1.5-Mile Run Time: _____ (min:sec); divide sec by 60 = _____ (min w/ decimal)

Estimated VO$_2$max: You will use the following equation to estimate VO$_2$max, where time = run time to the nearest hundredth of a minute. Plug in your time from above, compute the number in parentheses first, and complete the calculation to find your estimated VO$_2$max.

- VO$_2$max = [483 ÷ time (min)] + 3.5
- VO$_2$max = [483 ÷ _____(min)] + 3.5
- VO$_2$max = _____ + 3.5
- VO$_2$max = _____ (ml/kg·min)

Run Test VO$_2$max Fitness Rating: _____

Estimated VO$_2$max Fitness Ratings (ml/kg·min)						
Men	**Superior**	**Excellent**	**Good**	**Fair**	**Poor**	**Very Poor**
18–29 yrs	>56.1	51.1–56.1	45.7–51.0	42.2–45.6	38.1–42.1	<38.1
30–39 yrs	>54.2	48.9–54.2	44.4–48.8	41.0–44.3	36.7–40.9	<36.7
40–49 yrs	>52.8	46.8–52.8	42.4–46.7	38.4–42.3	34.6–38.3	<34.6
50–59 yrs	>49.6	43.3–49.6	38.3–43.2	35.2–38.2	31.1–35.1	<31.1
60–69 yrs	>46.0	39.5–46.0	35.0–39.4	31.4–34.9	27.4–31.3	<27.4
Women	**Superior**	**Excellent**	**Good**	**Fair**	**Poor**	**Very Poor**
18–29 yrs	>50.1	44.0–50.1	39.5–43.9	35.5–39.4	31.6–35.4	<31.6
30–39 yrs	>46.8	41.0–46.8	36.8–40.9	33.8–36.7	29.9–33.7	<29.9
40–49 yrs	>45.1	38.9–45.1	35.1–38.8	31.6–35.0	28.0–31.5	<28.0
50–59 yrs	>39.8	35.2–39.8	31.4–35.1	28.7–31.3	25.5–28.6	<25.5
60–69 yrs	>36.8	32.3–36.8	29.1–32.2	26.6–29.0	23.7–26.5	<23.7

Source: From *Physical Fitness Assessments and Norms for Adults and Law Enforcement.* Copyright © The Cooper Institute. Reprinted with permission from The Cooper Institute, Dallas, Texas. For more information: www.cooperinstitute.org

Name: _____

Date: _____

Instructor: _____

Section: _____

Materials: Results from cardiorespiratory fitness assessments, calculator, lab pages.

Purpose: To learn how to set appropriate cardiorespiratory fitness goals and create a personal cardiorespiratory fitness program designed to meet those goals.

Directions: Complete the following sections.

SECTION I: SHORT- AND LONG-TERM GOALS

Create short- and long-term goals for cardiorespiratory fitness. Be sure to use SMART goal-setting guidelines (specific, measurable, action-oriented, realistic, time-oriented). Select appropriate target dates and rewards for completing your goals.

SHORT-TERM GOAL (3–6 months)

_____

_____

_____

_____

Target Date: _____

Reward: _____

_____

LONG-TERM GOAL (12+ months)

_____

_____

_____

_____

Target Date: _____

Reward: _____

_____

SECTION II: CARDIORESPIRATORY FITNESS OBSTACLES AND STRATEGIES

1. What **barriers or obstacles** might hinder your plan to improve your cardiorespiratory fitness? Indicate your top three obstacles below:

a.

b.

c.

2. Overcoming these barriers/obstacles to change will be an important step in reaching your goals. Write down three **strategies** for overcoming the obstacles listed above:

a.

b.

c.

SECTION III: GETTING SUPPORT

1. List **resources** you will use to help you change your cardiorespiratory fitness:

Friend/partner/relative: _____

School-based resource: _____

Community-based resource: _____

Other: _____

2. How will you use these supportive resources to help you meet your cardiorespiratory fitness goals?

_____

_____

_____

_____

_____

_____

_____

_____

_____

_____

SECTION IV: CARDIORESPIRATORY FITNESS PROGRAM REFLECTIONS

1. How realistic are the short- and long-term target dates you have set for achieving your cardiorespiratory fitness goals?

2. How many days per week are you planning to work on your cardiorespiratory fitness program? _____

3. What types of workouts are you planning to try?

4. Do you have a workout partner? Do you plan to work with a workout partner, personal trainer, or instructor to help get you started?

SECTION V: CARDIORESPIRATORY TRAINING PROGRAM DESIGN

Plan a 4-week cardiorespiratory training program, using resources available to you (facility, instructor, text) and completing the following training calendar (A = activity, I = intensity, T = time).

4-Week Cardio Program						
Sun	**Mon**	**Tues**	**Wed**	**Thurs**	**Fri**	**Sat**
Date: _____ A: I: T:	Date: _____ A: I: T:	Date: _____ A: I: T:	Date: _____ A: I: T:	Date: _____ A: I: T:	Date: _____ A: I: T:	Date: _____ A: I: T:
Date: _____ A: I: T:	Date: _____ A: I: T:	Date: _____ A: I: T:	Date: _____ A: I: T:	Date: _____ A: I: T:	Date: _____ A: I: T:	Date: _____ A: I: T:
Date: _____ A: I: T:	Date: _____ A: I: T:	Date: _____ A: I: T:	Date: _____ A: I: T:	Date: _____ A: I: T:	Date: _____ A: I: T:	Date: _____ A: I: T:
Date: _____ A: I: T:	Date: _____ A: I: T:	Date: _____ A: I: T:	Date: _____ A: I: T:	Date: _____ A: I: T:	Date: _____ A: I: T:	Date: _____ A: I: T:

SECTION VI: TRACKING YOUR PROGRAM AND FOLLOWING THROUGH

1. **Goal and Program Tracking:** Use the following chart to monitor your progress. Change the activity, intensity, or time of your workout plan to reflect your progress as needed.

2. **Goal and Program Follow-up:** At the end of the course or at your short-term goal target date, reevaluate your cardiorespiratory fitness and answer the following questions:

   a. Did you meet your short-term goal or your goal for the course? If so, what positive behavioral changes contributed to your success? If not, which obstacles blocked your success?

   b. Was your short-term goal realistic? What would you change about your goals or cardiorespiratory training plan?

Dates	Activity	Time	Av. HR	RPE	Comments
Week _____ Day _____					
Day _____					
Day _____					
Day _____					
Day _____					
Week _____ Day _____					
Day _____					
Day _____					
Day _____					
Day _____					
Week _____ Day _____					
Day _____					
Day _____					
Day _____					
Day _____					
Week _____ Day _____					
Day _____					
Day _____					
Day _____					
Day _____					
Week _____ Day _____					
Day _____					
Day _____					
Day _____					
Day _____					

5-Week Cardiorespiratory Training Log

CHAPTER 5

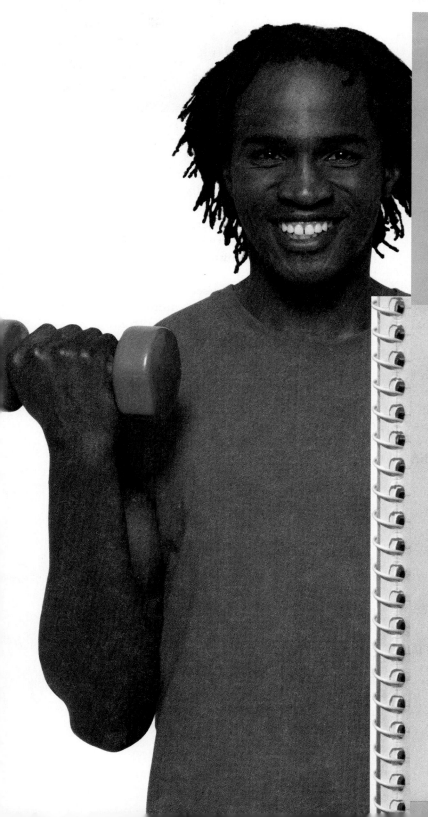

Building Muscular Strength and Endurance

OBJECTIVES

Define *muscular strength* and *muscular endurance* and describe the benefits of each.

Discuss the basic structure and function of skeletal muscle.

Outline the fitness and wellness improvements that occur with regular resistance training.

Assess your muscular strength and muscular endurance.

Set appropriate muscular fitness goals.

Describe common resistance-training methods and programs and create an exercise plan compatible with your goals and lifestyle.

Identify and observe precautions for safe resistance training.

Describe the risks associated with supplement use, including anabolic steroids.

CASE STUDY

Gina

"Hi, I'm Gina. I'm from San Francisco and I'm a sophomore majoring in economics. I'm taking a fitness and wellness class this semester, and this week we're starting the section on muscular fitness. I'm curious about it because I've never lifted weights before! I like to go hiking, and I take yoga classes from time to time, but I wouldn't call myself an athlete. Does it really make sense for someone like me to start a strength-training program?"

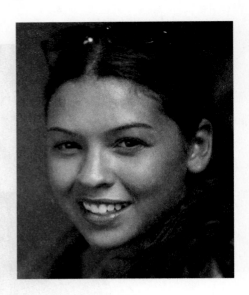

Whether you're a beginner like Gina or an athlete interested in conditioning, this chapter will answer common questions about muscular fitness, explain the many benefits of strength training, and give you the tools for designing a program that is custom-made for you.

Muscular fitness is the ability of your musculoskeletal system to perform daily and recreational activities without undue fatigue and injury. Muscular fitness involves having adequate muscular strength and endurance. **Muscular strength** is the ability of a muscle or group of muscles to contract with maximal force. It describes how strong a muscle is or how much force it can exert. Exercise professionals often measure muscular strength by determining the maximum weight a person can lift at one time. **Muscular endurance** is the ability of a muscle to contract repeatedly over an extended period of time. It describes how long you can sustain a given type of muscular exertion. One way that fitness professionals measure muscle endurance is by determining the maximum weight a person can lift 20 times consecutively.

You can build better muscular strength and endurance through resistance training. **Resistance training** is also referred to as *weight training* or *strength training* and can be done with measured weights, body weight, or other resistive equipment (i.e., exercise bands or exercise balls). Resistance exercises stress the body's musculoskeletal system, which enlarges muscle fibers and improves neural control of muscle function, resulting in greater muscular strength and endurance.

Are you already participating in a resistance-training program? If so, you are not alone. According to the National Health Interview Survey (NHIS), resistance training is the fourth most popular leisure-time activity for adults over the age of 18.[1] It is more popular than jogging, aerobics, and many other recreational sports (but is less popular than walking, working in the yard, or stretching.) In 2004, 17.5 percent of women and 21.5 percent of men reported regular resistance training.[2] However, these numbers still do not approach the *Healthy People 2010* national health objective: that 30 percent of adults participate in strength-training exercises at least two times per week. If you are not participating, now may be the perfect time to start because of readily

muscular fitness The ability of your musculoskeletal system to perform daily and recreational activities without undue fatigue and injury

muscular strength The ability of a muscle to contract with maximal force

muscular endurance The ability of a muscle to contract repeatedly over an extended period of time

resistance training Controlled and progressive stressing of the body's musculoskeletal system using resistance (i.e., weights, resistance bands, body weight) exercises to build and maintain muscular fitness

available facilities and classes at most colleges and universities.

Resistance training offers such varied benefits that exercise professionals recommend it in nearly all health-related fitness programs. Regular resistance training can make daily activities easier: carrying around a backpack full of heavy textbooks won't tire you as much; bringing in a bag of groceries will be less taxing; and taking the stairs will seem natural and feel better than riding in an elevator. No matter what your health and fitness goals may be, resistance training can be an important and rewarding wellness tool throughout your life.

HOW DO MUSCLES WORK?

The human body contains hundreds of muscles, each of which belongs to one of three basic types: (1) voluntary *skeletal muscle*, which allows movement of the skeleton and generates body heat; (2) involuntary *cardiac muscle*, which exists only in the heart and facilitates the pumping of blood through the body; and (3) involuntary *smooth muscle*, which lines some internal organs and moves food through the stomach and intestines. Together, resistance training and cardiorespiratory exercise will benefit all three muscle types. Here we will focus on skeletal muscles and the signals from the nervous system that coordinate and control their contraction.

AN OVERVIEW OF SKELETAL MUSCLE

Each skeletal muscle is surrounded by a sheet of connective tissue that draws together at the ends of the muscle, forming the **tendons** (see Figure 5.1). Muscular contractions allow for skeletal movement because muscles are attached to bones via tendons. These attached muscles pull the bones, which pivot at joints, creating a specific body movement.

Within each skeletal muscle are individual muscle cells called **muscle fibers.** Bundles of muscle fibers are called *fascicles.* Each muscle fiber extends the full length of the muscle. Within each muscle fiber are many **myofibril** strands, each containing contractile protein filaments. These filaments are made up of two kinds of protein—*actin* and *myosin*—which are arranged in alternating bands that give the whole cell a striped appearance. The microscopic structure

and function of actin and myosin allow them to slide across each other and shorten the muscle. You can picture this sliding and shortening as similar to the way your forearms can slide past each other inside the front pocket of a hooded sweatshirt, pulling your elbows closer together. Simultaneous shortening of the many fibers within a whole muscle causes the pattern of muscular tension we call *contraction*. It is this whole-muscle contraction that moves bones and surrounding body parts.

Every muscle fiber can be categorized as either *slow* or *fast,* depending on how quickly it can contract. **Slow-twitch muscle fibers** (Type I) are oxygen-dependent and contract relatively slowly, but can contract for longer periods of time without fatigue. **Fast-twitch muscle fibers** (Type II) are not oxygen-dependent and contract more rapidly than slow-twitch fibers, but tire relatively quickly (they also produce greater muscle power). In slow-twitch fibers, the energy for contraction comes from the breakdown of fat from the blood, muscle cells, and adipose tissue. Fat breakdown requires oxygen and minimal levels of glucose breakdown as well. In fast-twitch fibers, the energy for contraction comes from phosphocreatine and glycogen reserves within the muscles, glycogen stored within the liver, and glucose in the blood.

All fiber types exist in skeletal muscles, but some muscles within the body—such as postural trunk muscles—have more slow-twitch fibers, while other muscles (such as those in the calves) have more fast-twitch fibers. The proportion of muscle fiber types varies from person to person based on both genetics and training. Elite athletes have muscle fiber compositions that complement their sport. Marathoners,

tendon The connective tissue attaching a muscle to a bone

muscle fiber The cell of the muscular system

myofibril Thin strands within a single muscle fiber that bundle the skeletal muscle protein filaments and span the length of the fiber

slow-twitch muscle fiber Muscle fiber type that is oxygen-dependent and can contract over long periods of time

fast-twitch muscle fiber Muscle fiber type that contracts with greater force and speed but also fatigues quickly

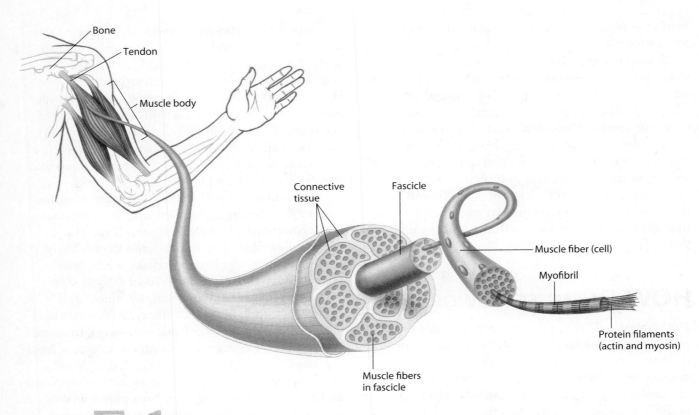

FIGURE 5.1

A muscle is attached to bones via tendons. Tendons are a continuation of the connective tissue that surrounds the entire muscle as well as each muscle bundle (fascicle). A fascicle is made up of many muscle cells (muscle fibers). Within each muscle fiber, myofibril strands contain actin and myosin proteins.

for instance, have higher levels of slow-twitch fibers that supply them with optimal muscular endurance. Power weight lifters, on the other hand, have more fast-twitch fibers that allow feats of enormous muscular strength over short periods of time. Sedentary individuals and people who do general resistance training typically have 50 percent slow-twitch and 50 percent fast-twitch fiber composition.

MUSCLE CONTRACTION
REQUIRES STIMULATION

For a voluntary skeletal muscle to contract, your nervous system must send a signal directly to the muscle. When you want to move any part of your body—for example, a finger on your right hand—your brain will send a signal down the spinal cord and through motor nerves to the skeletal muscle fibers in

motor unit A motor nerve and all the muscle fibers it controls

that finger. One motor nerve will stimulate many skeletal muscle fibers, together creating a functional unit called a **motor unit** (see Figure 5.2). A motor unit can be small or large, depending on the number of muscle fibers that it stimulates. Small motor units are comprised of slow-twitch fibers; larger motor units are comprised of fast-twitch fibers. The strength of a muscle contraction depends upon the intensity of the nervous system stimulus, the number and size of motor units activated, and the types of muscle fibers that are stimulated. For example, if you are getting ready to lift a heavy weight, your central nervous system will send a stronger signal. This will activate a greater number of large fast motor units, resulting in a more forceful muscle contraction than if you were merely picking up an apple.

THREE PRIMARY TYPES
OF MUSCLE CONTRACTIONS

Muscle contractions all result in an increase in tension or force within the muscle, but some contractions move body parts while others do not.

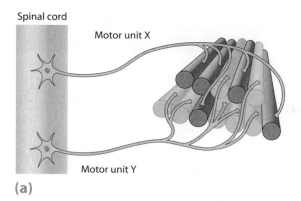

Spinal cord

Motor unit X

Motor unit Y

(a)

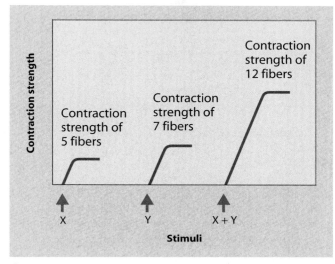

Contraction strength

Contraction strength of 5 fibers

Contraction strength of 7 fibers

Contraction strength of 12 fibers

X   Y   X + Y

Stimuli

(b)

FIGURE **5.2**

Motor Units and Muscle Contraction Strength
(a) Motor unit X is smaller (5 fibers) than motor unit Y (7 fibers). (b) The strength of a muscular contraction increases with increased fibers per motor unit (X vs. Y) and with more motor units activated (X + Y).

There are three primary types of contractions: isotonic, isometric, and isokinetic. **Isotonic** contractions are characterized by a consistent muscle tension as the contraction proceeds and a resulting movement of body parts (Figure 5.3a). An arm curl with a 10-pound hand weight involves isotonic contractions throughout your arm. **Isometric** contractions are characterized by a consistent muscle length throughout the contraction with no visible movement of body parts. An example of an isometric contraction is when you hold a hand weight at arm's length in front of you; your arm is not moving, but you feel tension in your arm muscles (Figure 5.3b). **Isokinetic** contractions are characterized by a consistent muscle contraction speed within a moving

CASE STUDY

Gina

"I love to go on short hikes. There are some gorgeous trails in the San Francisco Bay Area. Some of them are kind of hilly, but I don't mind—the views from the top are always worth it. My calves definitely get a workout! I'd like to be able to do longer hikes, but the truth is that I usually get tired after about three miles. I know there are some longer hikes with spectacular views, but I don't feel ready for them yet."

1. Given what you've learned so far, what would you tell Gina about how resistance training can benefit her?

2. Which type of muscle fibers would you guess that Gina has more of: slow-twitch fibers or fast-twitch fibers?

3. Name an outdoor activity that you enjoy. Can you give one or two examples of isotonic contractions that occur in your body during the course of that activity?

body part. In order to perform isokinetic contractions, you need specialized equipment that holds the speed of movement constant as your arm, leg, or other muscles contract with varying forces.

Isotonic contractions are the most common in exercise programs. Lifting free weights, working on machines, and doing push-ups are all examples of isotonic contractions. Isotonic contractions can be either concentric or eccentric. **Concentric** contractions occur when force is developed in the muscle as the muscle is shortening—for example, when you curl a free weight up toward your shoulder. In **eccentric** muscle contractions, force remains in

isotonic A muscle contraction with relatively constant tension

isometric A muscle contraction with no change in muscle length

isokinetic A muscle contraction with a constant speed of contraction

concentric A muscle contraction with overall muscle shortening

eccentric A muscle contraction with overall muscle lengthening

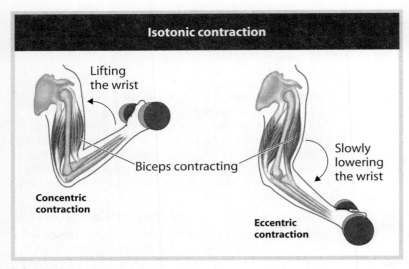

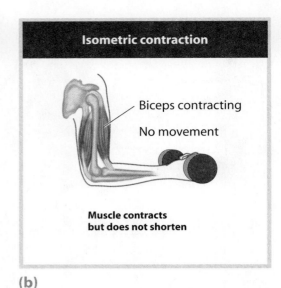

(a)

(b)

FIGURE **5.3**

(a) Isotonic contractions include concentric (shortening) and eccentric (lengthening) contractions.
(b) Isometric contractions produce force in the muscle with no movement.

the muscle while the muscle is lengthening. This occurs as you lower a free weight back to its original position. Figure 5.3a illustrates these muscular contractions, using a bicep-curl exercise as an example.

HOW CAN REGULAR RESISTANCE TRAINING IMPROVE YOUR FITNESS AND WELLNESS?

People used to think that weight lifting was solely a means of improving body shape and producing bigger muscles. We now know that, in addition to improving physical appearance, resistance training can also result in specific physiological changes that have significant fitness and wellness benefits. Table 5.1 summarizes these changes. We discuss the benefits of resistance training in detail in the section that follows.

REGULAR RESISTANCE TRAINING INCREASES STRENGTH

Regular resistance training with an adequate *load*, or amount of weight lifted, will result in an increase in muscle strength. Although men tend to realize

greater gains in muscle size due to higher testosterone levels, women can often have a larger capacity to improve strength.[3] Stronger lower- and upper-body muscles benefit both men and women.

TABLE **5.1**

Physiological Changes from Resistance Training	
Increased	**Decreased**
Muscle mass	Percentage of body fat
Muscular strength and/or muscular endurance	Time required for muscle contraction
Bone mineral density	Blood pressure (if high)
Basal metabolic rate	Blood cholesterol (if high)
Intramuscular fuel stores (ATP, PC, glycogen)	
Tendon, ligament, and joint strength	
Tendon strength	
Coordination of motor units	
Insulin sensitivity	

Neural Improvements When you start a resistance-training program, you will gain muscular *strength* before noticing any increase in muscle *size*. This is because internal physiological adaptations to training take place before muscle enlargement. The strength of a muscular contraction depends, in large part, on effective recruitment of the motor units needed for that contraction. The better your body gets at recruiting the necessary motor units through voluntary neural signaling, th stronger your muscles will be. In the first few weeks or months of a resistance-training program, most of the adaptation involves an increased ability to recruit motor units, which causes more muscle fibers to contract.

Increased Muscle Size After the initial improved neural activation, the amount of actin and myosin within your muscle fibers increases in response to resistance training. This results in an increase in the size or cross-sectional area of the protein filaments or **hypertrophy.** With more contractile proteins, a muscle can contract more forcefully; in other words, larger muscles are stronger muscles. While both slow- and fast-twitch muscles will increase in size with resistance training, greater increases in strength will result from hypertrophy changes in fast-twitch muscle fibers.

Muscle growth in response to resistance training takes longer than neural improvements. Nevertheless, muscle growth is the most important contributor to strength gains if your program is long-term and consistent. The degree of hypertrophy or enlargement you can expect with weight training depends upon your gender, age, genetics, and how you design your training program. Some individuals will develop larger muscles more quickly than others; some will experience only limited hypertrophy. In particular, women and men with smaller builds will realize less muscle development than those with larger builds, even with identical training programs (see the box **Understanding Diversity: Women and Weight Training**). The same is true for older individuals, though they can still see significant improvements.

A program with heavier weights, longer durations, or more frequent training can produce greater gains than a more standard fitness-training program. People who stop resistance training due to injury, life circumstances, or disinterest will experience some degree of **atrophy,** a shrinking of the muscle to its pretraining size and strength. To avoid atrophy, you need to make a long-term commitment to resistance training.

REGULAR RESISTANCE TRAINING INCREASES MUSCULAR ENDURANCE

Muscular endurance helps you complete daily tasks and take part in recreational activities without tiring easily. It helps you perform both cardiorespiratory activities, such as hiking and running, and muscular fitness activities, such as circuit or sports training. In fact, just doing these activities will improve your muscular endurance. Muscle endurance exercises trigger physiological adaptations that improve your ability to regenerate ATP efficiently and thus sustain muscular contractions for a longer period of time. The end result will be the ability to snowboard five runs in a row instead of two before having to rest; to walk up three flights of stairs with ease; or to rake leaves vigorously for an hour without difficulty.

REGULAR RESISTANCE TRAINING IMPROVES BODY COMPOSITION, WEIGHT MANAGEMENT, AND BODY IMAGE

Improved body composition is an important outcome of resistance training: the amount of lean muscle tissue will increase, the amount of fat tissue will decrease, and thus the ratio of lean to fat will improve. Research has demonstrated that such higher lean-to-fat ratios improve your overall health profile and reduce your risk of heart attack, stroke, and death from cardiovascular diseases.[4] Fat does not turn into muscle or vice versa; the number of fat and muscle cells remains the same, with cells merely enlarging or shrinking depending on food intake and activity levels.

More muscle means a faster metabolic rate, because pound for pound, muscle tissue expends more energy than fat tissue. With more total calories being expended during the day, weight control becomes easier and more effective. The most successful weight maintainers (those who lose weight and keep it off for long periods of time) incorporate

hypertrophy An increase in muscle cross-sectional area

atrophy A decrease in muscle cross-sectional area

UNDERSTANDING DIVERSITY

WOMEN AND WEIGHT TRAINING

While it is true that fewer American women are currently in strength-training programs than men, the benefits for women are just as great.

A common misconception is that women don't benefit much from resistance exercise because their muscles are generally smaller than those of men. On average, men's muscles *are* larger and more powerful than women's. Men produce 5 to 10 times more testosterone, which promotes muscle development. Men's nervous systems also signal muscle contraction more rapidly, producing greater power. Because they have *more* total muscle tissue, men's absolute strength is greater than women's—but when muscle mass is compared pound for pound, women are equally strong.

Another common misconception is that weight training will cause women to "bulk up." In truth, women who do regular resistance training rarely look heavily muscled. Women who train for competitive bodybuilding are self-selected to begin with, meaning they have a natural tendency toward muscle definition that they augment through hours in the gym every week. Very few women build large, bulky muscles without major effort (or the use of dangerous steroid drugs.)

Although the benefits of weight training are the same for both sexes, several of the advantages are especially appealing to women based on other life and health issues. These benefits include stronger bones and better

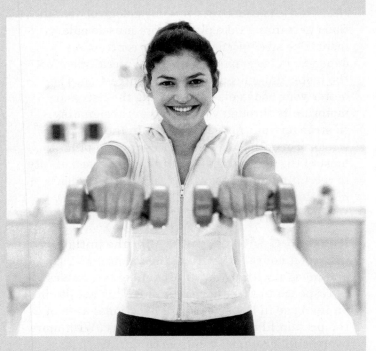

prevention of osteoporosis; reduced body fat and greater ability to control body weight; improved stamina and decreased fatigue; better sleep and less insomnia; and increased self-confidence, body image, and sense of well-being.

some type of resistance training into their overall fitness programs.[5] Resistance training during weight loss helps ensure that you will lose fat and not precious muscle tissue; your body can be lighter, stronger, and leaner (i.e., more toned) instead of just lighter (and potentially still flabby), as often happens with traditional diet-only weight-loss methods.

When you begin a resistance-training program, you may experience a slight initial weight gain as muscle tissue grows. If you focus only on the scale, this can be discouraging. It is better to focus on how much stronger and more toned your muscles feel. With a consistent fitness and nutrition program, fat loss will eventually "catch up" to muscle gain and will be reflected in weight loss as well. Since muscle tissue is more compact than fat tissue, your body size will gradually decrease over time as muscles become toned and fat tissues atrophy. Even without dieting, resistance training leads to more lean tissue and less fat tissue. This, in turn, can improve your

body image. In one study, college students realized measurable increases in overall body image after circuit weight training (a form of resistance training) for 6 weeks.[6]

REGULAR RESISTANCE TRAINING STRENGTHENS BONES AND PROTECTS THE BODY FROM INJURIES

Bone health is an important issue for everyone, from children to older adults. Osteoporosis-related fractures are common among older women and men and can cause dramatic decreases in a person's mobility, independence, and quality of life. By putting stress and controlled weight loads on the muscles, joint structures, and supporting bones, resistance training stimulates muscle tissue growth and the generation of harder, stronger bones, thereby reducing the risk of fracture.

Building strong bones is especially important in the period starting with childhood skeletal growth and development and ending at about age 30. The "reservoir" of bone tissue you lay down in those years and then maintain throughout life will help prevent weak, brittle bones as you age. Even the bones of older individuals can benefit from strength training. Several research studies have revealed a positive relationship between resistance training and bone density.[7]

Getting hurt will put you on the sidelines. Whether you exercise for fun, fitness, or competition, preventing injuries is a key to continued participation. Injury prevention tips are often specific to your chosen activity; however, strong muscles, bones, and connective tissues are the common denominator for preventing injury in any activity. Regular resistance training improves not only muscular strength and endurance, but also the strength of tendons, ligaments, and other supporting structures around each joint. As they grow stronger, the joints themselves are better protected from injury. A stronger body can handle the physical stresses of everyday life (carrying heavy books or groceries, lifting laundry baskets, moving furniture, etc.) with less chance of injury. A strong, pain-free back and proper posture are crucial to daily functioning without injury. Individuals who participate in regular resistance-training exercise have stronger postural muscles and report less low back pain.

Imbalanced muscles around a joint may result in a change in joint alignment with subsequent pain or injury. Muscular balance will reduce this risk. A well-designed muscle fitness program will work toward improving strength and muscle endurance in opposing muscular groups, promoting overall muscle balance.

REGULAR RESISTANCE TRAINING HELPS MAINTAIN PHYSICAL FUNCTION WITH AGING

Starting between the ages of 25 to 30, men and women begin to lose muscle mass. As they age, they lose up to one-third of their muscle mass due to changes in hormones, activity, nutrition, and chronic or acute illnesses. **Sarcopenia,** literally "poverty of flesh," is the term applied to this aging-related loss in skeletal muscle (see Figure 5.4). Sarcopenia reduces overall physical functioning by decreasing muscular strength and endurance and causing losses in **muscle power,** or the capacity to exert force rapidly. While no one is immune from the aging process, resistance training throughout one's life can significantly slow natural muscle loss. In fact, older individuals who do resistance training can show a rate of improvement equal to that of younger people. The increase in muscular fitness and the improvements it brings to everyday physical functioning help individuals live independently for a longer portion of their lives.

REGULAR RESISTANCE TRAINING HELPS REDUCE CARDIOVASCULAR DISEASE RISK

Regular resistance training can lower your risk of cardiovascular disease by increasing blood flow to working muscles and vital tissues throughout your body. In fact, people who perform regular resistance-training exercise have lower blood pressure and blood cholesterol readings than sedentary people. Since being *overfat* (having a higher than recommended percentage of body fat) increases your risk of cardiovascular disease and adult-onset diabetes, an improved body composition achieved through resistance training can help you lower your risk of both of these diseases.

REGULAR RESISTANCE TRAINING ENHANCES PERFORMANCE IN SPORTS AND ACTIVITIES

Achieving muscular fitness through resistance training has yet another benefit: A stronger body is more resistant to fatigue, moves more quickly, and recovers more quickly from illness or injury. All of these traits contribute to better performance in sports, recreational activities, and other fitness pursuits. Resistance training is often the common denominator among training programs for different sports and activities. Because of these benefits, physically active adults often incorporate some form of resistance training that builds strength and endurance in the muscle groups most crucial to their sport.

sarcopenia The degenerative loss of muscle mass and strength in aging

muscle power The ability of a muscle to quickly contract with high force

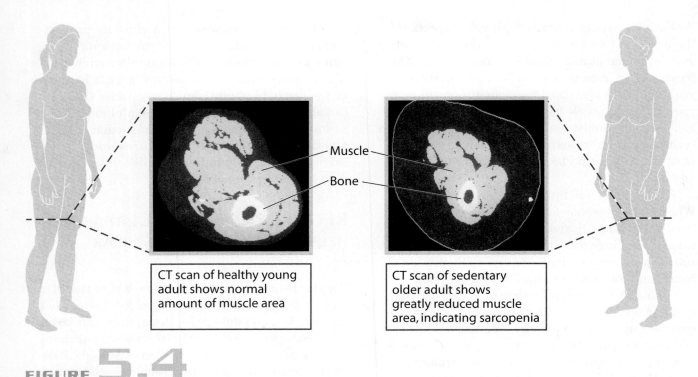

Muscle

Bone

CT scan of healthy young adult shows normal amount of muscle area

CT scan of sedentary older adult shows greatly reduced muscle area, indicating sarcopenia

FIGURE 5.4

CT scans showing the difference in muscle mass in a healthy young adult vs. an older adult with sarcopenia. Age-related muscle loss can be slowed down with resistance training.

HOW CAN YOU ASSESS YOUR MUSCULAR STRENGTH AND ENDURANCE?

Before you can plan an appropriate resistance-training program, it is important to assess your current muscular strength and endurance. You can then compare the results to norm charts for your age and gender, or simply use them as a starting point for designing your program. After you've followed your program for a while, follow-up assessments will help you evaluate your progress and make adjustments to stay on track.

TEST YOUR MUSCULAR STRENGTH

Tests of muscular strength gauge the maximum amount of force you can generate in a muscle.

People usually carry out these tests in a weight room where measured weights of all sizes are readily available.

1 RM Tests One repetition maximum (1 RM)

tests are the most common tool fitness instructors and personal trainers use to assess their clients' muscular strength. To participate in the tests safely, you must be medically cleared to lift heavier weights than you have in the past, have detailed instructions for the test procedure, know general weight-training guidelines, have a few weeks of weight-training experience, and have qualified **spotters** standing nearby to watch and assist if necessary. If you are weight training on campus or at a gym, an instructor will be able to help you through these preliminary steps.

One RM tests are performed by discovering the maximum amount of weight you can lift one time on a particular exercise. You need to accurately determine your 1 RM within three to five trials so that muscle fatigue from repetitions does not change your result. In general health and fitness classes or beginning weight-training programs, instructors often tell students to predict their 1 RM instead of actually attempting a maximum lift. This is particularly true when students

CASE STUDY

Gina

"I've always wanted to hike to the top of Nevada Falls in Yosemite National Park. I'm told that it can be done as a day hike, but it is about 7 miles round trip. There is also a steep section of rocks near another waterfall along the way—apparently you get completely soaked while hiking that part of the trail! I'm always extra careful hiking downhill, because I once sprained my ankle on a hike, which was not fun.

If resistance training can help me take on Nevada Falls, I'm interested. I've also always wished I had better muscle tone, but to be honest, I don't want to 'bulk up' . . ."

1. Name at least two ways that resistance training can help Gina realize her goal of safely hiking to the top of Nevada Falls.

2. How would you respond to Gina's concerns about "bulking up"?

3. What's your "Nevada Falls"—that is, what is something you have always wanted to do, but feel like you need to be in better physical shape to take on?

are new to resistance training and are unfamiliar with weight-training guidelines. To predict your 1 RM, you will lift, press, or pull a weight that will fully fatigue your upper- or lower-body muscles in 2 to 10 repetitions. You can then use a formula that converts your actual weight lifted and your real number of repetitions to a prediction of your 1 RM capacity for that exercise. In *Lab5.1* (at the back of this chapter), you will use bench-press and leg-press exercises to determine your 1 RM. You can perform these tests for any weight-training exercise and then convert to the predicted 1 RM value. Many weight-training programs use a percentage of your 1 RM or predicted 1 RM to determine a safe starting level for weight lifting.

Grip Strength Test
Another common test of muscle strength is the hand grip strength test using a piece of equipment called a *grip strength dynamometer*. As you squeeze the dynamometer (with one hand at a time), it measures the static or isometric strength of your grip-squeezing muscles in pounds or kilograms (kg).

TEST YOUR MUSCULAR ENDURANCE

Muscular endurance tests evaluate a muscle's ability to contract for an extended period of time. Some of these tests must be performed in a weight room, whereas others require only your body weight for resistance and can be performed anywhere.

20 RM Tests
You can use any weight-training exercise to find your **20 repetition maximum (20 RM).** This test determines the maximal amount of weight you can lift exactly 20 times in a row before the muscle becomes too fatigued to continue. Twenty repetition maximum tests are particularly useful for setting muscular endurance goals and then tracking your progress. Try to discover your 20 RM within one to three tries to avoid fatiguing your muscles and altering your results. *Lab5.2* walks you through the steps of finding your 20 RM for the bench-press and leg-press exercises.

Calisthenic Tests
Calisthenics are conditioning exercises that use your body weight for resistance. Calisthenic tests use sit-ups, curl-ups, pull-ups, push-ups, and flexed arm support/hang exercises to assess muscular endurance. The procedures for each test vary. You will learn how to perform the curl-up and push-up assessments in Lab 5.2. Calisthenic tests allow you to test yourself outside of a weight-training facility and to compare your results to well-established physical fitness norms.

20 repetition maximum (20 RM) The maximum amount of weight you can lift 20 times in a row

calisthenics A type of muscle endurance and/or flexibility exercise that employs simple movements without the use of resistance other than one's own body weight

HOW CAN YOU DESIGN YOUR OWN RESISTANCE-TRAINING PROGRAM?

Designing an effective resistance-training program takes some knowledge, and many people enlist the help of a personal trainer or fitness professional. You can become your own personal trainer, however, by using the guidelines in this section to plan a safe and effective muscular fitness program.

SET APPROPRIATE MUSCULAR FITNESS GOALS

Remember to use SMART goal-setting guidelines: Goals should be **s**pecific, **m**easurable, **a**ction-oriented, **r**ealistic, and have a **t**imeline. Your goals may be appearance-based, function-based, or a combination of the two.

Appearance-Based Goals
Many people have appearance-based goals for muscular fitness: they want larger muscles, or muscles that are more toned and less flabby. "Spot reduction" (i.e., trimming down just one area of the body) is another often-voiced goal—but is not realistic as the box **Facts and Fallacies: Does Spot Reduction Work?** explains.

In order to judge your progress toward appearance-based goals, be sure to include some sort of measure of progress in your resistance-training plan. For muscle size, measure the circumference of your biceps or calves, for example, then set a goal to increase or decrease this number. For overall body size, your goal may be to increase lean tissue weight but decrease fat tissue and percentage of body fat. If your goal is to become more "toned," quantify this in some way, too: look in the mirror and make notes about the way your body looks and moves. After you reach the target date for your plan, reread your notes, look in the mirror, and then reevaluate whether your muscle tone has improved.

Function-Based Goals
Include some specific goals for improving muscle function in your fitness plan. Function-based goals focus on your muscular capabilities and include gaining better muscular strength, greater muscular endurance, or both. *Lab5.3* will guide you in setting goals for realistic changes in muscle function, and then help you to assess your improvements.

EXPLORE EQUIPMENT OPTIONS

Should you use weight machines in your resistance-training program? Free weights? Other equipment?

FACTS AND FALLACIES

DOES SPOT REDUCTION WORK?

Have you ever thought, "I don't need a resistance-training program for my whole body. I just need to lose some fat off my hips (or thighs or abdomen)"? Indeed, why work on your whole body when you could just work off the fat in one offending area? Despite people's desire to spot-reduce and the multimillion-dollar industry it has spawned for ab-crunchers, thigh-slimmers, arm-toners, and cellulite creams, the answer is disappointingly simple: spot reduction doesn't work. Researchers have punctured the spot-reduction myth with several carefully controlled studies and have

verified that fat doesn't disappear through repeated exercise to one area. Instead, fat stores throughout the entire body dwindle when a negative caloric balance causes you to use up calories stored in fat tissue. In one study, researchers compared fat thickness in both arms of several tennis players. If anyone could work off fat selectively, it would be a tennis player, since he or she holds and swings the racquet thousands of times per week with his or her dominant hand and arm. The fat thickness, however, was identical in each arm.

Even though spot reducing won't work, as you exercise—particularly with resistance training—you simultaneously strengthen and build lean tissue. If your calorie balance is also negative and you lose fat body-wide, your muscle definition will show more clearly, both in the offending spots and elsewhere as well!

Source: American Council on Exercise (ACE). "Why Is the Concept of Spot Reduction Considered a Myth?" ACE FitnessMatters (January/February 2004). www.acefitness.org/fitfacts/ fitnessqa_display.aspx?itemid-341.

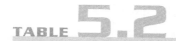
Machine Weight vs. Free Weight Training

Machine Weights	Free Weights
PROS	**PROS**
Safe and less intimidating for beginners	Can be tailored for individual workouts
Quicker to set up and use	Range of motion set by lifter, not machine
Spotters not typically needed	Some exercises can be done anywhere
Support of standing posture not needed	Standing and sitting postural muscles worked
Adaptable for those with limitations	Movements can transfer to daily activities
Variable resistance is possible	Good for strength and power building
Good isolation of specific muscle groups	Additional stabilizer muscles worked
Only good option for some muscle groups	Lower cost and more available for home use
CONS	**CONS**
Machine sets range of motion	More difficult to learn
May not fit every body size and type	A spotter may be needed
Some people lack access to weight machines	Incorrect form may lead to injuries
Core posture supporting muscles not used	More time may be needed to change weights
Limited number of exercises/machines	More training needed to create program

No equipment at all? These are important decisions, and they depend on your fitness goals, the type of equipment available to you, your experience with weight-training exercises, and your preferences.

Machines If you are new to resistance training, weight machines can be very useful. Systems such as Cybex, Nautilus, Life Fitness, and many others allow you to isolate and strengthen specific muscle groups as well as to train without a spotting partner. Table 5.2 compares machine weight training and free weight training.

Free Weights Personal trainers and exercise physiologists consider free-weight exercises to be a more advanced approach to weight training than machine-weight exercises. Free-weight exercises use **dumbbells; barbells;** incline, flat, or decline benches; squat racks; and related equipment. Free-weight exercises allow your body to move through its natural range of motion instead of the path predetermined by a weight machine. This both requires and promotes development of more muscle control. Some athletes prefer free-weight exercises because the balance and movement patterns needed to successfully lift free weights are closer to their sport movement patterns, whether that be tossing a football, putting a shot, or doing the breaststroke. Since workout facilities often have both free weights and weight machines, many people start their resistance-training program exclusively with machine-weight exercises and then progress to free weights within the first few months.

Alternate Equipment You can increase resistance on your body with equipment other than machines or free weights. *Resistance bands* made of tubing or flat strips of rubber allow you to simultaneously increase resistance throughout a range of motion and to improve muscular endurance. You can perform many different exercises with these bands. They also fold up and pack perfectly in a suitcase or

dumbbell A weight intended for use by one hand; typically one uses a dumbbell in each hand

barbell A long bar with weight plates on each end

gym bag for a portable workout. *Stability balls* (also called Swiss, fitness, or exercise balls) are 18–30 inch diameter vinyl balls that have various uses for muscular fitness, endurance, and balance. Ball routines involve performing exercises while sitting, lying, and/or balancing on the ball. The ball exerciser must use core trunk muscles to counteract the natural instability of the ball, which enhances overall body function. People sometimes use heavily weighted balls called *medicine balls* to increase resistance, either individually, with a partner, or in a group. You can hold a medicine ball while doing calisthenic or free-weight exercises or pass a ball from partner to partner for a functional increase in muscle endurance.

No-Equipment Training Calisthenics such as push-ups, pull-ups, lunges, squats, leg lifts, and curl-ups do not involve equipment. Instead, they use your body weight to provide the resistance. Like resistance bands, they are perfect for maintaining muscular strength and endurance while traveling.

UNDERSTAND THE DIFFERENT TYPES OF RESISTANCE-TRAINING PROGRAMS

You can plan a resistance-training program with various types of equipment and numerous exercise routines. Choosing the right program will depend upon your goals, experience, and personal preference.

Traditional Weight Training Traditional weight training takes place in a weight room and usually includes a combination of machine-weight, free-weight, and calisthenic exercises. Individuals may work alone or with a partner and will usually perform multiple **sets** and **repetitions**

set A single attempt at an exercise that includes a fixed number of repetitions

repetitions The number of times an exercise is performed within one set

plyometric exercise An exercise that is characterized by a rapid deceleration of the body followed by a rapid acceleration of the body in the opposite direction

of a particular exercise before moving on to the next exercise.

Circuit Weight Training Circuit weight training is done in a specialized circuit-training room, a general workout room, or a weight room. Exercisers move from one station to another in a set pattern (the "circuit") after a certain amount of time at a station or after performing a certain number of repetitions of an exercise such as a biceps curl, leg press, or chest press. Some circuits include only resistance-training exercises and have the single goal of improving muscular fitness. Some circuits involve cardiorespiratory or aerobic training equipment, such as stair-steppers or stationary bicycles, mixed in with the resistance exercises to improve both cardiorespiratory and muscular fitness.

In circuit training, it is important to remember the *specificity* training principle: in order to get optimal muscle fitness benefits, you must focus on the resistance exercises, and in order to realize added cardiorespiratory benefits, you must spend a minimal amount of time on the cardio machines (20 to 30 minutes total per exercise session).

Circuit exercises should be organized properly in order to ensure a safe and effective exercise session. For example, multijoint exercises (bench press, leg press) are often performed before single-joint exercises (bicep curl, leg extension), muscle groups worked are spread out to allow recovery between sets, and exercises that stress the core postural muscles are reserved for the end of the workout.

Plyometrics and Sports Training
Resistance-training programs designed to support specific sports can be quite different from general resistance training. Athletes may use many of the general weight-training exercises illustrated in this chapter, but they usually also perform exercises or exercise methods that specifically benefit their sports performance. Plyometrics, power lifts, and speed and agility drills are examples.

A **plyometric exercise** program incorporates explosive exercises that mimic the quick, percussive movements needed in many sports (i.e., basketball, wrestling, and gymnastics). These exercises are characterized by a landing and slowing down of the body mass followed immediately by a rapid jump in the opposite direction (for instance, jumping down off of a box and then immediately jumping back up as high as you can). Plyometrics is a highly specialized training method that should be performed under proper direction and only by individuals who have achieved a high level of muscular fitness.

Power lifting is a type of resistance training in which an individual lifts a heavy weight quickly. Examples include the Olympic lifts such as the clean and jerk, snatch, front squat, and push press. Sports that require high levels of explosive movement and power (football, wrestling, gymnastics, and track-and-field events) may require power-lifting training to build strength with speed. Power lifting is also a competitive sport in itself. Like plyometrics, power lifting should be practiced only by experienced athletes or those with comparable weight-training experience. Spotters and proper form are necessary for safety.

The training regimens for certain athletes may include **speed** and **agility** drills. These drills are also making their way into mainstream sports training and boot-camp-style group exercise classes. Speed and agility drills improve muscle responsiveness, speed, footwork, and coordination. Typical speed and agility drills include line sprints, high-knee runs, fast foot turnover running, and hopping quickly through varying foot patterns (using agility dots or other markers). Speed and agility drills can be performed by anyone who is physically fit enough to learn and perform the skills. Proper instruction and modification of the drills for differing ability levels is essential to prevent injuries.

LEARN AND APPLY FITT PRINCIPLES

FITT stands for *frequency, intensity, time,* and *type.* The acronym represents a checklist for determining how often, how hard, and how long to exercise, and what types of exercise to choose at your current level of muscular fitness.

Frequency of Training
Your goals and your schedule determine how often you will train each week. At a minimum, you should work each muscle group twice per week, and if you do a full-body muscle workout, that means two sessions in the weight room each week. If you split your muscle workouts (for example, into upper/lower body), then you would go to the weight room four times per week. Table 5.3 presents American College of Sports Medicine (ACSM) guidelines for muscle strength and muscle endurance programs.

Try It NOW! Many people find group exercise classes to be motivating. • If you are among them, find a class that will help you meet your muscular fitness goals (such as Pilates, fitness "boot camp," muscle pump, etc.). • Some classes are designed solely for muscular fitness, while others address both muscular fitness and cardiovascular training. • Be sure to use enough resistance or weight to elicit a muscle training response.

It is important to let each muscle group rest for 48 hours before taxing it again with resistance training. Therefore, especially when you are just beginning, schedule your workouts so that they are at least 2 days apart.

When you perform an intense weight-training session, microdamage occurs within the muscle cells and rest time is needed for muscle repair and adaptation. Your muscles will adapt by constructing new actin and myosin contractile proteins and other supporting structures. Over time, this adaptation results in stronger, leaner, larger muscles. Intense workouts of the same muscle group on subsequent days will disrupt the repair and adaptation process. Rather than faster muscle development, this overtraining is more likely to cause injuries, muscle fatigue, and weakening. An exception can be made for lower intensity muscular fitness classes or calisthenics, which can be done daily as long as they are not overly fatiguing.

Muscle soreness that sets in within a day or two is called *delayed-onset muscle soreness* (DOMS)

speed The ability to rapidly accelerate; exercises for speed will increase stride length and frequency

agility The ability to rapidly change body position or body direction without losing speed, balance, or body control

Table **5.3**

ACSM's Resistance-Training Guidelines for Muscular Strength and Endurance

Recommendations for the General Adult Population

Frequency (days/week)	2–3
Intensity (how hard)	Lift to fatigue
Time (sets/reps)	1 set; 3–20 repetitions
Type (exercises)	Machines, free weights, and/or calisthenics; 8–10 exercises to work all major muscles of the hips, thighs, lower legs, back, chest, shoulders, arms, and abdomen

Strength, Endurance, and Progression Guidelines for Healthy Adults

Muscular Strength	Frequency	Intensity	Time (sets/reps) (1–3 min rest between sets)
Novice	2–3 days/week	60%–70% 1 RM	1–3 sets, 8–12 reps
Intermediate	2–4 days/week	70%–80% 1 RM	Multiple sets, 6–12 reps
Advanced	4–6 days/week	80%–100% 1 RM	Multiple sets, 1–12 reps
Muscular Endurance	Frequency	Intensity	Time (sets/reps) (30 sec–2 min rest between sets)
Novice	2–3 days/week	50%–70% 1 RM	1–3 sets, 10–15 reps
Intermediate	2–4 days/week	50%–70% 1 RM	Multiple sets, 10–15 reps
Advanced	4–6 days/week	30%–80% 1 RM	Multiple sets, 10–25 reps

Sources: American College of Sports Medicine. *ACSM's Guidelines for Exercise Testing and Prescription.* 7th Edition. Baltimore, MD: Lippincott Williams & Wilkins, 2006; and Kraemer W. J., Adams K., Cafarelli E., et al. "Writing Group for the ACSM Position Stand. Progression Models in Resistance Training for Healthy Adults," *Medicine and Science in Sports and Exercise* 34, no. 2 (2002): 364–380. Used by permission of Wolters/Kluwer.

and is a sign that your body was not ready for the amount of overload you applied. Contrary to popular belief, it is not lactic acid that causes DOMS; accumulated lactic acid is cleared from the muscle cells within hours of exercise. If you choose weight amounts correctly, your muscles will sustain small amounts of microdamage that do not result in soreness and that your body can repair within 48 hours after the workout.

Intensity of Training The **intensity** of a weight-training program refers to the amount of

intensity The resistance level of the exercise

resistance The amount of effort or force required to complete the exercise

resistance you apply through any given exercise. **Resistance** here means the weight that you are moving. For each exercise, the intensity you choose will depend on your fitness goals for that particular muscle group or your body as a whole. The ACSM guidelines in Table 5.3 for muscle strength and muscle endurance can help you choose weight-training intensities (shown as a percentage of your 1 RM or predicted 1 RM).

Each choice for each exercise should be enough to *overload* the muscle group you are working; that means you should feel slight discomfort or muscle fatigue near the end of your exercise set. If you feel no fatigue during the entire set of repetitions and feel you could lift the weight another 3 to 10 times, then the intensity is too low. If you choose the right intensity for building muscular strength, you will be almost completely fatigued by the end of each set of repetitions. The right intensity for building muscle endurance will leave the muscle group fatigued but not near maximal exhaustion as with strength building.

Resting between sets will affect your weight-training intensity and performance on subsequent exercises. The greater the weight you lift for strength building, the longer the rest period you need between sets. Resting periods should be shorter for muscular endurance building exercises. In fact, shorter rests will help build better muscular endurance. Table 5.3 provides guidelines for determining appropriate rest periods between sets.

Time: Sets and Repetitions
Choosing the appropriate number of repetitions or lifts within each set is yet another important part of setting up your resistance-training program. Once again, your fitness goals help determine the number of sets you will execute for each exercise and the number of repetitions within each set. Your weight-training experience and the time you have available to work out will affect your planning as well. ACSM recommends that to start with, you perform one set of each exercise during a given workout session (see Table 5.3). If you are new to resistance training, you will see progress with just one set per muscle group. Although you will gain additional benefits from extra sets, two sets will not translate into double the benefits of one. If you are pressed for time, one is sufficient. As you progress in your resistance-training program, you can increase your sets from one to two, and eventually to three or more. Evidence suggests that three sets will produce twice the strength gains of one set.[8] You can execute one, two, or three sets for all your exercises, or perform one set of certain exercises, two of others, and so on. Keep in mind, however, that overtraining one particular muscle group can lead to muscle imbalance and injury.

If your muscular fitness goals include improvement to both muscular strength *and* endurance, choose a number of sets and repetitions that falls between the ACSM recommendations for strength and endurance in Table 5.3. Intensity and repetitions have an inverse relationship relative to muscular strength and endurance (see Figure 5.5): for muscular strength development, you will lift heavier weights and do fewer repetitions. For muscular endurance, you will lift lighter weights with more repetitions. A good starting point for a balanced strength/endurance program is one to two sets of 10 repetitions per exercise. Table 5.4 outlines sample resistance-training programs.

Type: Choosing Appropriate Exercises
Which exercises should you do during each session? The final part of designing a muscular fitness program is deciding on appropriate exercises, remembering to work toward muscle balance within all of the major muscle groups. Create

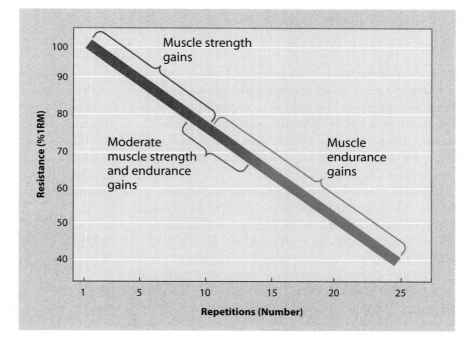

FIGURE 5.5
Fewer repetitions with higher resistance will produce gains in muscular strength. More repetitions with lower resistance will produce gains in muscular endurance. An overlap between the two kinds of development is reflected in the strength and endurance continuum.

TABLE **5.4**

Sample Designs for Resistance Training Programs

		Beginning	Intermediate
Frequency		2 days/week (all exercises done each day)	4 days/week (1/2 of upper/lower done each day; trunk done all days)
Intensity		55%–65% 1 RM	70%–80% 1 RM
Time		1 set, 10 reps (1–2 min rest)	2–3 sets, 5–12 reps (2–3 min rest)
Exercises			
Lower body		Leg press	Squats or lunges
		Leg extension	Leg extension
		Leg curl	Leg curl
		Heel raise	Heel raise
Upper body		Bench press	Bench press
		Chest flys	Chest flys
		Lat pull down	Lat pull down
		Seated row	Seated row
		Lateral raise	Upright row
		Biceps curl	Overhead press
		Triceps extension	Lateral raise
			Biceps curl
			Triceps extension
Trunk		Abdominal curl	Abdominal curl
		Oblique curl	Oblique curl
		Back extension	Side bridge
			Back extension

your own muscular fitness goals in Lab 5.2 and use Figure 5.6 to start planning your resistance-training program. The next step is deciding which exercises will help you attain your muscular fitness goals: complete *Lab5.4* to plan a muscular fitness program using Figures 5.7 and 5.8 to assist you in exercise selection.

Muscle balance requires a selection of upper-body exercises, trunk exercises, and lower-body exercises. Choose exercises from Figure 5.8 that allow you to work muscles on both the front and back of your body. For a starting program, choose between 8 and 15 exercises, remembering that each additional exercise will add time to your exercise session; with too many exercises, you may need to split your

workout into alternating selections of exercises on different days (see Table 5.4). In choosing exercises, you may select weight machines, free weights, calisthenics, or a combination of all three. Most weight-training programs will include all three and will also depend upon the equipment available to you. As mentioned earlier, focus on weight-training machines if you are new to resistance training.

WHAT IF YOU DON'T REACH YOUR GOALS?

Once you've applied FITT principles, chosen training levels, designed a program, and set target dates,

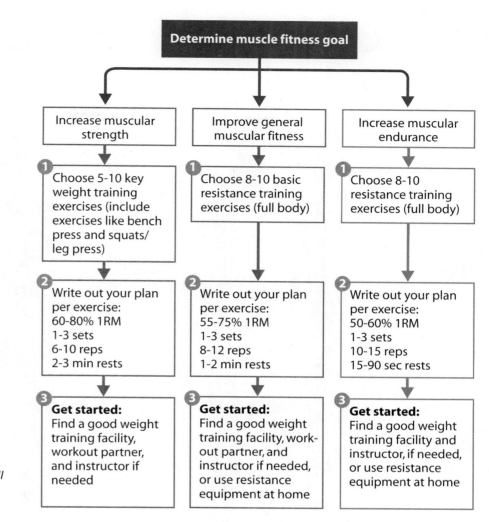

```
                    Determine muscle fitness goal


    Increase muscular          Improve general          Increase muscular
       strength               muscular fitness             endurance


  ① Choose 5-10 key        ① Choose 8-10 basic       ① Choose 8-10
     weight training          resistance training       resistance training
     exercises (include       exercises (full body)     exercises (full body)
     exercises like bench
     press and squats/
     leg press)


  ② Write out your plan    ② Write out your plan     ② Write out your plan
     per exercise:            per exercise:             per exercise:
     60-80% 1RM               55-75% 1RM                50-60% 1RM
     1-3 sets                 1-3 sets                  1-3 sets
     6-10 reps                8-12 reps                 10-15 reps
     2-3 min rests            1-2 min rests             15-90 sec rests


  ③ Get started:           ③ Get started:            ③ Get started:
     Find a good weight       Find a good weight        Find a good weight
     training facility,       training facility, work-  training facility and
     workout partner,         out partner, and          instructor, if needed,
     and instructor if        instructor if needed,     or use resistance
     needed                   or use resistance         equipment at home
                              equipment at home
```

FIGURE 5.6

Use this flowchart as you design your muscular fitness program. Just starting? Begin at the lower end of all recommended ranges (except rest period—begin at the upper end).

you may find that your muscular development is not keeping up with your ambitions, or you cannot follow through consistently with training sessions. What other steps can you take to ensure success in your muscular fitness program?

Track Your Progress Use a weight-training log or a notebook to track your progress. Lab 5.4 provides you with a log that allows you to (1) see your week-to-week progress, (2) stay motivated, (3) detect problems with your program design or goals, and (4) know where to redesign your program if needed.

Evaluate and Redesign Your Program as Needed Periodically reevaluate your muscular fitness program. Common times to reassess are

at your target completion date, when you feel you aren't making progress, when your improvement rate is faster than anticipated, and when you feel overtraining fatigue or injury. First, retake the initial tests for muscular strength and endurance. Second, reassess your goals: accomplished or not? Third, evaluate your overall program and write out what you like and don't like about it. If you have met your goals and enjoy your program, continue but set more challenging goals based on FITT parameters. If you have not met your goals or don't like your program, rewrite the goals and target dates, redesigning to solve your issues. In addition, get help from an exercise professional if needed. Evaluating and redesigning should allow you, once again, to move toward your muscular fitness goals successfully. Lab 5.4 provides practice at evaluation and redesign.

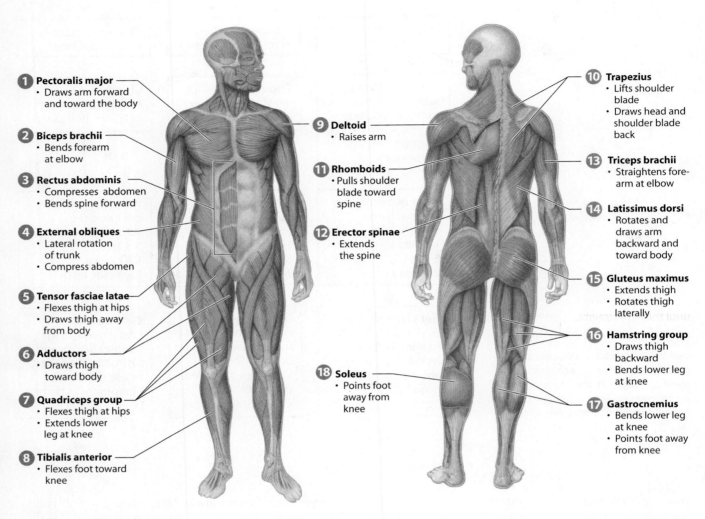

1 Pectoralis major
• Draws arm forward and toward the body

2 Biceps brachii
• Bends forearm at elbow

3 Rectus abdominis
• Compresses abdomen
• Bends spine forward

4 External obliques
• Lateral rotation of trunk
• Compress abdomen

5 Tensor fasciae latae
• Flexes thigh at hips
• Draws thigh away from body

6 Adductors
• Draws thigh toward body

7 Quadriceps group
• Flexes thigh at hips
• Extends lower leg at knee

8 Tibialis anterior
• Flexes foot toward knee

9 Deltoid
• Raises arm

11 Rhomboids
• Pulls shoulder blade toward spine

12 Erector spinae
• Extends the spine

18 Soleus
• Points foot away from knee

10 Trapezius
• Lifts shoulder blade
• Draws head and shoulder blade back

13 Triceps brachii
• Straightens forearm at elbow

14 Latissimus dorsi
• Rotates and draws arm backward and toward body

15 Gluteus maximus
• Extends thigh
• Rotates thigh laterally

16 Hamstring group
• Draws thigh backward
• Bends lower leg at knee

17 Gastrocnemius
• Bends lower leg at knee
• Points foot away from knee

FIGURE 5.7

These muscles or muscle groups are commonly used in resistance-training exercises. Figure 5.8 illustrates exercises you can use to work the muscle groups shown.

FIGURE 5.8 RESISTANCE TRAINING EXERCISES*

Lower-Body Exercises

1. Squat

(a) Free weight squat and

(b) Machine squat: Place the barbell (or pad, if using machine) on your upper back and shoulders. Stand with feet shoulder-width apart, toes pointing forward, hips and shoulders lined up, abdominals pulled in. Looking forward and keeping your chest open, bend your knees and press your hips back. Lower until you have between a 45- and 90-degree angle between your thigh and calf. Keep your knees behind the front of your toes. To return to the start position, contract your abdominals, press hips forward, and extend your legs until they are straight.

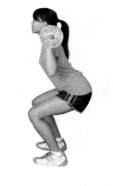
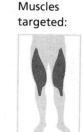

(a)

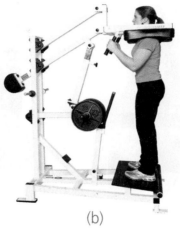
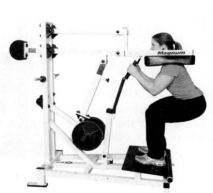

(b)

Muscles targeted:

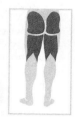

7 Quadriceps

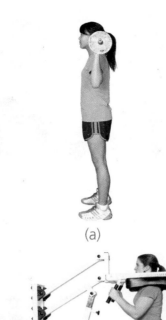

15 Gluteus maximus
16 Hamstrings

2. Leg Press

Sit with your back straight or firmly against the back-rest. Place your feet on the foot pads so that your knees are at a 60- to 90-degree angle. Stabilize your torso by contracting your abdominals and holding the hand grips or seat pad. Press the weight by extending your legs slowly outward to a straight position without locking your knees. Return the weight slowly back to the starting position. If your buttocks rise up off of the seat pad, you may be lifting too much weight.

*Videos for many of these exercises are available at www.aw-bc.com/hopson

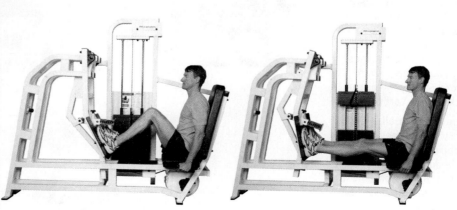

Muscles targeted:

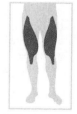

7 Quadriceps

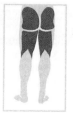

15 Gluteus maximus
16 Hamstrings

3. Lunges

Stand with feet shoulder-width apart. Step forward and transfer weight to the forward leg. Lower your body straight down with your weight evenly distributed between the front and back legs. Keep your front knee in line with your ankle by striding out far enough. Make sure the front knee does not extend over your toes. Repeat with other leg.

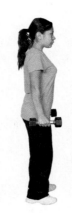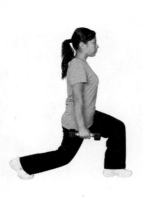

Muscles targeted:

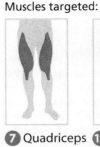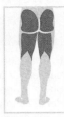

7 Quadriceps **15** Gluteus maximus
16 Hamstrings

4. Leg Extension

Sit with your back straight or firmly against the backrest and place your legs under the foot pad. Stabilize your torso by contracting your abdominals and holding the handgrips or seat pad. Lift the weight by extending your legs slowly upward to a straight position without locking your knees. Return the weight slowly back down to the starting position. If your buttocks rise up off the seat pad, you may be lifting too much weight.

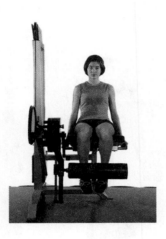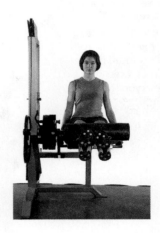

Muscles targeted:

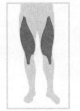

7 Quadriceps

5. Leg Curl

(a) Machine: Lie on your stomach so that your knees are placed at the machine's axis of rotation and the roller pad is just above your heel. Keep your head on the machine pad. Grasping the hand grips for support, lift the weight by contracting your hamstrings and pulling your heels toward your buttocks. Slowly lower the weight back to the start position.

(b) Calisthenics with ball: Lie on your stomach with knees bent and place the ball between your feet. Keep your head on the mat. Lower the ball to the ground and lift it back up by contracting your hamstrings and pulling your heels toward your buttocks.

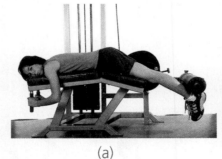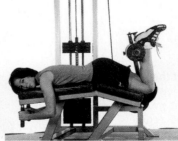

(a)

Muscles targeted:

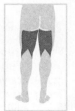

16 Hamstrings

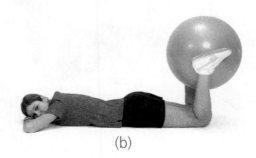

(b)

6. Hip Abduction

(a) Machine: Sit with your back straight or firmly against the back-rest and place your legs behind the pads. Grasping the hand grips or seat pad for support, press your legs outward slowly by contracting your outer thighs or hip abductors. Be careful not to extend the legs further than your normal range of motion. Slowly lower the machine weight by bringing your legs back together.

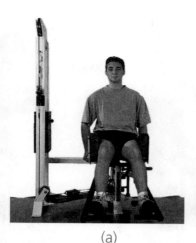 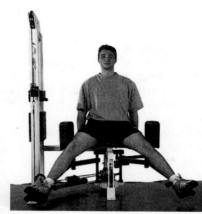

(a)

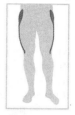

Muscles targeted:

5 Tensor fasciae latae

(b) Calisthenics with resistance band: Connect the resistance band to a low point on a machine and attach the free end to your outside leg. Stand with good posture and hold onto a wall or machine for support. Contract your hip abductors and extend your leg out to the side of your body. Slowly release the outside leg back to the starting position beside or crossed slightly in front of the standing leg.

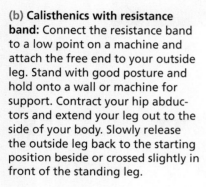

(b)

7. Hip Adduction

(a) Machine: Sit with your back straight or firmly against the backrest and place your legs behind the pads set at a comfortable range of motion. Grasping the hand grips or seat pad for support, press your legs together slowly by contracting your inner thighs or hip adductors. Slowly return your legs to the starting position.

(b) Calisthenics with ball: Lie on your back with a ball pressed between your knees. Press your knees firmly together, squeezing the ball. Hold the squeeze for 3–10 seconds and release.

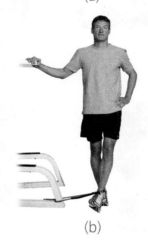 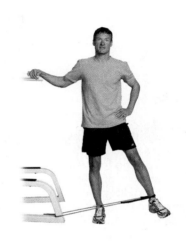

(a)

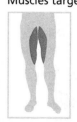

Muscles targeted:

6 Adductors

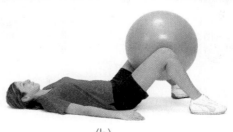

(b)

8. Hip Extension

Stand tall with your working leg extended in front of you. Support yourself by contracting your abdominals and holding onto the machine or handrails. Press the working leg behind you, contracting the gluteals and hamstrings. Hold the end position for 1–3 seconds before slowly returning to the starting position.

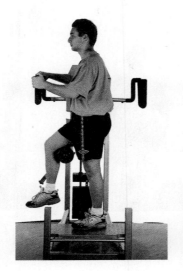 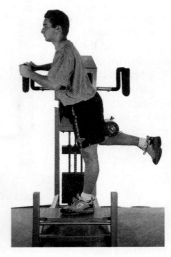

Muscles targeted:

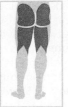

15 Gluteus maximus
16 Hamstring

9. Straight Leg Heel Raise

Stand tall with good posture and place your heels lower than the toes (you should feel just a slight stretch in the calf muscle). Looking forward and contracting your trunk muscles for balance and support, lift your heels up by contracting your gastrocnemius muscle. Be sure to do a full range of motion and slow, controlled repetitions.

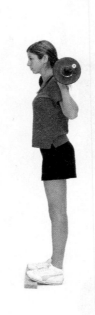 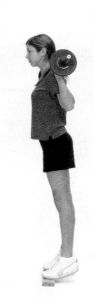

Muscles targeted:

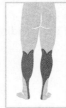

17 Gastrocnemius

10. Bent Leg Heel Raise

Place your body in the machine with your heels lower than the toes and the weight pad placed comfortably on your thighs. Lift your heels up slightly and release the weight support bar with your hand. Slowly lower and lift the weight by contracting your soleus calf muscle through its full range of motion.

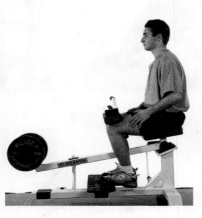 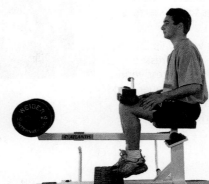

Muscles targeted:

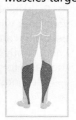

18 Soleus

Upper-Body Exercises

11. Chest Press

(a) Free-weight: Lie down on the bench and position yourself with the weight bar directly above your chest. Stabilize your legs and back by placing your feet firmly on the ground, a step, or the bench and keeping your lower back flat. Grasp the bar with your hands slightly wider than shoulder-width apart and lift the bar off the rack. Slowly lower the bar to just above your chest. Press the weight up to a straight arm position and return the bar to the rack when your set of repetitions is complete. Use a spotter when lifting heavier free weights.

(b) Machine: Place yourself on the chest press machine and adjust the seat height so that the hand grips are at chest height. Stabilize your torso by firmly pressing your back against the seat back and planting your feet on the ground or foot supports. Press the hand grips away from the body until the arms are straight. Slowly return your hands to the starting position.

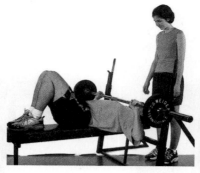 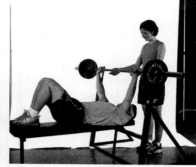
(a)

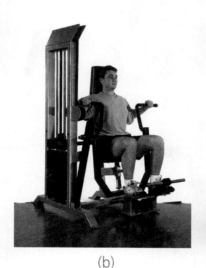 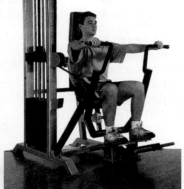
(b)

Muscles targeted:

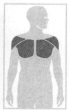

1 Pectoralis major
9 Deltoids (anterior)

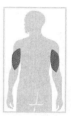

13 Triceps brachii

12. Push-Ups

(a) Full push-ups and

(b) Modified push-ups: Support yourself in push-up position (from the knees or feet) by contracting your trunk muscles so that your neck, back, and hips are completely straight. Place hands slightly wider than shoulder width apart. Slowly lower your body down toward the floor, being careful to keep a straight body position. Your elbows will press out and back as you lower to a 90-degree elbow joint angle. Press yourself back up to the start position. Be careful not to let your trunk sag in the middle or your hips lift up during the exercise. Continually contract the abdominals to keep a strong, straight body position.

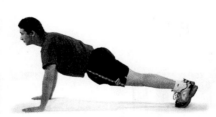 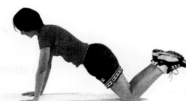

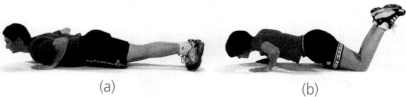
(a)   (b)

Muscles targeted:

1 Pectoralis major
9 Deltoids (anterior)

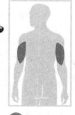

13 Triceps brachii

13. Chest Flys

(a) Machine: Sit with your back straight or firmly against the back-rest, plant your feet on the ground, and place your arms behind the machine pads. Your arms should be directly to the side but not behind your body. Press your arms together slowly by contracting your chest and shoulder muscles. Slowly return your arms to the starting position.

(b) Bench chest flys: Lie down on the bench and position yourself with the dumbbells directly above your chest. Stabilize your legs and back by placing your feet firmly on the ground, a step, or the bench and keeping your lower back flat against the bench. Holding the dumbbells with a slight bend in the elbow joint, slowly lower the dumbbells out to the side until your upper arms are parallel with the floor. Be careful not to extend the arms beyond this position. Return your arms to the starting position by contracting your chest and shoulder muscles.

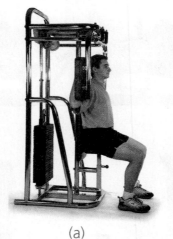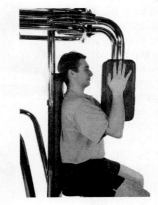

(a)

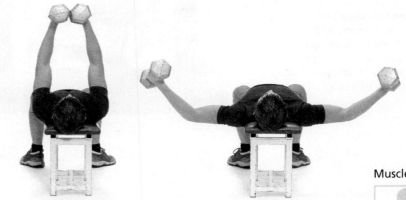

(b)

14. Lat Pull Down

Position the seat and leg pad on the lat pull down machine so that your thighs are snug under the pad while your feet are flat on the ground. Grab the pull down bar with a wide overhand grip on your way down to a seated position. Sitting directly under the cable, pull the bar down to your upper chest. Focus on contracting the mid-back first and then the arms by pulling the shoulder blades and elbows back and down. Slowly straighten your arms back to the start position.

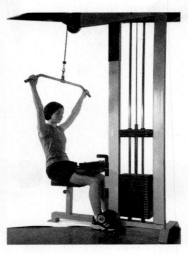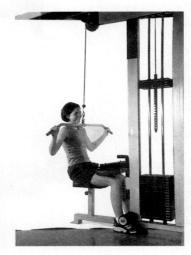

Muscles targeted:

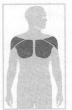

1 Pectoralis major
9 Deltoids (anterior)

Muscles targeted:

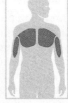

1 Pectoralis major
2 Biceps brachii

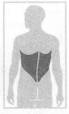

14 Latissimus dorsi

15. Assisted Pull-Up

Grab the pull-up bar with a wide overhead grip. Contract the back and arms in order to pull your body up until the bar is at chin height. Slowly straighten your arms back to the start position.

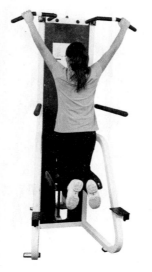
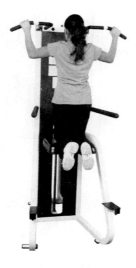

Muscles targeted:

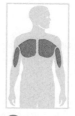
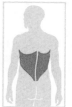

1 Pectoralis major

2 Biceps brachii

14 Latissimus dorsi

16. Rows

(a) Machine compound row: Grab the handgrips and pull your elbows back until you have reached the end position (pictured.) Hold this position for 1–3 seconds, then slowly return to the start position.

(b) Free-weight dumbbell: Position right hand and right knee on bench as shown. Pull dumbbell up with left hand, leading with your elbow. Return to start position and repeat on other side.

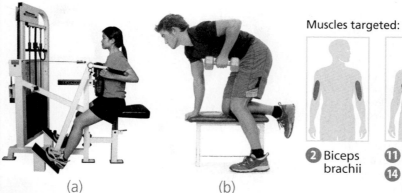

(a)　　　　(b)

Muscles targeted:

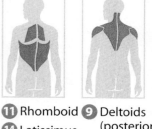

2 Biceps brachii

11 Rhomboid

14 Latissimus dorsi

9 Deltoids (posterior)

10 Trapezius

17. Upright Row

Stand with your feet either in a stride or a shoulder-width position. Keep your hips and shoulders in line with each other and your abdominals pulled in. Hold a barbell down in front of the body with straight arms and your hands positioned slightly narrower than shoulder-width. Lift the weight to chest height keeping your elbows above the bar. Remember to lift without shrugging the shoulders up toward the ears.

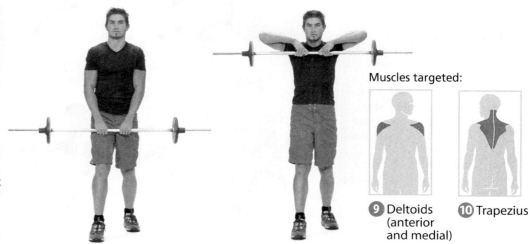

Muscles targeted:

9 Deltoids (anterior and medial)

10 Trapezius

18. Overhead Press

(a) Machine and

(b) Free-weight dumbbell:
Sit with your back straight or firmly against the backrest, plant your feet firmly on the ground, and pull in your abdominals. Position your hands just wider than shoulder width and just above the shoulders. Carefully press the weight over your head until your arms are straight but your elbows are not locked out. Slowly return the weight to the start position and repeat.

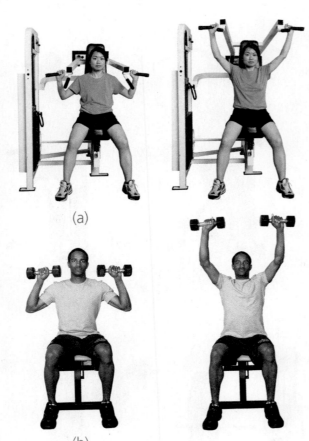

(a)

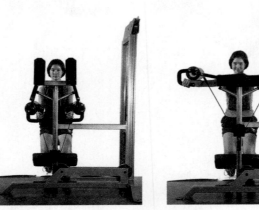

(b)

Muscles targeted:

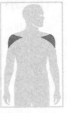 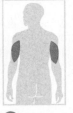

9 Deltoids (anterior and medial) **13** Triceps brachii

19. Lateral Raise

(a) Machine: Position yourself in the machine and sit with a tall, straight back. Contract your shoulders and lift your arms out to your sides until they are parallel with the ground. Slowly lower your arms back down to your sides.

(b) Free-weight dumbbell: Stand with your feet shoulder-width apart. Hold the dumbbells to your sides or slightly in front of you. Lift your arms out to your sides until they are parallel with the ground. While lifting, your elbows should have a slight bent to avoid over-extension of the elbow joint. Keep the weights even with or slightly lower than your elbows and keep your shoulders down. Slowly return the dumbbells back down to the start position.

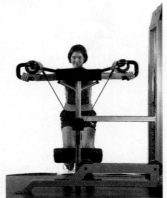

(a)

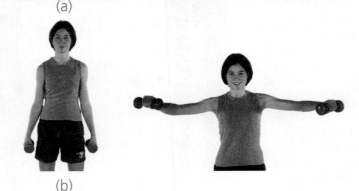

(b)

Muscles targeted:

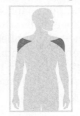

9 Deltoids (anterior and medial)

20. Biceps Curl

(a) Machine: Position yourself in the machine so that your feet are on the ground and your elbows are placed at the axis of rotation for the exercise. Grab the hand grips and start with your arms straight but not over-extended. Lift your hands toward your head until your biceps are fully contracted. Slowly lower the weight back down to the starting position.

(b) Free-weight barbell: Stand with your feet either in a stride or a shoulder-width position and your knees slightly bent. Keep your hips and shoulders in line with each other and your abdominals pulled in. Hold a barbell down in front of the body with an underhand grip, straight arms, and your hands at shoulder-width. Lift the weight up to your shoulders while keeping your back straight and abdominal muscles tight. If you are leaning back to perform the lift, you may be lifting too much weight. Return the weight back down to the starting position slowly and repeat.

(c) Free-weight dumbbell: For one-arm concentration curls, sit on a bench and hold a dumbbell in one hand. Start with the working arm extended toward the ground and your elbow pressed into your inner thigh. Lift the dumbbell up to the shoulder and then return slowly back to the starting position.

(d) Calisthenics with resistance band: Place the center of a resistance band under one foot and grab the free ends of the band with a straight arm on the same side. Stand tall with your feet either in a stride or a side to side position and your knees soft. Keep your hips and shoulders in line with each other and your abdominals pulled in. Lift the resisted hand toward your shoulder until the biceps are fully contracted. Slowly lower the hand back down to the starting position and repeat.

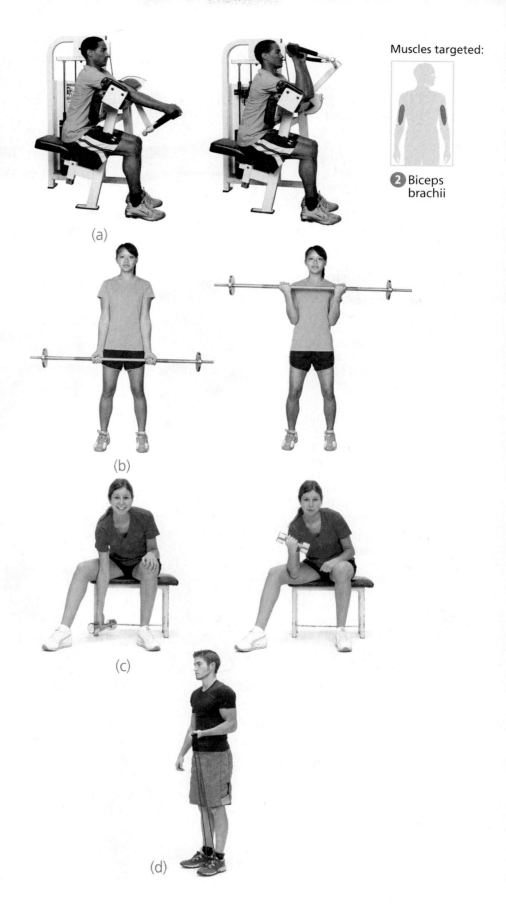

Muscles targeted:

2 Biceps brachii

(a)

(b)

(c)

(d)

21. Pullover

In the starting position your upper arms should be just above your ears and your elbows slightly bent. Pull the weight back up and over the body without changing your elbow angle. Stop when the weight bar is directly over the chest.

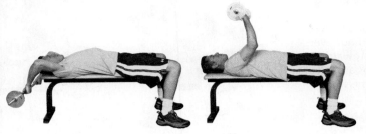

Muscles targeted:

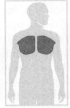 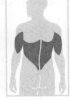

1 Pectoralis major   **13** Triceps brachii

            14 Latissimus dorsi

22. Triceps Extension

(a) **Machine:** Grab the hand grips and start with your arms bent to at least 90 degrees. Press your hands away and down until your elbows are straight but not locked out. Slowly release the weight back up to the start position.

(b) **Free-weight dumbbell:** Start with the weight behind your head and your elbows lifted to the ceiling. Contract the tricep muscles to lift the weight over the head until the arms are straight. Slowly return to the start position and repeat.

(c) **Calisthenics with resistance band:** Grasp the middle of a resistance band with one band and the free ends with the other hand. Place one hand behind you and "anchor" the band at your hips or low back. Extend the arm until straight by contracting the tricep muscle. Slowly return the working arm to the start position and repeat.

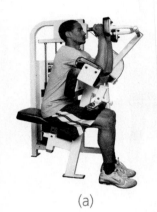 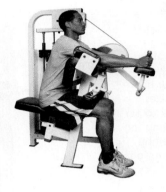

(a)

Muscles targeted:

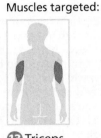

13 Triceps brachii

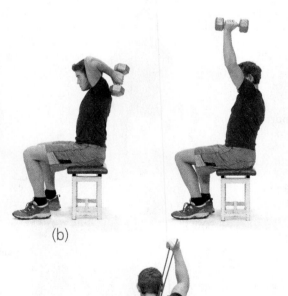

(b)

(c)

Trunk Exercises

23. Back Extension

(a) Calisthenics on a mat: Start in a prone position with arms and legs extended and your forehead on the mat. Lift and further extend your arms and legs using your back and hip muscles. If you are free of low-back problems, you can lift a little further up for increased intensity. Hold the position for 3–5 seconds and then slowly lower back down to the mat.

(b) Calisthenics on a ball: Lie with your stomach over the ball, anchoring your feet and knees on the ground. Place your hands behind your head or extend the arms out straight for increased exercise intensity. Lift the head, shoulders, arms, and upper back until you have a slight curve in the back. Hold this position for 3–5 seconds and then lower back down over the ball.

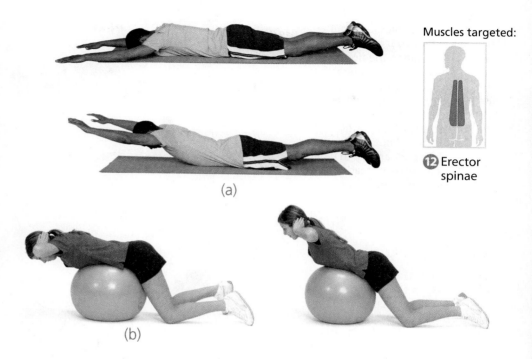

(a)

(b)

Muscles targeted:

12 Erector spinae

24. Abdominal Curl

(a) Machine: Place yourself in the sitting or lying abdominal machine per the machine instructions. Place your feet on the ground or foot pads and press your back firmly against the backrest. Grab the hand grips overhead and/or place your arms behind the arm pads. Contract your abdominals, pulling them in, while you flex your upper torso forward. Slowly return to the starting position and repeat.

(b) Calisthenics on a ball: Lie back with the ball placed at your low to mid-back region. Place your feet shoulder-width on the ground so that your knees are bent at about 90 degrees. Cross your hands at your chest or place lightly behind the head. Contract your abdominals, pulling them in, while you flex your upper torso forward. Slowly return to the starting position and repeat.

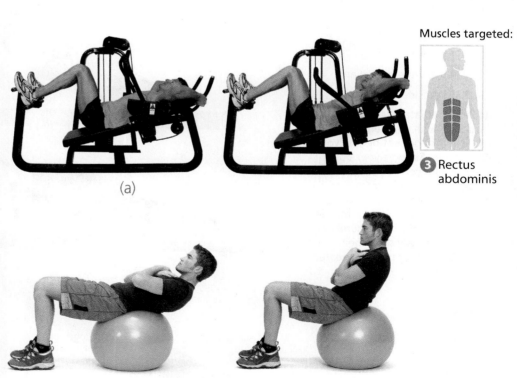

(a)

(b)

Muscles targeted:

3 Rectus abdominis

25. Reverse Curl

Lie on your back and place your hands near your hips. Lift your legs up so that your hips are at a 90-degree angle to the floor. Your knees may be bent or straight for this exercise. Contract your abdominals, pulling them in, while you lift your hips up off the mat. Slowly return to the starting position and repeat. Be careful not to rock the hips and legs back and forth when doing this exercise; instead perform a controlled lifting of the hips upward.

26. Oblique Curl

Lie on your back with your hip and knee joints bent to 90 degrees and your hands lightly supporting the head. Contract your oblique abdominals and lift one shoulder toward the opposite knee. Keep the other arm and elbow on the floor and refrain from pulling on the head and neck. Return to the starting position slowly and repeat to the other side.

27. Side Bridge

(a) Modified side bridge and

(b) Forearm side bridge and

(c) Intermediate side bridge: Lie on your side with your legs together and straight or bent behind you at 90 degrees. Support your body weight with your forearm or a straight arm. Lift your torso to a straight body position by contracting your abdominal and back muscles. Hold this position for a number of seconds or slowly drop the hip to the mat and lift back up for repeated repetitions.

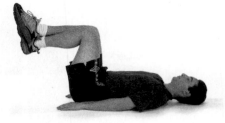

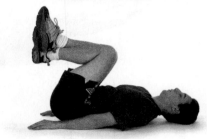

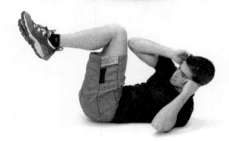

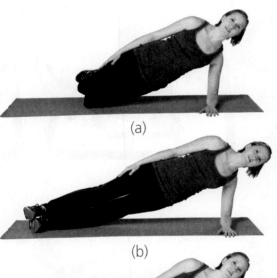

(a)

(b)

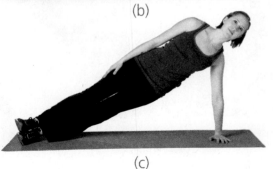

(c)

Muscles targeted:

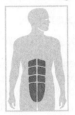

3 Rectus abdominis

Muscles targeted:

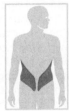

4 External obliques

Muscles targeted:

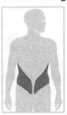

4 External obliques

28. Plank

(a) **Forearm plank** and

(b) **Push-up position plank:** Lie on your stomach and support yourself in plank position (from the forearms or hands) by contracting your trunk muscles so that your neck, back, and hips are completely straight. Your forearms or hands should be under your chest and placed slightly wider than shoulder-width apart. Hold this position for 5–60 seconds, working up in length as you gain muscular endurance.

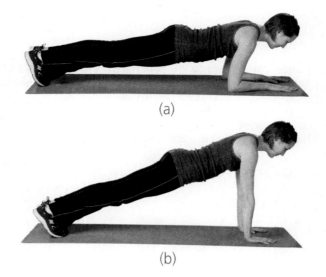

(a)

(b)

Muscles targeted:

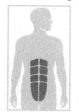

❸ Rectus abdominis

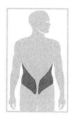

❹ External obliques

WHAT PRECAUTIONS
SHOULD YOU TAKE TO AVOID RESISTANCE-TRAINING INJURIES?

The greater muscular fitness achieved through resistance training helps prevent general injury during sports or daily activity. However, weight training itself can cause injuries such as muscle or tendon strains, ligament sprains, fractures, dislocations, and other joint problems. This is especially true if the lifter pushes for an unrealistic overload. Injuries tend to occur while using free weights, but you can prevent them by getting proper instruction and guidance, and by heeding a few basic suggestions.

FOLLOW BASIC WEIGHT-TRAINING GUIDELINES

When starting your resistance-training program, be conservative: Do not begin with too many exercises, sets, or too much weight! Before increasing your resistance-training intensity or duration, observe how your body responds to the training over a few weeks. After that, you can safely increase the number of repetitions and/or amount of weight. The safest approach is to follow the "10 percent rule." Do not increase exercise frequency, intensity, or time more than 10 percent per week. Gentle increases will help prevent injury, overtraining, or soreness.

Break this rule only if the initial intensity you selected was very low or a certified fitness professional instructs you to do otherwise.

BE SURE TO WARM UP AND COOL DOWN PROPERLY

Weight-training guidelines include a warm-up and a cool-down before and after training sessions. A proper weight-training warm-up includes a *general warm-up* and a *specific warm-up*. The general warm-up consists of 3 to 10 minutes of cardiorespiratory exercises—walking, jogging (on or off a treadmill), biking, stationary biking, elliptical trainer use, or any activity that increases body temperature (breaking a light sweat) and blood flow to muscles. The specific warm-up should include range-of-motion exercises that mimic (without weight added) the resistance exercises you'll be performing. Move your limbs through a full range of motion before using a given weight machine or lifting free weights. Then, do a warm-up set with very light resistance. Now you are ready to perform your serious sets.

Some people also like to stretch before weight training. If you want to add stretching to your warm-up, do so only after a general warm-up where the body has been adequately warmed up in preparation for stretching. The pre-exercise stretching should be light, and you should hold each stretch no more than 10 to 20 seconds. A proper cool-down for resistance training

CASE STUDY

Gina

"My main goals in resistance training are to improve my muscle endurance so that I can go on longer hikes and to strengthen my muscles and joints so that I can lower the chances of getting injured on the trail. I live close to campus and there is a gym with weight equipment available, but how do I decide what equipment to use and what exercises to focus on?"

1. Describe to Gina the benefits of using free weights versus machines.

2. Explain to Gina the differences between traditional weight training, circuit weight training, and plyometrics programs. Which would you advise her to begin with?

3. Think about your own resistance-training goals. Are they appearance based or function based?

4. How would you apply the FITT principles to your own resistance-training goals?

---

includes general range-of-motion exercises and stretches for the muscle groups applied during the weight-training session.

KNOW BASIC WEIGHT-TRAINING SAFETY TIPS

Learn the proper use of weights and weight machines. When lifting free weights, use a spotter to watch, guide, and assist you. Ask the spotter to keep your free-weight movements slow and controlled, not fast, jerky, or bouncy. Spotters typically assist a weight lifter who is attempting to lift a weight near his or her maximal fatigue level and the lift requires full-body balance. Exercises such as squats and the bench press require the weight to be lifted over the head or in a position that could present a danger to the lifter. A personal trainer can help you learn the proper head and body position for lifting each type of weight (with or without the help of a spotter) and for using weight machines of each type. Learning to adjust the machines properly is part of this training.

Muscle strains are common among people who use improper lifting techniques and machine setups. Eccentric contractions, in particular, tend to cause microtears in the muscle fibers and connective tissue within and surrounding the muscles. Since eccentric contractions typically take place during the "lowering" of a weight, it is important not to "drop" a weight to its starting position, whether lifting free weights or using a machine. Lift the weight slowly and lower it at a slow, controlled rate. Some personal trainers recommend using a count of two up and four down to control the weight-lowering phase.

The box **Tools for Change: Safety Tips for Weight Training** gives you additional important safety tips.

GET ADVICE FROM A QUALIFIED EXERCISE PROFESSIONAL

Seek out people qualified to provide accurate resistance-training information, especially if you are just getting started. How can you recognize a qualified exercise professional? Ask any potential personal trainer or instructor questions such as the following:

- Are you certified as a personal trainer or fitness instructor by a reputable, nationally recognized organization such as ACSM, National Strength and Conditioning Association (NSCA), and the American Council on Exercise (ACE)?

- Do you have a certificate or degree in exercise science from an accredited two- or four-year college?

- What types of experience have you had as an instructor or personal trainer?

- How long have you been working in the field of fitness and wellness?

- What are your references from employers and past/present clients?

- How current are you with the changing guidelines and emerging trends in exercise and fitness, and how can you demonstrate this currency?

You'll want to look at practical details such as how much the personal trainer charges, whether or not he or she has liability insurance, and how well his or her

TOOLS FOR CHANGE

SAFETY TIPS FOR WEIGHT TRAINING

Always observe the general guidelines for safe resistance training (see Table 5.3), as well as these safety tips:

- Get a proper introduction to weight training before beginning. Learn the proper grips and postures; the right way to isolate muscle groups and stabilize others; the correct way to adjust machines for your height; and the safe way to sit, stand, and move during weight lifting to prevent injury.

- Wear gym shoes to protect your feet and wear gloves to improve your grip and protect your hands.

- When using free weights, ask a spotter to make sure you are lifting safely and can return the bar safely after the lift.

- Work out with a friend or partner to spot your lifts and point out any positional errors, equipment problems, and so on.

- Use safety collars at the end of weight bars to secure the weights on the bar.

- Perform all exercises through a full range of motion. With free weights, you must determine the range yourself and may need extra training and attention.

- Perform all exercises in a slow and controlled manner. Some trainers recommend counting as you lift: two up and four down. The object is to avoid fast, jerky, or bouncy motions that can injure your muscles or allow the weight to get away from you and cause injury.

- Stay balanced: Set up in a relaxed, balanced position and maintain that after a lift or set of lifts. Getting off balance is an easy way to create strain on one side

and to pull or tear a muscle. Balance your exercise as well so that you build equal strength on both sides and from front to back.

- Breathe in deeply in preparation for a lift and breathe out continuously as you lift. Some weight lifters use a **Valsalva maneuver** (that is, they exhale forcibly with a closed throat so no air exits) as a way to stabilize the trunk during a lift. However, holding your breath this way can cause an unhealthy blood pressure increase and slow blood flow to the heart, lungs, and brain. Breathe out during the push or pull part of a lift, particularly while lifting heavy weights, to avoid doing the Valsalva maneuver.

- Use lighter weights when attempting new lifts or after taking time off from your routine. You can build up by 3 to 5 percent per session or 10 percent per week. Don't assume you can pick up where you left off before a break in your training; that's asking for muscle strain or injury.

- Do not continue resistance training if you are in pain. Learn to differentiate the effort of lifting from the pain of an injury, particularly to a joint.

- Seek the advice of a qualified fitness professional before significantly changing these aspects of your routine: amount of weight, number of repetitions, speed of movement, or body posture.

Source:
American College of Sports Medicine. "Building Strength Safely." Fit Society Page (Fall 2002): www.acsm.org.
Georgia State University, Strength Training Main Page. www2.gsu.edu/~wwwfit/strength.html#safety.

---

schedule will accommodate yours. Intangibles are equally important: How well do you get along with this potential trainer, and how motivated does he or she help you feel? Consider enrolling in a specific weight-training class at your college or university. Instructors in such courses are already screened for the above-listed qualifications, and the cost will be significantly lower than hiring your own personal trainer.

PERSONS WITH DISABILITIES MAY HAVE DIFFERENT WEIGHT-TRAINING GUIDELINES

Weight-training programs benefit virtually everyone, including people with some limitations or disabilities. Resistance training can decrease pain and increase mobility in people with joint and muscle

disabilities and orthopedic conditions such as arthritis, multiple sclerosis, or osteoarthritis.

Safety guidelines and appropriate exercises will vary for different individuals and depend on the disability or limitation of each person. Everyone will need medical clearance before beginning a resistance-training program, and those with certain chronic conditions and muscle disorders may need specific exercise recommendations and directions from their physicians. If your gym lacks specialized equipment,

> **Valsalva maneuver** The process of holding one's breath while lifting heavy weight. This practice can increase chest cavity pressure and result in light-headedness during the lift; excessively increased blood pressure can result after the lift and breath are released.

look for a trainer who can help you perform modified exercises on the available machines. Wheelchair exercisers can perform many seated resistance-training exercises in the gym or at home. Visit this book's website to view demonstrations of easily adaptable resistance-training exercises for people of all abilities.

IS IT RISKY TO USE SUPPLEMENTS FOR MUSCULAR FITNESS?

Dietary supplements marketed as promoters of muscle conditioning are called *performance aids* or dietary **ergogenic aids.** Some supplements are safe but ineffective; some are both unsafe and ineffective. Few, if any, are worth the risk, making this an area to tread lightly into, if at all. Manufacturers of nutritional supplements need not prove their products are safe or effective before offering them on the open market. The FDA may remove unsafe products, but this occurs after the product is "tested" on the buying public. To avoid being an inadvertent subject in an uncontrolled experiment, look into the risks of any supplement very carefully before considering its use. Some ergogenic aids, such as anabolic steroids, are also controlled substances. This means they require a prescription for legal use and should not be used for nonprescription purposes. In addition, their use can get you banned from athletic competitions.

ANABOLIC STEROIDS

Anabolic steroids are synthetic drugs that are chemically related to the hormone testosterone. Physicians sometimes prescribe small doses within a medical setting for people with muscle diseases, burns, some cancers, and pituitary disorders. However, some athletes and recreational weight trainers take anabolic steroids—illegally, outside of a medical setting, without a prescription—to increase muscle mass, strength, and power. Anabolic steroids can produce some of these results in some users—but not without overwhelmingly negative side effects that far outweigh the benefits. Besides being illegal, steroids increase the risk of liver and heart disease, cancer,

acne, breast development in men, and masculinization in women. Anabolic steroid use can also promote connective tissue and bone injuries because dramatically stronger muscles may exert more force than the body can handle. Steroid use can also be habit forming, lead to other drug addictions, and even cause death, as explained in the box **Spotlight: Behind the Steroid Warnings.**

CREATINE

Creatine is a legal nutritional supplement containing amino acids. It is most often sold as creatine monohydrate in powder, tablet, capsule, or liquid form. The body's natural form of creatine (phosphocreatine) is generated by the kidneys and stored in muscle cells. You can also consume creatine in the diet by eating meat products.

Creatine taken at recommended levels can improve performance by temporarily increasing the body's normal muscle stores of phosphocreatine. Since this natural energy substance powers bursts of activity lasting less than 60 seconds, creatine users sometimes find they can train more effectively in power activities and may be able to maintain higher forces during lifting. This can result in increased training adaptations such as strength and muscle size. Creatine intake also causes a temporary retention of water in muscle tissue that produces a small temporary increase in size, strength, and ability to generate power. Creatine has no effect on performance of aerobic endurance exercise.

So far, there have been few serious side effects reported in studies of people using creatine for up to 4 years. Since the long-term effects of creatine use are unknown, however, potential users should proceed with caution.

ADRENAL ANDROGENS
(DHEA, ANDROSTENEDIONE)

Dehydroepiandrosterone (DHEA) is the body's most common hormone and acts as a weak steroid chemical messenger (a conveyor of internal control signals and information). Although DHEA occurs naturally in the body, manufacturers produce and sell it as a supplement in a synthetic concentrated form despite no definitive proof of its safety or effectiveness. DHEA proponents claim that it increases muscle mass and strength, lowers body fat, alters natural hormone levels, slows aging, and boosts immune functions. However, research

ergogenic aid Any nutritional, physical, mechanical, psychological, or pharmacological procedure or aid used to improve athletic performance

CASE STUDY

Gina

"I'm a big baseball fan. Growing up in San Francisco, I used to go to Giants and A's games all the time. So I was kind of shocked to hear about the allegations of steroid and drug use among professional baseball players. I'm confused about the health risks of steroids and supplements. Are they all dangerous? What about the products you can buy in a health store, like creatine?"

1. How would you answer Gina's questions about steroids and creatine?

2. Give two other examples of ergogenic supplements. How safe are they?

3. Have you ever taken an ergogenic supplement? If so, how much do you know about the pros and cons of taking that supplement?

studies have produced conflicting results on DHEA and overall do not provide strong evidence of a large positive effect on muscle mass and strength, or on body fat levels.

Androstenedione (nickname "andro") is another naturally occurring steroid hormone with a structure related to both DHEA and testosterone. It is found naturally in meats and some plants. Even though manufacturers claim "andro" will increase testosterone levels, one pivotal study found that it actually lowers the body's natural production of testosterone, did not increase the body's adaptations to resistance training, and increased heart disease risk in men.[9] Androstenedione was ordered off the market by the FDA in 2004, and its use is dwindling. Both DHEA and androstenedione appear to decrease HDL or "good" cholesterol,[10] which helps explain why these substances increase heart attack risks and other cardiovascular problems. Both also increase the risk of developing certain cancers and accelerating the growth of existing cancers. These serious side effects strongly argue against the use of DHEA or "andro."

GROWTH HORMONE (GH)

Your body's pituitary gland produces human growth hormone (GH), which promotes bone growth and muscle growth and decreases fat stores. Drug manufacturers produce GH synthetically for medical use in children and young adults with abnormally slow or reduced growth and related disorders. Although the FDA regulates growth hormone, athletes wanting to gain an edge over their competitors sometimes obtain and use it illegally. Marketers claim that growth hormone supplementation will counteract the muscle mass lost with disuse and aging, among other alleged benefits. However,

GH side effects include irreversible bone growth (acromegaly/gigantism); increased risk of cardiovascular disease and diabetes; and decreased sexual desire, among others.

Marketers of oral GH supplements (GH promoters, not actual GH) claim the same positive benefits to lean muscle mass and fat mass, but this is not borne out in tests or actual use. Oral GH, in fact, cannot even be absorbed from your digestive tract into your bloodstream! A far better way to increase natural levels of growth hormone is to perform regular exercise. In a study of women who ran for exercise, baseline resting GH levels increased by 50 percent in those training at higher compared to lower intensities.[11]

AMINO ACID AND PROTEIN SUPPLEMENTS

Many bodybuilders and weight lifters take amino acid supplements because they believe that consuming protein or its building blocks (amino acids) will lead to enhanced muscle development. However, evidence is mixed that high intake of protein or taking protein-based supplements will improve training, exercise performance, or build muscle mass beyond the levels achieved through normal dietary protein. When combined with resistance training, moderate increases in protein intake may lead to small increases in lean muscle mass and strength beyond resistance training alone.[12] In contrast, supplementation with the amino acid glutamine produced no beneficial effect above and beyond resistance training itself.[13] Taking moderate doses of these supplements has no dramatic side effects, but large doses of either the supplements or protein itself can create amino acid imbalances, alter protein and bone metabolism, and be dangerous to individuals with liver or kidney disease.[14]

SPOTLIGHT

BEHIND THE STEROID WARNINGS

The National Institute on Drug Abuse (NIDA) publishes two postcards for young men and women with a potent message on the dangers of anabolic steroids. Each card lists the risks and side effects of steroid use, ranging from cancer and heart disease to HIV infection, behavioral problems, and unwelcome body changes. Why are government drug regulators—not to mention parents, educators, and coaches—so worried about steroid use in young people?

Steroid use in teens and young adults is a problem for several major reasons:

1. Use of these drugs is surprisingly common. More than half a million 8th and 10th graders have used anabolic steroids, as have tens of thousands of high school seniors. According to NIDA, steroid use is also "probably widespread among athletes and would-be sports competitors at all levels."

2. Steroid use can lead to the abuse of other drugs. Some of the side effects of steroid use—insomnia, fatigue, restlessness, depression—are so disruptive that people turn to opiate drugs such as cocaine and heroin to relieve their distress.

3. Anabolic steroids can permanently disrupt normal development. A person's body and brain are still developing during adolescence and into their early 20s. Steroids interfere with the normal maturational effects of sex hormones. In males, this interference can shrink the testes and reduce sperm production, stunt normal height, induce breast development, and cause baldness. In females, steroids can reduce breast size, deepen the voice, and induce excessive body hair growth while thinning the head hair. Most of these changes are irreversible.

4. Steroid use can lead to behavioral changes, including irritability, hostility, aggression, and depression. Researchers injected adolescent hamsters with commonly used steroids, then observed as their playful fighting—wrestling and nibbling—turned to outright attacking and biting at levels 10 times higher. This aggression went on even after the drugs were withdrawn and stayed throughout half of the hamsters' remaining adolescence. The researchers found increased levels of a neurotransmitter called *vasopressin* coming from one brain region that closely resembles the same structure in the human brain. The same may be true of a region that produces serotonin and is involved in depression. Such changes during teenage brain development could mean lifelong changes in a person's aggression and depression levels, even after he or she stops using steroids.

5. Steroids disrupt the way the body processes cholesterol. As a result, steroids promote heart disease, heart attacks, and strokes, even in athletes younger than 30. The liver and kidneys must detoxify and remove steroids from the body, and both organs are more prone to cancerous tumors in steroid users. The drugs also cause blood-filled cysts in the liver that can burst and cause serious internal bleeding.

6. Injecting steroids, rather than taking them orally, and sharing needles with other users can lead to dangerous infections transmitted through dirty needles. The disease risks include hepatitis; HIV; and endocarditis, a bacterial infection of the heart.

Sources:

American Psychological Association (APA). "Animal Models Show that Anabolic Steroids Flip the Adolescent Brain's Switch for Aggressive Behavior." Press release. February 26, 2006. www.apa.org/releases/steroids0226.html.

Grimes, J. M. et al. "Plasticity in Anterior Hypothalamic Vasopressin Correlates with Aggression during Anabolic-Androgenic Steroid Withdrawal in Hamsters," *Behavioral Neuroscience* 120, no. 1 (2006): 115–124.

National Institute on Drug Abuse (NIDA). Research Report Series—Anabolic Steroid Use September–November, 2006. www.drugabuse.gov/researchreports/steroids/anabolicsteroids.html

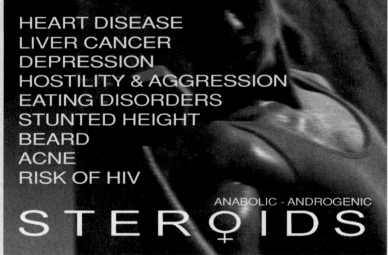

HEART DISEASE
LIVER CANCER
DEPRESSION
HOSTILITY & AGGRESSION
EATING DISORDERS
STUNTED HEIGHT
BEARD
ACNE
RISK OF HIV

ANABOLIC - ANDROGENIC
STEROIDS

REVIEW QUESTIONS

1. Muscular strength is the ability to
   a. contract your muscles repeatedly over time.
   b. run a 6-minute mile.
   c. look "toned" in a swimsuit.
   d. contract your muscle with maximal force.

2. Which of the following benefits of resistance training will reduce your risk of cardiovascular diseases?
   a. Increased bone density
   b. Increased muscle power
   c. Reduced body fat levels
   d. Better sports recovery

3. What is a single muscle cell called?
   a. Muscle fiber
   b. Muscle fascia
   c. Fascicle
   d. Contractile bundle

4. Which of the following will result in a stronger muscle contraction?
   a. Eating more protein before your workout
   b. Activating slow, smaller motor units
   c. Taking DHEA before your workout
   d. Activating more motor units overall

5. Sitting down in a chair and standing up again is an example of this type of exercise:
   a. Isotonic
   b. Isokinetic
   c. Isometric
   d. Isostatic

6. Muscle strength improvements in the first few weeks of a program are due to:
   a. Increased size of muscle fibers
   b. Increased activation and coordination of motor units
   c. Increased ability of muscles to move through a full range of motion
   d. Increased blood flow to working muscles

7. A good test of muscular endurance includes
   a. a 1 RM test.
   b. a grip-strength test.
   c. a 20 RM test.
   d. a pull-up test.

8. One disadvantage of using machines for resistance-training exercises is
   a. the machine takes time to adjust for your height and desired resistance level.
   b. the machine does not promote the use of postural and stabilizing muscles during the exercise.
   c. spotters are needed.
   d. it can be hard to isolate specific muscle groups.

9. Which of the following is NOT part of the criteria you should use when selecting a personal trainer?
   a. Certified by ACSM, NSCA, or ACE
   b. Good references by former and current clients
   c. Number of years in the field
   d. The number of dietary supplements they can help you obtain at a reduced cost

10. Which of the following supplements/drugs have irreversible bone growth, cardiovascular disease, diabetes, and decreased sexual desire among its negative side effects?
    a. Anabolic steroids
    b. Creatine
    c. Growth hormone
    d. Androstenedione

CRITICAL THINKING QUESTIONS

1. Why is weight training a popular activity among college students and adults of all ages?

2. Define *sarcopenia* and discuss how it can be reversed through exercise. How are sarcopenia and atrophy different?

3. Which fiber type is activated most during a sprint? What is the predominant fiber type in the postural trunk muscles?

4. Discuss the role of resistance training in preventing injuries.

5. How does circuit weight training differ from regular weight training? What are the specific benefits of doing circuit weight training?

ONLINE RESOURCES

Please visit this book's website at **www.aw-bc.com/hopson** to view videos of strength training exercises and to access links related to topics in this chapter.

REFERENCES

1. National Health Interview Survey (NHIS), "U.S. Physical Activity Statistics: 1998 U.S. Physical Activity Statistics: Participation in Select Physical Activities," http://www.cdc.gov/nccdphp/dnpa/physical/stats/pasports.htm. (accessed December 11, 2006).

2. Centers for Disease Control (CDC), "Trends in Strength Training—United States, 1998–2004." *Morbidity and Mortality Weekly Report* 55, no. 28 (2006): 769–72.

3. M. J. Hubal and others, "Variability in Muscle Size and Strength Gain after Unilateral Resistance Training," *Medicine and Science in Sports and Exercise* 37, no. 6 (2005): 964–72.

4. S. Calling and others, "Effects of Body Fatness and Physical Activity on Cardiovascular Risk: Risk Prediction Using the Bioelectrical Impedance Method," *Scandinavian Journal of Public Health* 34, no. 6, (2006): 568–75.

5. B. L. Marks and others, "Fat-free Mass is Maintained in Women Following a Moderate Diet and Exercise Program," *Medical Science Sports Exercise* 27, no. 9 (1995): 1243–51.

6. P. A. Williams and T. F. Cash, "Effects of a Circuit Weight Training Program on the Body Images of College Students," *International Journal of Eating Disorders* 30, no. 1 (2001): 75–80.

7. G. A. Kelley, K. S. Kelley, and Z. V. Tran, "Resistance Training and Bone Mineral Density in Women: A Meta-Analysis of Controlled Trials," *American Journal of Physical Medicine and Rehabilitation* 80 (2001): 65–77.

8. J. Munn and others, "Resistance Training for Strength: Effect of Number of Sets and Contraction Speed," *Medicine and Science in Sports and Exercise* 37, no. 9 (2005): 1622–26.

9. C. E. Brodeur and others, "The Andro Project: Physiological and Hormonal Influences of Androstenedione Supplementation in Men 35–65 Years Old Participating in a High-Intensity Resistance Training Program," *Archives of International Medicine* 160, no. 20, (2000): 3093–104.

10. M. L. Kohut and others, "Ingestion of a Dietary Supplement Containing Dehydroepiandrosterone (DHEA) and Androstenedione has Minimal Effect on Immune Function in Middle-Aged Men," *Journal of American College of Nutrition* 22, no. 5 (2003): 363–71.

11. A. Weltman and others, "Endurance Training Amplifies the Pulsatile Release of Growth Hormone: Effects of Training Intensity," *Journal of Applied Physiology* 72, no. 6 (1992): 2188–96.

12. D. G. Candow and others, "Effect of Whey and Soy Protein Supplementation Combined with Resistance Training in Young Adults," *International Journal of Sport Nutrition and Exercise Metabolism* 16, no. 3 (2006): 233–44.

13. D. G. Candow and others, "Effect of Glutamine Supplementation Combined with Resistance Training in Young Adults," *European Journal of Applied Physiology* 86, no. 2 (2001): 142–49.

14. E. L. Knight and others, "The Impact of Protein Intake on Renal Function Decline in Women with Normal Renal Function or Mild Renal Insufficiency," *Annals of Internal Medicine* 138 (2003): 460–67.

Name: _____   Date: _____

Instructor: _____   Section: _____

Materials: Calculator, leg press machine, bench press machine

Purpose: To assess your current level of muscular strength.

NOTE: This lab should be performed in the presence of an instructor to ensure proper form and safety.

MUSCULAR STRENGTH ASSESSMENT

One Repetition Maximum (1 RM) Prediction Assessment

The "gold standard" for measuring muscular strength is using a one repetition maximum (1 RM) to determine the maximum amount of weight that you can lift one time only. This lab will <u>estimate</u> 1 RM for the bench press and leg press by finding the amount of weight you can maximally lift 2 to 10 times.

1. Warm-up. Complete 3 to 10 minutes of light cardiorespiratory activity to warm the muscles. Perform range-of-motion exercises and light stretches for the joints and muscles that you will be using.

2. Use proper form while executing the bench press and leg press exercises. For the bench press, position yourself so the bar or handles are across the middle of your chest. Spread your hands slightly wider than shoulder width. Bring the handles/bar to just above your chest and then press upward/outward until your arms are straight. For the leg press, position yourself so that your knees are at a 90-degree angle. Press the weight away from your body until your legs are straight.

3. Perform one light warm-up set. Set the machine at a very light weight and lift this weight about 10 times as a warm-up for your assessment.

4. Find the appropriate strength-assessment weight and number of repetitions. Set a weight that you think you can lift at least 2 times but no more than 10 times. Perform the lift as many times as you can (to complete fatigue) up to 10 repetitions. If you can lift more than 10 repetitions, try again, using heavier weight. Repeat until you find a weight you cannot lift more than 2 to 10 times. In order to prevent muscle fatigue from affecting your results, attempt this assessment no more than three times to find the proper weight and number of repetitions. If you experience muscle fatigue, rest and perform the test again on another day. Record your results in the Muscular Strength Results section (see step 7).

5. Find your predicted 1 RM. Predict your 1 RM based upon the number of repetitions you performed. If the weight you lifted was between 20 and 250 pounds, use the 1 RM Prediction Table to find your predicted 1 RM. If you lifted over 250 pounds, use the Multiplication Factor Table to find your predicted 1 RM. You can find these tables at the end of this lab.

6. Find your strength-to-body weight ratio. Divide your predicted 1 RM by your body weight for your strength-to-body-weight ratio (S/BW). Since heavier people often have more muscle, this is a better indicator of muscular strength than just the weight lifted alone. Record your results in the Muscular Strength Results section.

7. **Find your muscle strength rating by using the Strength-to-Body Weight Ratio chart provided on the last page of this lab.** Finding your rating tells you how you compare to others who have completed this test in the past. Record your results below.

Muscular Strength Results

Bench Press: Weight lifted _____ Repetitions _____

_____ × _____ = _____

Weight lifted (lb)   Multiplication factor*   Predicted 1 RM (lb)

_____ ÷ _____ = _____

Predicted 1 RM (lb)   Body weight (lb)   S/BW ratio

Rating _____

Leg Press: Weight lifted _____ Repetitions _____

_____ × _____ = _____

Weight lifted (lb)   Multiplication factor*   Predicted 1 RM (lb)

_____ ÷ _____ = _____

Predicted 1 RM (lb)   Body weight (lb)   S/BW ratio

Rating _____

*Multiplication factor from the Multiplication Factor Table on the last page of this lab.

1 RM Prediction Table

Wt (lb)	Repetitions									
	1	2	3	4	5	6	7	8	9	10
20	20	21	21	22	23	23	24	25	26	27
25	25	26	26	27	28	29	30	31	32	33
30	30	31	32	33	34	35	36	37	39	40
35	35	36	37	38	39	41	42	43	45	47
40	40	41	42	44	45	46	48	50	51	53
45	45	46	48	49	51	52	54	56	58	60
50	50	51	53	55	56	58	60	62	64	67
55	55	57	58	60	62	64	66	68	71	73
60	60	62	64	65	68	70	72	74	77	80
65	65	67	69	71	73	75	78	81	84	87
70	70	72	74	76	79	81	84	87	90	93
75	75	77	79	82	84	87	90	93	96	100
80	80	82	85	87	90	93	96	99	103	107
85	85	87	90	93	96	99	102	106	109	113
90	90	93	95	98	101	105	108	112	116	120
95	95	98	101	104	107	110	114	118	122	127
100	100	103	106	109	113	116	120	124	129	133
105	105	108	111	115	118	122	126	130	135	140
110	110	113	116	120	124	128	132	137	141	147
115	115	118	122	125	129	134	138	143	148	153
120	120	123	127	131	135	139	144	149	154	160
125	125	129	132	136	141	145	150	155	161	167
130	130	134	138	142	146	151	156	161	167	173
135	135	139	143	147	152	157	162	168	174	180
140	140	144	148	153	158	163	168	174	180	187
145	145	149	154	158	163	168	174	180	186	193
150	150	154	159	164	169	174	180	186	193	200
155	155	159	164	169	174	180	186	192	199	207
160	160	165	169	175	180	186	192	199	206	213
165	165	170	175	180	186	192	198	205	212	220
170	170	175	180	185	191	197	204	211	219	227
175	175	180	185	191	197	203	210	217	225	233
180	180	185	191	196	203	209	216	223	231	240
185	185	190	196	202	208	215	222	230	238	247
190	190	195	201	207	214	221	228	236	244	253
195	195	201	206	213	219	226	234	242	251	260
200	200	206	212	218	225	232	240	248	257	267
205	205	211	217	224	231	238	246	255	264	273
210	210	216	222	229	236	244	252	261	270	280
215	215	221	228	235	242	250	258	267	276	287
220	220	226	233	240	248	256	264	273	283	293
225	225	231	238	245	253	261	270	279	289	300
230	230	237	244	251	259	267	276	286	296	307
235	235	242	249	256	264	273	282	292	302	313
240	240	247	254	262	270	279	288	298	309	320
245	245	252	259	267	276	285	294	304	315	327
250	250	257	265	273	281	290	300	310	322	333

Multiplication Factor Table for Predicting 1 RM

Repetitions	1	2	3	4	5	6	7	8	9	10
Multiplication Factor	1.0	1.07	1.11	1.13	1.16	1.20	1.23	1.27	1.32	1.36

Table and multiplication factors generated using the Bryzcki equation: **1 RM = weight (kg) /[1.0278 − (0.0278 × repetitions)]**.
Source: Adapted from Bryzcki, M. "Strength Testing: Predicting a One-Rep Max from a Reps-to-Fatigue," *J Phys Educ Recreation Dance* 64 (1993): 88–90.

Strength-to-Body Weight Ratio Ratings

Bench Press						
Men	**Superior**	**Excellent**	**Good**	**Fair**	**Poor**	**Very Poor**
<20 yrs	>1.75	1.34–1.75	1.19–1.33	1.06–1.18	0.89–1.05	<0.89
20–29 yrs	>1.62	1.32–1.62	1.14–1.31	0.99–1.13	0.88–0.98	<0.88
30–39 yrs	>1.34	1.12–1.34	0.98–1.11	0.88–0.97	0.78–0.87	<0.78
40–49 yrs	>1.19	1.00–1.19	0.88–0.99	0.80–0.87	0.72–0.79	<0.72
50–59 yrs	>1.04	0.90–1.04	0.79–0.89	0.71–0.78	0.63–0.70	<0.63
>60 yrs	>0.93	0.82–0.93	0.72–0.81	0.66–0.71	0.57–0.65	<0.57
Women	**Superior**	**Excellent**	**Good**	**Fair**	**Poor**	**Very Poor**
<20 yrs	>0.87	0.77–0.87	0.65–0.76	0.58–0.64	0.53–0.57	<0.53
20–29 yrs	>1.00	0.80–1.00	0.70–0.79	0.59–0.69	0.51–0.58	<0.51
30–39 yrs	>0.81	0.70–0.81	0.60–0.69	0.53–0.59	0.47–0.52	<0.47
40–49 yrs	>0.76	0.62–0.76	0.54–0.61	0.50–0.53	0.43–0.49	<0.43
50–59 yrs	>0.67	0.55–0.67	0.48–0.54	0.44–0.47	0.39–0.43	<0.39
>60 yrs	>0.71	0.54–0.71	0.47–0.53	0.43–0.46	0.38–0.42	<0.38
Leg Press						
Men	**Superior**	**Excellent**	**Good**	**Fair**	**Poor**	**Very Poor**
<20 yrs	>2.81	2.28–2.81	2.04–2.27	1.90–2.03	1.70–1.89	<1.70
20–29 yrs	>2.39	2.13–2.39	1.97–2.12	1.83–1.96	1.63–1.82	<1.63
30–39 yrs	>2.19	1.93–2.19	1.77–1.92	1.65–1.76	1.52–1.64	<1.52
40–49 yrs	>2.01	1.82–2.01	1.68–1.81	1.57–1.67	1.44–1.56	<1.44
50–59 yrs	>1.89	1.71–1.89	1.58–1.70	1.46–1.57	1.32–1.45	<1.32
>60 yrs	>1.79	1.62–1.79	1.49–1.61	1.38–1.48	1.25–1.37	<1.25
Women	**Superior**	**Excellent**	**Good**	**Fair**	**Poor**	**Very Poor**
<20 yrs	>1.87	1.71–1.87	1.59–1.70	1.38–1.58	1.22–1.37	<1.22
20–29 yrs	>1.97	1.68–1.97	1.50–1.67	1.37–1.49	1.22–1.36	<1.22
30–39 yrs	>1.67	1.47–1.67	1.33–1.46	1.21–1.32	1.09–1.20	<1.09
40–49 yrs	>1.56	1.37–1.56	1.23–1.36	1.13–1.22	1.02–1.12	<1.02
50–59 yrs	>1.42	1.25–1.42	1.10–1.24	0.99–1.09	0.88–0.98	<0.88
>60 yrs	>1.42	1.18–1.42	1.04–1.17	0.93–1.03	0.85–0.92	<0.85

Name: _____   Date: _____

Instructor: _____   Section: _____

Materials: Leg press machine, bench press machine, exercise mat, yardstick or ruler, tape

Purpose: To assess your current level of muscular endurance.

NOTE: This lab should be performed in the presence of an instructor to ensure proper form and safety.

SECTION I: MUSCULAR ENDURANCE WEIGHT-LIFTING ASSESSMENT

Twenty Repetition Maximum (20 RM) Assessment

The 20 RM assessment is a weight-lifting assessment of your muscular endurance. By performing the assessments before and after completing 8 to 12 weeks of muscular fitness exercises, you can measure your improvement.

1. **Prepare for the muscle endurance assessments.** If you have just completed the muscular strength assessments in Lab 5.1, you will already be warmed up. If not, perform a warm-up similar to the one described in Lab 5.1. Follow the position, form, and warm-up instructions for bench press and leg press in Lab 5.1.

2. **Find your 20 RM for bench press and leg press.** Set a weight that you think you can lift a maximum of 20 times. Perform the lift to see if you were correct. If not, increase or decrease the weight and try again until you find your 20 RM. In order to make sure that muscle fatigue does not affect your results, try to find your 20 RM within three tries. If it takes longer, rest and perform the test again on another day. Record your results below.

Muscular Endurance Weight Lifting Results

Bench Press: 20 RM weight lifted _____

Leg Press: 20 RM weight lifted _____

SECTION II: MUSCULAR ENDURANCE CALISTHENIC ASSESSMENT

Push-Up Assessment

In this muscular endurance assessment, you will perform as many push-ups as you can. This test will assess the muscular endurance of your pectoralis major, anterior deltoid, and triceps brachii muscles. If you work with a partner, your partner can check your positioning, form, and count your repetitions.

1. **Get into the correct push-up position on an exercise mat.** Support the body in a push-up position from the knees (women) or from the toes (men). The hands should be just outside the shoulders and the back and legs straight.

2. **Start in the "down" position** with your elbow joint at a 90-degree angle, your chest just above the floor, and your chin barely touching the mat. Push your body up until your arms are straight and then lower back to the starting position (count one repetition). Complete the push-ups in a slow and controlled manner.

3. **Complete as many correct technique push-ups** as you can without stopping and record your results in the Muscular Endurance Calisthenic Results section on the next page.

4. **Find your muscle endurance rating** for push-ups in the chart at the end of this lab and record your results.

Curl-Up Assessment

In this muscular endurance assessment, you will perform as many curl-ups as you can (up to 25). This test will assess the muscular endurance of your abdominal muscles.

1. **Lie on a mat** with your arms by your sides, palms flat on the mat, elbows straight, and fingers extended. Bend your knees at a 90-degree angle. Mark the start and end positions with tape. Your instructor or partner will mark your starting finger position with a piece of tape under each hand. He or she will then mark the ending position 10 cm or 3 in away from the first piece of tape—one ending position tape for each hand. Your goal is to rise far enough on the curl-up to achieve a 30-degree trunk elevation.

2. **Your instructor or partner will set a metronome to 50 beats/min** and you will complete the curl-ups at this slow, controlled pace: one curl-up every 3 seconds (25 curl-ups per minute).

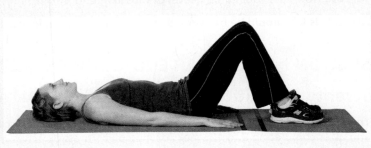

3. **To start the test,** curl your head and upper back upward, reaching your arms forward along the mat to touch the ending tape. Then curl back down so that your upper back and shoulders touch the floor. During the entire curl-up, your fingers, feet, and buttocks should stay on the mat. Your partner will count the number of correct repetitions you complete. Any curl-ups performed without touching the ending position tape will not be counted in the final results.

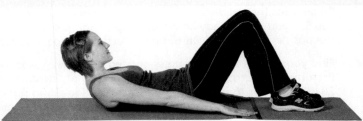

4. **Perform as many curl-ups as you can** without pausing, to a maximum of 25. Record your score below. Determine your muscular endurance rating for curl-ups using the chart below and record your results.

**Alternative: One minute timed curl-ups. Your instructor may choose to have you complete as many curl-ups as you can within 1 minute (without the metronome pacing). Use the same start and end positions, perform controlled repetitions of curl-ups for 1 minute, and record your results below.

Muscular Endurance Calisthenic Results

Push-Ups: Repetitions _____   Rating _____

Curl-Ups: Repetitions _____   Rating _____

**Alternative – 1 min timed curl-ups: Repetitions _____

SECTION III: REFLECTION

1. What was surprising about your muscular fitness results, if anything? _____

_____

2. Based upon your assessment results, which aspect of muscular fitness will your program focus on—muscular

strength or muscular endurance? _____

Muscle Endurance Rating

PUSH-UPS						
Men	**Superior**	**Excellent**	**Good**	**Fair**	**Poor**	**Very Poor**
20–29 yrs	>36	31–36	24–30	21–23	16–20	<16
30–39 yrs	>30	24–30	19–23	16–18	11–15	<11
40–49 yrs	>25	19–25	15–18	12–14	9–11	<9
50–59 yrs	>21	15–21	12–14	9–11	6–8	<6
60–69 yrs	>18	13–18	10–12	7–9	4–6	<4
Women	**Superior**	**Excellent**	**Good**	**Fair**	**Poor**	**Very Poor**
20–29 yrs	>30	22–30	16–21	14–15	9–13	<9
30–39 yrs	>27	21–27	14–20	12–14	7–11	<7
40–49 yrs	>24	16–24	12–15	10–11	4–9	<4
50–59 yrs	>21	12–21	8–11	6–8	1–5	<1
60–69 yrs	>17	13–17	6–12	4–6	1–3	<1

CURL-UPS						
Men	**Superior**	**Excellent**	**Good**	**Fair**	**I. Poor**	**Very Poor**
20–29 yrs	>25	22–25	16–21	13–15	10–12	<10
30–39 yrs	>25	19–25	15–18	13–14	10–12	<10
40–49 yrs	>25	19–25	13–18	8–12	5–7	<5
50–59 yrs	>25	18–25	11–17	9–10	7–8	<7
60–69 yrs	>25	17–25	11–16	8–10	5–7	<5
Women	**Superior**	**Excellent**	**Good**	**Fair**	**Poor**	**Very Poor**
20–29 yrs	>25	19–25	14–18	7–13	4–6	<4
30–39 yrs	>25	20–25	10–19	8–9	5–7	<5
40–49 yrs	>25	20–25	11–19	6–10	3–5	<3
50–59 yrs	>25	20–25	10–19	8–9	5–7	<5
60–69 yrs	>25	18–25	8–17	5–7	2–4	<2

Source: Adapted from Canadian Society for Exercise Physiology. *The Canadian Physical Activity, Fitness & Lifestyle Approach: CSEP-Health & Fitness Program's Health-Related Appraisal & Counseling Strategy,* 3rd ed. Canadian Society for Exercise Physiology: 2003.

Name: _____ **Date:** _____

Instructor: _____ **Section:** _____

Purpose: To learn how to set appropriate muscular fitness goals (short- and long-term).

SECTION I: SHORT- AND LONG-TERM GOALS

Create short- and long-term goals for muscular strength and muscular endurance. Be sure to use SMART (**s**pecific, **m**easurable, **a**ction-oriented, **r**ealistic, **t**imed) goal-setting guidelines. Apply information from the Chapter 5 text and use your results from Labs 5.1 and 5.2. Remember that aiming to improve your assessment scores is a highly measurable way to set goals. Select appropriate target dates and rewards for completing your goals.

Short-Term Goals (3–6 months)

1. Muscular Strength Goal:

_____

Target Date: _____

Reward: _____

2. Muscular Endurance Goal:

_____

Target Date: _____

Reward: _____

Long-Term Goals (12+ months)

1. Muscular Strength Goal:

_____

Target Date: _____

Reward: _____

2. Muscular Endurance Goal:

_____

Target Date: _____

Reward: _____

SECTION II: MUSCULAR FITNESS OBSTACLES AND STRATEGIES

What barriers or obstacles might hinder your plan to improve your muscular fitness? Indicate your top three obstacles below and list strategies for overcoming each obstacle.

a. _____

b. _____

c. _____

SECTION III: GETTING SUPPORT

1. List resources you will use to help change your muscular fitness:

Friend/partner/relative: _____   School-based resource: _____

Community-based resource: _____   Other: _____

SECTION IV: REFLECTION

1. How realistic are the short- and long-term target dates you have set for achieving your muscular fitness goals?

_____

_____

_____

_____

2. Are there any other strategies not listed above that could assist you in reaching your goals?

_____

_____

_____

3. Think about all of the opportunities that present themselves in your daily life to work toward muscular fitness. List as many of these as you can think of:

_____

_____

_____

_____

Name: _____   Date: _____

Instructor: _____   Section: _____

Purpose: To create a basic, personal resistance-training workout plan. Forms for following up and tracking your muscular fitness and your resistance-training program are included.

Directions: Complete the following sections.

SECTION I: MUSCULAR FITNESS PROGRAM QUESTIONS AND MOTIVATIONS

1. How many days per week are you planning to work on your muscular fitness program? _____

2. How experienced are you at resistance training? (circle one below)

Novice   **Intermediate** (training 1 to 2 years)   **Advanced** (training 3+ yrs)

3. Which will you focus on first? (circle one)   **Muscular strength**   **Muscular endurance**

4. The best muscular fitness programs are well-rounded and work the entire body. However, some people want to focus more heavily on one area than another. Which muscle groups do you want to focus on?

_____

5. Which type of equipment do you plan to use and why? (check all that apply)

☐ **Weight machines**

☐ **Free weights**

☐ **No equipment (calisthenic exercises)**

6. How much time do you plan to spend each day on your resistance-training program? _____

7. Do you have a workout partner? Do you plan to work with a partner, trainer, or instructor to help you get started?

_____

SECTION II: RESISTANCE-TRAINING PROGRAM DESIGN

Plan your resistance-training program using resources available to you (facility, instructor, text). Complete one line for each exercise you have chosen to do in your program.

Exercise	Frequency (days/week)	Intensity (weight in lb)	Sets (number)	Reps (number per set)	Rest (time between sets)
LOWER BODY					
1.					
2.					
3.					
4.					
5.					
6.					
7.					
8.					
UPPER BODY					
1.					
2.					
3.					
4.					
5.					
6.					
7.					
8.					
9.					
10.					
11.					
12.					
TRUNK					
1.					
2.					
3.					
4.					
5.					

SECTION III: TRACKING YOUR PROGRAM AND FOLLOWING THROUGH

1. **Goal and program tracking:** Use the following resistance-training chart to monitor your progress. Change the amount of resistance, sets, or repetitions frequently to accommodate your stronger musculature and ensure continuing progress toward your goals.

2. **Goal and program follow-up:** At the end of the course or at your short-term goal target date, reevaluate your muscular fitness and answer the following questions:

   a. Did you meet your short-term goal or your goal for the course?

   b. If so, what positive behavioral changes contributed to your success? If not, which obstacles blocked your success?

   c. Was your short-term goal realistic? After evaluating your progress during the course, what would you change about your goals or resistance-training plan?

DATE																						
EXERCISE	Wt.	Sets	Reps	Wt.	Sets	Reps	Wt.	Sets	Reps	Wt.	Sets	Reps	Wt.	Sets	Reps	Wt.	Sets	Reps	Wt.	Sets	Reps
1.																					
2.																					
3.																					
4.																					
5.																					
6.																					
7.																					
8.																					
9.																					
10.																					
11.																					
12.																					
13.																					
14.																					

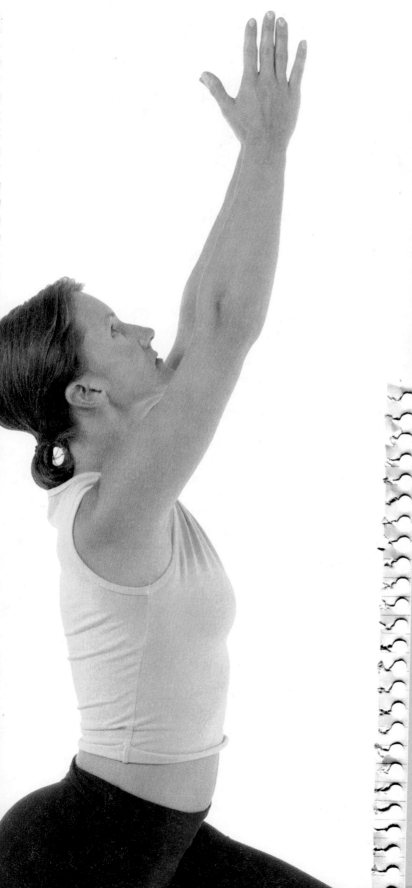

CHAPTER 6

Maintaining Flexibility and Back Health

OBJECTIVES

Describe the benefits of stretching and flexibility.

Discuss the factors that determine a person's flexibility.

Identify safe and effective stretching exercises.

Describe ways to lower your risk of stretching-related injuries.

Create a personalized program for improving your flexibility.

Explain the primary causes of lower-back pain.

Describe ways to reduce your risk of lower-back pain.

Mark

"Hi, I'm Mark. I live in Colorado Springs, at the foothills of the Rocky Mountains. I love the outdoors. I've been a backpacker, fisherman, and skier my whole life. My girl-friend is a fitness instructor and has been telling me that I should really stretch more, but I'm skeptical. What's so important about stretching? Will it help me be a better hiker or skier? How do I figure out what kind of stretches I should do? And when and how often should I stretch?"

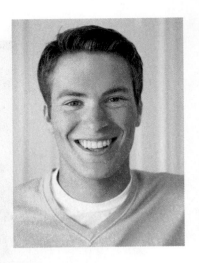

Flexibility is the ability of joints to move through a full **range of motion.** When you are young, it is easy to take your flexibility for granted—that is, until you start to lose it, which tends to happen as you get older. A complete fitness program should include **stretching** and range-of-motion exercises to help you maintain flexibility and prevent joint problems.

In this chapter, we will cover the benefits of stretching and maintaining your flexibility. We will discuss the factors that determine how flexible a person is, present strategies for stretching safely and effectively, and provide guidelines for developing a personalized stretching program. We will also discuss the common problem of lower-back pain and present strategies for incorporating a back-health component into your regular fitness plan.

WHAT ARE THE BENEFITS OF STRETCHING AND FLEXIBILITY?

Like Mark from our case study, many people are not in the habit of stretching and are not sure why stretching is important. There are many benefits to

stretching, but the most compelling reason is simple: maintaining and developing your flexibility will help you to move about freely and carry out everyday activities with greater ease over the course of your lifetime.

IMPROVED MOBILITY, POSTURE, AND BALANCE

A regular stretching program helps you maintain joint mobility throughout your body. Your joints allow you to *move*—whether you are bending your knees to tie a shoelace, riding a bicycle around campus, or reaching for a bowl on the top shelf of a cupboard. A reduction in your flexibility can result in a reduction in your ability to move about freely as you perform daily activities. Likewise, an improvement in your flexibility can result in greater freedom of movement.

Regular stretching can also help you maintain a balance of muscle strength and muscle flexibility, which is important for proper joint alignment and posture. For example, if the muscles on the front of your hips get too tight, your pelvis can get pulled forward and cause a larger sway in your lower back. This will alter your posture and could even affect your balance. Good flexibility, developed through stretching, can help you keep your joints and spine aligned, maintain your balance, and promote overall body stability.

HEALTHY JOINTS AND PAIN MANAGEMENT

Almost one-third of adults over the age of 18 (and over one-half of adults 65 years and older) report regular pain, aching, and stiffness in their knees, shoulders, fingers, or hips.[1] Many adults also have or will develop **arthritis** at some point in their

---

flexibility The ability of a joint (or joints) to move through a full range of motion

range of motion The movement limits of a specific joint or group of joints

stretching Exercises designed to improve or maintain flexibility

arthritis An umbrella-term for over 100 conditions characterized by inflammation of a joint

lives. Regular exercise, including range-of-motion and flexibility exercises, is essential for people with arthritis to maintain function and manage joint pain.[2] Even in people without arthritis, stretching will increase joint flexibility, improve joint function, and decrease periodic joint pain.[3]

MUSCLE RELAXATION
AND STRESS RELIEF

After sitting at a computer for hours working on a term paper, doesn't it feel great to stand up and stretch? Staying in one position for too long, repetitive movement, and other stressors can result in stiff and "knotted" muscles. Gentle stretching and relaxation increases blood flow to tight muscles, stimulates the nervous system to decrease stress hormones, and ultimately helps relax areas of tension in your body.

> **Try it NOW!** Sitting hunched over a pile of books for an extended period of time can be a pain in the neck! • Every 20 minutes or so, try doing shoulder rolls, shrugs, and neck stretches.

POSSIBLE REDUCTION
OF LOWER-BACK PAIN

Having an adequate level of flexibility *may* reduce your risk of lower-back pain; however, research on the subject is inconclusive. While poor flexibility has been linked to lower-back pain in adolescents, these relationships are less clear in adults.[4,5,6] Despite the mixed evidence, most experts agree that having a minimal level of joint mobility and flexibility through the hips and back is one of the strategies for reducing the risk of developing chronic lower-back pain.[7] We will discuss lower-back pain in more detail later in this chapter.

WHAT DETERMINES
YOUR FLEXIBILITY?

Flexibility can be classified as **static** or **dynamic.** Static (or passive) flexibility is a measure of the limits of a joint's overall range of motion. Dynamic (or active) flexibility is a measure of overall joint stiffness during movement (i.e., with muscular contraction). Active movement such as swinging a tennis racket or leaping over a hurdle on a track requires good dynamic flexibility.

So, what determines how flexible you are? Is it genetic, or can it be attributed entirely to the amount of stretching that you do? Many factors can affect your individual level of flexibility. Your joints, muscles, tendons, and nervous system—along with other characteristics such as age, gender, genetics, and activity level—can all influence your flexibility.

JOINT STRUCTURES, MUSCLES AND TENDONS, AND THE NERVOUS SYSTEM

The range of motion possible in a particular **joint** is limited by the structures that comprise that joint, the muscles and tendons that cross over the joint, and the nervous system.

Joint Structures The individual components of a joint all affect the joint's mobility and stability (Figure 6.1). *Cartilage* is a strong, smooth tissue that cushions the ends of the bones, preventing them from rubbing directly against one another and providing impact protection. *Ligaments* are fibrous, connective tissues that connect bone to bone. Some ligaments form the outer layer of the *joint capsule* to provide a reinforcing structure to the overall joint. Other ligaments, not part of the joint capsule, provide further stability to the joint. The *synovial membrane* forms the inner layer of the joint capsule and secretes *synovial fluid* into the *joint cavity*. Synovial fluid lubricates and protects the joint. *Bursae (singular, bursa)* are small fluid-filled sacs that lubricate the movement of muscles over one another or muscles over bone.

Overall joint structure accounts for 47 percent of the resistance to movement around a joint, while individual *soft tissues* (muscles, connective tissue, ligaments, tendons, and skin) account for 53 percent of the resistance to movement.[8]

static flexibility The joint range-of-motion limits with an external force applied

dynamic flexibility The joint range-of-motion limits with muscular contraction applied

joint The articulation or point of contact between two or more bones

AN EXAMPLE OF THE STRETCH REFLEX

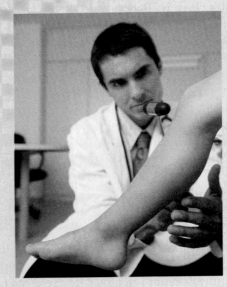

Have you ever had a doctor tap your knee and watch your leg kick out in response? The doctor was striking your *patellar tendon.* This rapidly stretches your quadriceps muscle, which triggers stretch receptors in the quadriceps to signal your nervous system. Your leg then kicks out because of a reflex contraction of your quadriceps muscle stimulated by the nervous system.

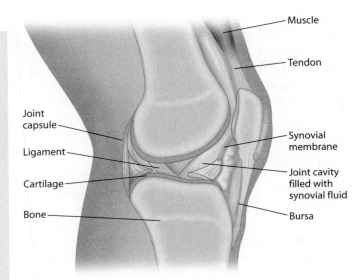

FIGURE 6.1

Joints are surrounded by a supportive joint capsule made of ligaments and synovial membranes. The joint cavity is filled with synovial fluid that (along with cartilage and bursa sacs) cushion and protect bones during movement. The stability of a joint is strengthened by muscle-tendon insertions surrounding the joint.

Muscles and Tendons Much of your flexibility range is determined by the muscles, **tendons,** and connective tissues around a joint. With regular activity and stretching, connective tissues within muscles remain supple and able to easily lengthen. With disuse and age, connective tissues become stiffer and shorter, limiting flexibility. Temperature can also affect the flexibility of soft tissues. When muscle temperature rises, connective tissues become softer and allow muscles to more easily lengthen.

tendons Connective tissues that attach muscle to bone

golgi tendon organs Muscle tension receptors located in tendons that are responsible for triggering muscle relaxation to relieve excessive muscle tension

muscle spindles (stretch receptors) Muscle length receptors located within muscle fibers that trigger muscle contractions in response to rapid, excessive muscle lengthening

stretch reflex The reflex contraction of a muscle triggered by stretch receptors (muscle spindles) in response to a rapid overextension of that muscle

The Nervous System As you learned in Chapter 5, your nervous system is responsible for stimulating muscle contractions. It also triggers muscle relaxation. Muscles and tendons contain nervous-system receptors that interpret information about the tension and length of muscles at any given moment. These receptors protect the muscle from damage caused by excessive amounts of tension or by stretching too far. If there is too much tension or force within a muscle, receptors in the tendon (called **golgi tendon organs**) will trigger your muscle to relax. If your muscle is stretching too far, receptors in the muscle fibers (called **stretch receptors** or **muscle spindles**) will trigger your muscle to contract. This reflexive contraction is called the **stretch reflex.** Reducing the stretch reflex and activating the golgi tendon organs allows your muscles to relax, elongate, and gain improvements in flexibility. The box **Spotlight: An Example of the Stretch Reflex** illustrates the reflex contraction in action.

INDIVIDUAL FACTORS

Beyond the anatomical structures and physiological mechanisms that we all share, individual factors such as genetics, gender, age, body type, and activity level also affect flexibility.

Genetics Most people have a moderate level of flexibility. They have flexible and less-flexible areas of their bodies and need to work to maintain their present level of flexibility. However, some people are extremely flexible by nature, while others are exceptionally inflexible. Genetic differences in body structure and the elasticity of soft tissues help account for the wide variety of flexibility levels.

Gender Although it is widely assumed that females are more flexible than males, this may only be true for specific joints, as discussed in the box **Understanding Diversity: Men, Women, and Flexibility.**

Age Flexibility typically improves from childhood through the preteen years and can even continue to improve throughout a person's twenties. At some point during adulthood, however, flexibility begins to decrease with age, due to physical changes in muscles and connective tissues. These changes are joint-specific and are primarily related to inactivity and disuse.

The good news is that with regular exercise, people of all ages can improve their current level of flexibility. In a study of men over 65 years of age, researchers observed flexibility improvements when the men participated in a regular resistance-training program.[9] These improvements disappeared when the men stopped training, reinforcing the notion that regular and sustained exercise is the key to maintaining and improving flexibility.

Body Type Body type can affect flexibility but typically only at the extremes of body shape and size. For example, body type may affect range of motion if an excessive amount of muscle or fat physically interferes with full joint movement. That said, genetics and training are far more influential factors in determining flexibility than is body type. There are people with long, lean bodies who you might expect to be flexible but who actually are not due to genetics or inactivity. Meanwhile, there are people with stocky, muscular builds who are exceptionally flexible, including many gymnasts.

Activity Level Inactivity can result in low levels of flexibility as muscles and connective tissues

UNDERSTANDING DIVERSITY

MEN, WOMEN, AND FLEXIBILITY

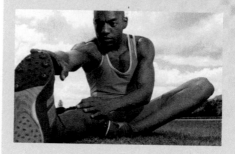

The conventional wisdom is that women are more flexible than men. Generally, females *are* more flexible in the hip joint and hamstrings, which are the most common sites for flexibility testing.[1] Females may have greater flexibility in these areas than males due to their wider hips, hormonal influences, and tendency to participate in activities that develop greater flexibility.

In other joints and areas of the body, however, there is not a large difference between males and females. In fact, males may even have greater flexibility in certain areas. For example, the ability to perform trunk flexion and trunk extension is typically the same in both males and females, but males may have greater trunk rotation capabilities.[2]

Sources:
1. J. W. Youdas, D. A. Krause, J. H. Hollman, and others, "The Influence of Gender and Age on Hamstring Muscle Length in Healthy Adults," *Journal of Orthopaedic and Sports Physical Therapy* 35, no. 4 (2005): 246–52.
2. S. A. Plowman, and D. L. Smith, *Exercise Physiology for Health, Fitness, and Performance.* 2nd ed. (Baltimore, MD: Lippincott Williams & Wilkins, 2007).

tighten and shorten with disuse. Overly repetitive physical activity can also result in muscle "stiffness." However, when done properly, stretching and regular physical activity can improve flexibility. We will introduce effective stretches and exercises later in this chapter.

Health Status Certain medical conditions can affect your joint health and range of motion. Diseases that affect your **collagen** and connective tissues can produce overly mobile or exceptionally inflexible joints. In pregnant women, the release of the hormone *relaxin* can result in more flexible joints. Injuries or scar tissue can also affect your ability to move your joints through their full range of motion.

collagen The primary protein of connective tissues (cartilage, tendons, ligaments, skin, bones) throughout the body

CASE STUDY

Mark

"I've heard that physical activity is actually supposed to improve your flexibility. If that's the case, why do my muscles feel really stiff after a long day of skiing or hiking? I've noticed that this happens especially when I've gone for my first ski or hike of the season, when the weather's right. Are my muscles just out of shape?"

1. What might explain Mark's muscle stiffness?

2. Identify at least five different factors that might play a role in Mark's flexibility.

HOW CAN YOU ASSESS YOUR FLEXIBILITY?

Flexibility levels vary from joint to joint. As a result, most flexibility tests are designed to measure the flexibility of specific muscles and joints, not to measure your body's overall level of flexibility. However, if you take a variety of flexibility tests, you can get a sense of how your body's overall level of mobility is measuring up to recommended target ranges.

PERFORM THE "SIT-AND-REACH" TEST

One of the most common measures of flexibility is the "sit-and-reach" test. This test measures the flexibility of your lower back, hip, and hamstring muscles. These areas are often tight in individuals who are inactive. This muscular imbalance can negatively influence posture, balance, and risk of back pain. *Lab 6.1* provides instructions for the sit-and-reach test.

PERFORM RANGE-OF-MOTION TESTS

Having an adequate range of motion in your joints and maintaining that range over time should be the primary goal of a flexibility fitness program. Lab 6.1 provides instructions for performing range-of-motion tests on joints located in your neck, shoulders, trunk, hips, and ankles. By performing these tests, you can evaluate how the range of motion of your joints compares to those of the general population and can determine whether your joints are more flexible or less flexible than average. This information will help you design a personalized program for developing flexibility and will allow you to measure your progress over time (by retaking the tests after months of training).

HOW CAN YOU PLAN A GOOD STRETCHING PROGRAM?

Regardless of whether or not you already stretch regularly, keep in mind the following guidelines to ensure a safe and effective program.

SET APPROPRIATE FLEXIBILITY GOALS

Decide up front what your goal is. Do you want to *maintain* your current level of flexibility (which is all that many people want to do), or do you want to *improve* your flexibility? Complete the sit-and-reach test and the range-of-motion tests described in Lab 6.1 before making this decision.

Once you've decided on your overall goal, follow the SMART guidelines for setting more specific goals. Recall that SMART stands for specific, measurable, action-oriented, realistic, and time-oriented. An example of a SMART goal designed to *maintain* your flexibility is, "My goal for the next year is to maintain the joint flexibility and range-of-motion levels recorded on my flexibility assessments by incorporating stretching into my workouts at least four times per week." An example of a SMART goal designed to *improve* your flexibility is, "My goal is to regularly stretch so that I can increase my lower-back, hip, and hamstring flexibility from 'poor' to 'good' on the sit-and-reach test by the end of the school semester."

For most people, the primary goal should be the ability to move their joints through a normal range of motion. Achieving exceptionally high levels of flexibility may be desirable for some sports and activities but is not necessary for the average person.

TABLE 6.1

ACSM's Training Guidelines for Flexibility

	Guidelines for Healthy Adults*
Frequency	2–3 days/week minimum; 5–7 days/week ideal
Intensity	Stretch to tightness at the end of the range of motion but not pain
Time	15–30 seconds per stretch repetition 2–4 repetitions of each stretching exercise
Type	Static stretching of all major muscle groups

*Older adults should stretch at least 2 days/week and include exercises to maintain or improve balance if they are at risk for falls.
Sources: American College of Sports Medicine, *ACSM's Guidelines for Exercise Testing and Prescription.* 7th edition. (Baltimore, MD: Lippincott Williams & Wilkins, 2006); M. E. Nelson, W. J. Rejeski, S. N. Blair, and others, "Physical Activity and Public Health in Older Adults: Recommendation from the American College of Sports Medicine and the American Heart Association," *Circulation* 116 (2007): 1094–1105. Available at: http://circ.ahajournals.org/cgi/reprint/CIRCULATIONAHA.107.185650 (accessed August 11, 2007).

APPLY THE FITT PROGRAM DESIGN PRINCIPLES

Recall that FITT stands for frequency, intensity, time, and type. Use the FITT principles to design your own personalized stretching program. Table 6.1 provides general guidelines from the American College of Sports Medicine. Refer to this table as a starting point for designing your own program.

Frequency: How Often Should You Stretch?

Notice that the ACSM guidelines in Table 6.1 recommend stretching anywhere from 2 to 3 days/week to 5 to 7 days/week. If you've determined that your current level of flexibility is already within "normal" ranges and merely want to maintain that level, you should stretch at least 2 to 3 days/week. If you've determined that your current level of flexibility needs improvement in order to reach a "normal" range, you should stretch more frequently.

Should you stretch before a workout, after a workout, or both? The box **Facts and Fallacies: Common Misconceptions about Stretching** explores these questions and others.

Intensity: How Far Should You Stretch?

The ACSM guidelines state that you should "stretch to tightness at the end of the range of motion, but not pain." Stretches should always be done just to the point of mild discomfort. If you are feeling pain, you are stretching too far and risking injury. Pay close attention to your body whenever you stretch—your flexibility level may vary slightly from day to day.

Time: How Long Should You Hold a Stretch? How Many Times Should You Repeat a Stretch?

The ACSM guidelines state that you should hold stretches for 15 to 30 seconds each, and repeat stretches 2 to 4 times per session. As soon as you start to stretch, your stretch reflex will activate: You can feel this as a slight increase in muscle tension when you move into a stretch position. By holding your stretches for at least 15 seconds, you are giving the stretch reflex time to lessen. You are also giving your golgi tendon organ time to activate and allowing your muscles to lengthen farther.

By repeating stretches multiple times, you enable your muscles to relax and lengthen a little bit more each time (up to four repetitions). If you are beginning a stretching program for the first time and feel uncomfortable with multiple repetitions, you can perform one repetition of each stretch and still obtain benefits. After a few weeks of stretching consistently, increase the number of repetitions to the recommended range of 2 to 4 times/session.

Type: What Kind of Stretches Should You Do?

There are numerous kinds of stretching techniques. The most common are highlighted below.

- **Static stretching** involves moving slowly into a stretch and holding it for a prescribed amount of time. This is the simplest and safest method for individuals who are just starting a stretching

static stretching Stretching characterized by slow and sustained muscle lengthening

FACTS AND FALLACIES

COMMON MISCONCEPTIONS ABOUT STRETCHING

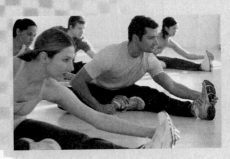

Below are answers to some common questions (and misconceptions) about stretching.

Should I stretch before a workout, after a workout, or both?

In general, it is better to perform static stretches after a workout, when your muscles have warmed up and your joint structures are more receptive to stretching. However, if you are in the habit of stretching before a workout, that is fine, too—so long as you thoroughly warm up before you stretch and stick to *light* stretching. What you want to avoid is overstretching cold muscles, which can result in injury. If you warm up properly first, you can stretch at any time of day and improve your flexibility.[1]

I have heard that pre-exercise stretching can actually hurt performance in some instances. Is this true?

Research has found that extensive static stretching results in a reduction in muscle strength and power

that can last 30 minutes or more.[2] Therefore, serious athletes may want to avoid static stretching before a competition or workout. For most individuals, however, pre-exercise static stretches of 30 seconds or less will not negatively affect exercise or recreational performance.

Does pre-exercise stretching reduce my chances of injury or muscle soreness?

Contrary to popular belief, there is no conclusive evidence that pre-exercise stretching helps prevent sports injuries or muscle soreness.[3] In fact, there is no definitive support for *or* against stretching anytime (before or after a workout) to reduce injury. Although more research needs to be done, the recommendations now include stretching for maintaining mobility in joints, but not as a primary means to reduce injury or enhance performance.

Sources:
1. G. G. Haff (ed.), "Round Table Discussion: Flexibility Training," *Strength and Conditioning Journal* 28, no. 2 (2006): 64–85.
2. T. Yamaguchi, and K. Ishii, "Effects of Static Stretching for 30 Seconds and Dynamic Stretching on Leg Extension Power," *Journal of Strength and Conditioning Research* 19, no. 3 (2005): 677–83.
3. S. B. Thacker and others, "The Impact of Stretching on Sports Injury Risk: A Systematic Review of the Literature," *Medicine and Science in Sports and Exercise* 36, no. 3 (2004): 371–78.

program. Static stretching is effective, because the activity of slow stretching and holding reduces the activation of stretch receptors. After a workout, static stretching can help muscles recover and help you to maintain or improve your flexibility.

- **Dynamic stretching** involves stretching through movement. During dynamic stretching, you mimic the motions of your workout or sports activity with slow, fluid movements. Dynamic stretching increases dynamic flexibility and can enhance muscle power.[10] The warm-up

phase of an exercise session is a good time to implement dynamic stretching, because it helps prepare the body for the more intense physical activity to come.

- **Ballistic stretching** is a stretching method characterized by bouncing, sometimes jerky, movements and high momentum. Ballistic stretching increases dynamic flexibility and can benefit trained athletes in sports requiring fast, explosive movements such as wrestling, gymnastics, tennis, and basketball. However, the bouncing movements in ballistic stretching rapidly activates the stretch receptors, making this method less effective at increasing static flexibility and increasing the risk of stretching-related injuries. For these reasons, ballistic stretching is not recommended for the average exerciser.

- **Proprioceptive neuromuscular facilitation (PNF)** uses the voluntary contraction of muscle groups to help facilitate relaxation and stretching in target muscles. The most common method of PNF stretching is called *contract-relax PNF*. In contract-relax PNF, the exerciser experiences an isotonic or isometric contraction of the target

dynamic stretching Stretching characterized by controlled, full-range-of-motion movements that mimic exercise session movements

ballistic stretching Stretching characterized by bouncing, jerky movements and momentum to increase range of motion

proprioceptive neuromuscular facilitation (PNF) Stretching that is facilitated or enhanced by the voluntary contraction of the targeted muscle group or contraction of opposing muscles

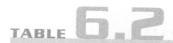

Pros and Cons of Common Stretching Methods

Stretching Method	Pro	Con
Static	Safe, simple to use, effective at increasing static flexibility	Can reduce muscle strength and power immediately after stretching, can be time-consuming
Dynamic	Increases dynamic flexibility, functional, safer than ballistic stretching	Potential for injury, time to learn correct movement patterns
Ballistic	Can be beneficial for ballistic sports, increases dynamic flexibility	Large potential for injury, not as effective at increasing overall flexibility
PNF	Effective at increasing flexibility levels	Need a partner or equipment to perform, potential for injury, complicated method

muscle just prior to slow, passive stretching of that muscle. For an example of contract-relax PNF in action, lie on your back, bend the knee of one leg, and lift your other leg toward the ceiling. Have a partner hold your lifted leg and provide resistance as you try to lower your leg to the ground. Your partner can either resist enough to allow no movement at all (resulting in an isometric contraction) or just enough to allow slow, gradual movement (resulting in an isotonic contraction). The muscle contraction stimulates the golgi tendon organs in the muscle to activate and promote muscle relaxation. Immediately following the 5- to 10-second contraction, have your partner move your leg up and toward your chest into a **passive stretch** for the hamstrings and hips. Hold this stretch for 15 to 30 seconds and release.

Table 6.2 lists some of the pros and cons of each stretching method.

CONSIDER TAKING A CLASS

If you would like more structure and instruction in your stretching program, consider enrolling in a class. Yoga (Figure 6.2), tai chi, Pilates, and dance classes can be fun, effective ways to maintain or improve your flexibility.

Yoga originated in India about 5,000 years ago and has become a highly popular activity in the United States. The practice of yoga requires a combination of mental focus and physical effort while performing a variety of postures, or *asanas*. The physical aspect of yoga results in improvements in flexibility, posture, agility, balance, stamina, muscle endurance, and coordination. The mental aspect of yoga promotes attention, controlled breathing, relaxation, a union of mind and body, and an overall psychological sense of well-being.

Tai chi is a martial art that was developed in ancient China by monks wanting to defend themselves. Tai chi practice involves a slow-moving, smooth, and continuous series of positions or forms. These exercises increase balance, muscle endurance, flexibility, and coordination; they also reduce anxiety and stress. Tai chi has become popular with many people, but older individuals in particular are drawn to this safe and effective way to exercise.

Pilates was developed by Joseph Pilates in New York City in the 1920s. Pilates involves performing a sequence of exercises on a mat or specialized equipment designed to stretch and strengthen muscles. Specific breathing patterns are combined with stretching and resistance exercises to increase flexibility and muscle endurance, particularly in the core trunk-supporting muscles.

Dance is a fantastic way to improve your flexibility and your overall fitness level. A group exercise

passive stretch A stretch that involves an outside force (such as a partner, your arms, weight, or gravity) to stretch targeted muscle groups. In contrast, an **active stretch** involves the contraction of the opposing muscle groups to stretch targeted muscle groups.

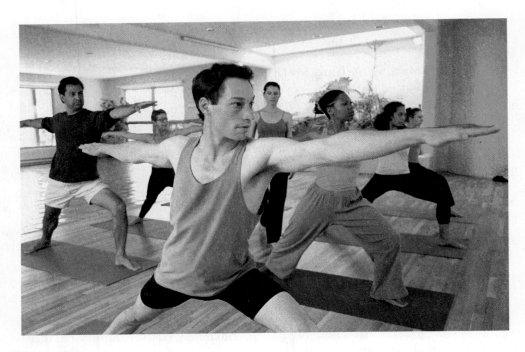

FIGURE 6.2

Yoga classes can be a great way to improve flexibility.

class, like aerobic dance, will usually give you a chance to work on your flexibility during the cooldown phase. Whether you play a dance-moves video game, hit the dance clubs at night, or take a dance class, you can regularly "stretch" your body and your creative spirit.

All of the activities described above require instruction by a trained professional, especially since some exercises can be risky for the untrained or novice participant.

If you prefer to stretch on your own, Figure 6.3 provides several common stretching exercises you can select from, and Table 6.3 provides sample exercise programs for you to follow. *Lab6.3* walks you through the process of designing your own program.

CASE STUDY

Mark

"The ski season just started again, and out of curiosity, I asked a ski instructor for his opinions on stretching. He was surprised that I have been skiing my whole life but wasn't in the habit of stretching! He explained how stretching can help reduce muscle tension, improve my ability to make quick turns, and help prevent strains and stiffness. He recommended quadricep and hamstring stretches, for starters. He also suggested some stretching exercises that mimic the motion of skiing, in case I ever wanted to try skiing at a more advanced level."

1. Look at the quadricep and hamstring stretches in Figure 6.3. Are these static or dynamic stretches? Explain the difference.

2. Assume that Mark wants to begin a general stretching program in the "off" season when he is not skiing, with the goal of improving his flexibility. Given the ACSM guidelines you have learned, what would you recommend that he do?

FIGURE **6.3** STRETCHES TO MAINTAIN OR INCREASE FLEXIBILITY*

All standing stretches should be started or performed from a good posture position (abs pulled in, feet facing forward, knees slightly bent). All one-arm or one-leg stretches should be performed on both sides. Hold stretches for 15 to 30 seconds. Refer to Figure 5.7 in Chapter 5 for the full-body muscle diagram.

*Videos for many of these exercises are available at www.aw-bc.com/hopson.

Upper-Body Stretches

1. Neck Stretches

(a) **Head turn:** Gently turn your head to look over one shoulder, keeping both of your shoulders down.

(b) **Head tilt:** Keeping your chin level and your shoulders down, tilt your head to one side.

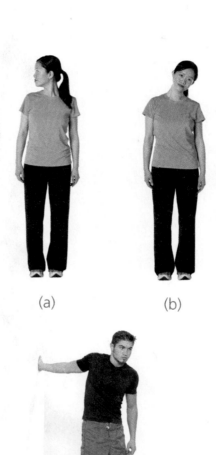

(a)   (b)

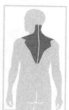

Muscles targeted:

10 Trapezius; various neck muscles

2. Pectoral and Bicep Stretch

Stand arm's length away from a wall. Reach your arm out to the side and place your palm flat on the wall. Turn your body away from the wall until you feel a comfortable stretch.

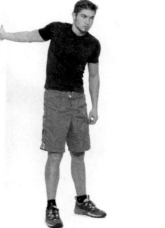

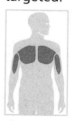

Muscles targeted:

1 Pectoralis major
2 Biceps brachii

3. Upper-Back Stretch

Reach your arms out in front of you and clasp your hands while rounding out your back and lowering your head.

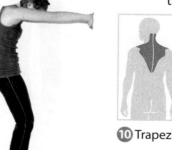

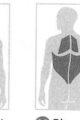

Muscles targeted:

10 Trapezius
11 Rhomboids
14 Latissimus dorsi

4. Side Stretch

Reach one straight arm over your head and bend sideways at the waist. Focus on the reaching up and over with your arm. The opposite hand can reach for the floor or be placed at your hip.

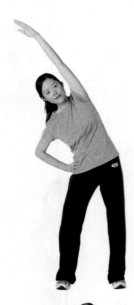

Muscles targeted:

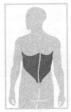
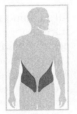

14 Latissimus dorsi   **4** External obliques

5. Shoulder Stretch

Reach one arm across the chest and hold it above or below the elbow with the other hand.

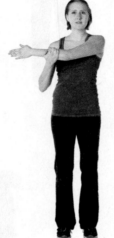

Muscles targeted:

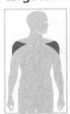

9 Deltoids

6. Tricep Stretch

Lift your arm overhead, reaching the elbow toward the ceiling and the hand down the back. Assist the stretch by using your other hand to either (a) press the arm back from the front or (b) reach over your head, grasp your arm just below the elbow, and pull back and toward your head.

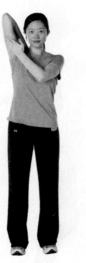
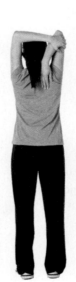

(a)   (b)

Muscles targeted:

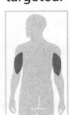

13 Triceps brachii

Lower-Body Stretches

7. Low-Back Knee-to-Chest Stretch

Lie on your back on a mat and lift either (a) one knee or (b) two knees toward the chest, grasping the leg(s) from behind for support.

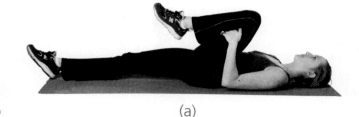

(a)

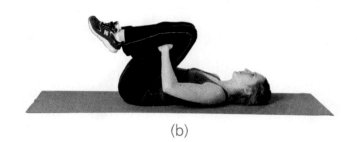

(b)

Muscles targeted:

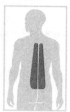

12 Erector spinae; various hip muscles

8. Torso Twist and Hip Stretch

(a) Seated twist: Sit on a mat with your legs straight out in front of you. Bend one knee and cross that leg over your other leg. Turn your body toward the bent knee and twist your body to look behind you. Place the opposite arm on the bent leg to gently press into the stretch further.

(b) Lying cross-leg twist: While lying on your back, bend both knees and cross one over the other. Gently lower your legs sideways toward the knee that is closest to you.

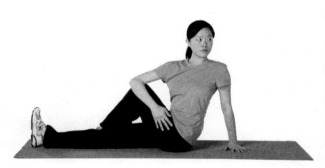

(a)

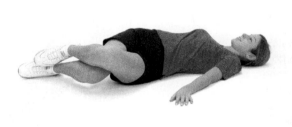

(b)

Muscles targeted:

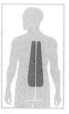

12 Erector spinae

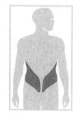

4 External obliques

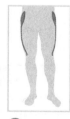

5 Tensor fasciae latae

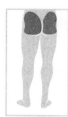

15 Gluteus maximus

9. Hip Flexor Stretch

(a) Standing stretch: Stand tall with one foot forward and one foot back in a lunge position. Lift up the heel of the back leg and press your hips forward.

(b) Low lunge stretch: Lunge forward and gently place your back knee on a mat and release your foot to point back. Lean forward into the hip and thigh stretch but make sure that your front ankle is directly under your front knee and not in front of it.

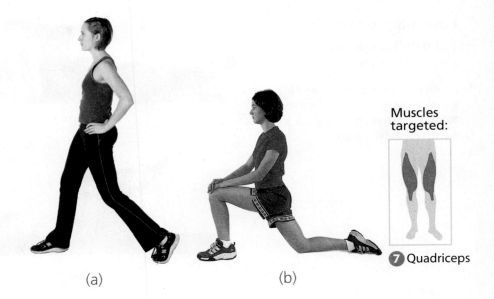

(a) (b)

Muscles targeted:

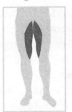

7 Quadriceps

10. Inner-Thigh Butterfly Stretch

Sitting on a mat, bring the bottoms of your feet together and pull your feet gently toward you. Actively contract your hip muscles to lower your knees closer to the ground.

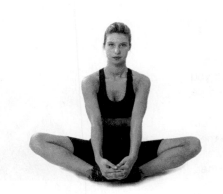

Muscles targeted:

6 Adductors

11. Outer-Thigh Stretch

Stand arm's length next to a wall. Place your outside foot on the floor closer to the wall, crossing over the inside leg. Lean your hip closer to the wall while you lean your upper body away from the wall for balance.

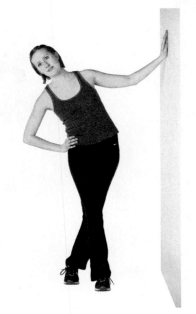

Muscles targeted:

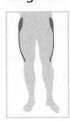

5 Tensor fasciae latae

12. Quadriceps Stretch

Grab your foot from behind and pull it back toward your rear until you feel a stretch in the front of your thighs. Maintain straight body alignment and keep your thighs parallel to one another. When (a) standing, assist your balance by holding a wall, chair, or another form of support. The stretch can also be done from a (b) lying down position.

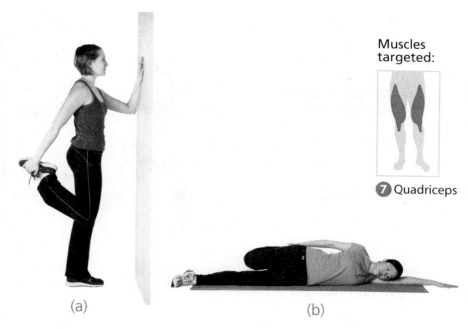

(a)

(b)

Muscles targeted:

7 Quadriceps

13. Hamstrings Stretch

(a) Modified hurdler stretch: Sit with one leg extended and the other leg bent. The bent leg should have the knee facing sideways and the foot placed next to the extended leg near the calf, knee, or thigh. Keeping your back as straight as possible, lean your body forward, moving your chest closer to your extended leg. Your hands can be placed on the floor next to your knee, calf, or ankle for support. If you are moderately flexible, you can reach for and hold your foot but only if this does not cause pain.

(b) Supine lying: Lying on your back, bend one knee and extend the other toward the ceiling. Support the stretch by placing your hands or a towel above or below the knee. As you become more flexible, work at bringing your leg closer to your chest.

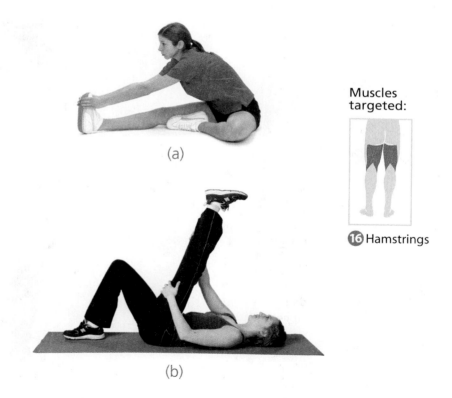

(a)

(b)

Muscles targeted:

16 Hamstrings

14. Calf Stretches

(a) Gastrocnemius lunge: Lean into a wall in a lunge position, extending one leg straight behind you. Press the heel of your straight leg into the floor as you lean your body and hips into the wall.

(b) Gastrocnemius heel drop: Stand tall and place your toes on a raised surface (mat or step) that will not tip over. Balance by holding on to a wall for support, as you lower your heels toward the floor.

(c) Soleus stretch: Starting in a lunge position (a), bend the back knee until you feel a stretch in the soleus muscle.

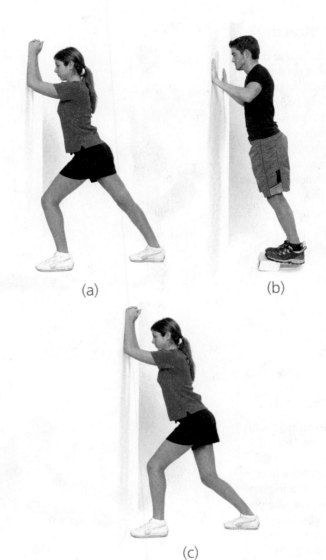

(a)

(b)

(c)

Muscles targeted:

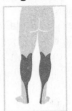

17 Gastrocnemius

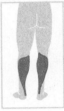

18 Soleus

15. Shin Stretch

Reach one leg behind you and place the tips of your toes on the ground. Bend both knees and lower the body slightly as you press the top of your back foot toward the ground. You can use a wall for support if needed.

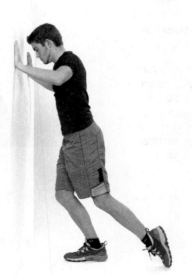

Muscles targeted:

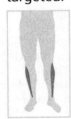

8 Tibialis anterior

TABLE 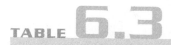 6.3

Sample Stretching Programs

Beginner Stretching Program

Exercise	Muscles Targeted	Length (sec)	Reps	Total Time (sec)
Head Tilt	Trapezius and neck muscles	15	2	30
Side Stretch	Latissimus dorsi, external obliques	20	2	40
Shoulder Stretch	Deltoids	15	2	30
Low-Back Knee-to-Chest Stretch	Erector spinae and various hip muscles	15	3	45
Standing Hip Flexor Stretch	Quadriceps and hip flexors	20	2	40
Seated Hamstring Stretch	Hamstrings	15	3	45
Lunge Calf Stretch	Gastrocnemius	15	2	30

Intermediate Stretching Program

Exercise	Muscles Targeted	Length (sec)	Reps	Total Time (sec)
Head Tilt	Trapezius and neck muscles	15	3	45
Upper-Back Stretch	Trapezius, rhomboids, latissimus dorsi	20	3	60
Side Stretch	Latissimus dorsi, external obliques	20	3	60
Shoulder Stretch	Deltoids	20	3	60
Tricep Stretch	Triceps	15	3	45
Torso Twist and Hip Stretch	Erector spinae, external obliques, tensor fasciae latae, and the gluteus maximus	20	3	60
Low Lunge Hip Flexor Stretch	Quadriceps and hip flexors	20	3	60
Outer-Thigh Stretch	Tensor fasciae latae	15	3	45
Quadriceps Stretch	Quadriceps	20	3	60
Lying Hamstring Stretch	Hamstrings	25	3	75
Heel Drop Calf Stretch	Gastrocnemius	20	3	60
Soleus Calf Stretch	Soleus	15	3	45

HOW CAN YOU AVOID STRETCHING-RELATED INJURIES?

Although we used to think of stretching as a way to avoid injury, we now know that stretching can actually *cause* injury if done improperly. To avoid a stretching-related injury, adhere to the following guidelines.

STRETCH ONLY WARM MUSCLES

An increase in body temperature prepares the joint fluid and structures for stretching and improves muscle elasticity. These changes allow you a greater range of motion while stretching. Static stretches, in particular, should be performed *after* a workout, when the muscles have been sufficiently warmed up.

PERFORM STRETCHES SAFELY

One of the keys to safe and effective stretching is to avoid activating stretch receptors when you want a muscle to relax. Stretch receptors are activated when muscles are lengthened rapidly. Muscle injury can occur from quick, bouncing movements, because

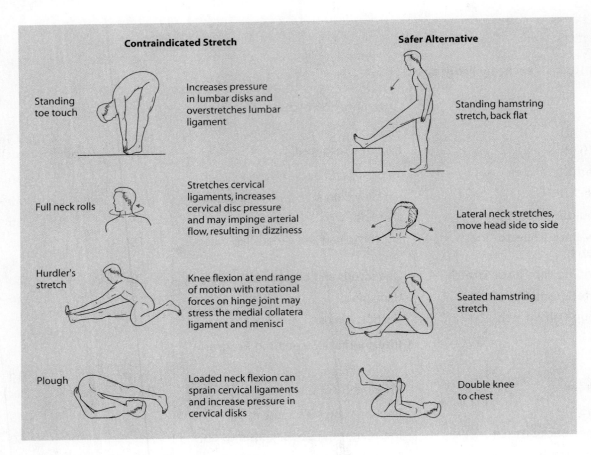

Contraindicated Stretch		Safer Alternative	
Standing toe touch	Increases pressure in lumbar disks and overstretches lumbar ligament	Standing hamstring stretch, back flat	
Full neck rolls	Stretches cervical ligaments, increases cervical disc pressure and may impinge arterial flow, resulting in dizziness	Lateral neck stretches, move head side to side	
Hurdler's stretch	Knee flexion at end range of motion with rotational forces on hinge joint may stress the medial collatera ligament and menisci	Seated hamstring stretch	
Plough	Loaded neck flexion can sprain cervical ligaments and increase pressure in cervical disks	Double knee to chest	

FIGURE 6.4

Avoid these common higher-risk contraindicated stretches and perform the safer alternatives instead.

Source: ACSM's Guidelines for Exercise Testing and Prescription, 7/e. Copyright © ACSM. Reprinted by permission of Wolters/Kluwer.

the muscle is lengthening too far too quickly, and the stretch reflex is creating tension at the same time. Avoid the stretch reflex by stretching carefully and slowly. Holding your stretches for up to 30 seconds will allow the stretch receptors and golgi tendon organ receptors to make nervous system adjustments. These adjustments will allow further relaxation and lengthening of the muscles involved.

KNOW WHICH EXERCISES
CAN CAUSE INJURY

Figure 6.4 shows common high-risk or **contraindicated** stretches with safer alternatives. Note that this figure is *not* an all-inclusive list. Choosing safe exercises is a highly individual process. Consider your personal limitations and

contraindicated Not recommended for everyone

health issues when deciding which exercises are best for your body.

BE ESPECIALLY CAUTIOUS
IF YOU ARE A HYPERFLEXIBLE
OR INFLEXIBLE PERSON

If you are really flexible, you may need to be more careful while stretching than the average exerciser. Excessive hypermobility increases joint laxity or looseness, decreases joint stability, and can lead to permanent changes in connective tissue. Take precautions to avoid overstretching, which may lead to injury or decreases in exercise performance. For example, if you are taking a yoga class, let your instructor know that you are hyperflexible and ask if there are any modified poses that would reduce your risk of overstretching.

Inflexibility is common in many people. If you have limited range of motion in one or more joints, avoid stretching beyond your abilities. Work gradually to improve your range of motion and overall flexibility. People with a very limited range of motion may be more susceptible to sudden acute injuries during sports, to activity-related injuries during daily-living tasks, and to lower-back injuries.

HOW CAN YOU PREVENT OR MANAGE BACK PAIN?

While you are young, back pain is probably the furthest thing from your mind. However, lower-back pain affects at least 80 percent of the general U.S. population at some point in life, and affects 20 to 30 percent of Americans at any given moment.[11] Research has shown that college students are not immune to back-health issues. In one study, 71 percent of students reported regular lower-back pain, most reported poor flexibility and posture, and a majority reported being unsure of what to do for back care.[12] Lower-back pain is the most common cause of job-related disability, and Americans spend over $50 billion each year treating its symptoms.[13]

Factors that increase your risk of lower-back pain include obesity, smoking, pregnancy, stress, inactivity, weak and inflexible muscles, and poor posture. In addition, a number of events can trigger back pain or cause a back injury, including accidents, sports injuries, repetitive movements, work trauma, and excessive sitting—especially if you already have other risk factors.

In the next sections, we will cover the causes of back pain, explain how the spine is structured and supported, and present strategies to reduce your risk of back pain. For those who already experience regular episodes of back pain, the next sections will also discuss ways to effectively manage, resolve, and prevent future recurrences of back pain.

UNDERSTAND THE PRIMARY CAUSES OF BACK PAIN

You experience back pain when your movement causes a sprain, strain, or spasm in one of the muscles, tendons, or ligaments in the back. You may also feel pain when your spine structures become misaligned or injured and the spinal nerves become compressed or irritated. Back pain can also result from age- or disease-related degeneration of the bones and joints of the spine. Ultimately, most back pain is caused by a *sedentary lifestyle,* which results in muscle weakness, inflexibility, and imbalance—all conditions that can lead to poor posture and body mechanics and to a higher risk of back pain and injury.

Muscular Weakness, Inflexibility, and Imbalance
Most back pain is related to muscle or tendon injuries. The supporting musculature of the spine is important for maintaining healthy posture, mobility, and spine structures. Weakness and inflexibility in key muscles can lead to muscular imbalances that affect the alignment of your spine. Weak abdominals, for instance, can cause your pelvis to rock forward and create a greater curvature in your lower back. This puts more pressure on spine structures and other spine-supporting muscles, potentially leading to back pain. Inflexible, tight hip flexor muscles can also cause a forward tilt of the pelvis and an increased curvature of the lower back.

Muscles become weak when they are not used on a regular basis. Repetitive movements or long hours of sitting can also cause muscles to shorten and tighten up. Some people have muscles of differing strength and flexibility levels around the spine and other joints. If your spine-supporting musculature does not have a muscle balance that promotes good posture and body mechanics, you may have back pain or injury in the future.

Improper Posture and Body Mechanics
Improper posture can lead to increased forces within the spine structures and eventually to back pain. Altered body mechanics resulting from improper posture puts you at risk for injury during all of your daily activities, but especially during exercise and sports activities.

Acute Trauma, Risky Occupations, and Medical Issues
Acute trauma to the back can happen to anyone at any age. Trauma could be the result of a car accident, a sports and recreation injury, or any other accident that affects the spine. Avoiding risky sports and recreational activities will reduce your chance of trauma.

Jobs that involve a lot of bending, twisting, and repeated lifting of heavy objects put workers at especially high risk of developing back pain. Jobs that involve a great deal of sitting every day are also considered high risk. Occupations with a high incidence of back pain include truck driving, nursing, firefighting, construction, and some professional sports (e.g., football, power lifting, golf, and wrestling). Occupations that are highly stressful and require long hours also increase the risk of back pain. Stress is a risk factor for back injury, but long hours at work can reduce the time you have to exercise and relax, further increasing the risk of developing back pain.

Medical issues and individual health factors can also significantly increase your chance of developing lower-back pain. For instance, smokers have an increased risk of low-back pain due to vascular damage, which facilitates disc degeneration.[14] Obesity and weight gain during pregnancy can increase lower-back pain due to greater loads on the spine, misalignment of the pelvis and low back, and muscular weakness. Pain can also result from degenerative conditions such as arthritis or disc disease, osteoporosis or other bone diseases, congenital abnormalities, viral infections, and general conditions that cause irritation to joints or discs.[15]

UNDERSTAND HOW THE BACK IS SUPPORTED

The back is comprised of bones, muscles, and other tissues that form the back side of your trunk. The trunk contains your essential organs and bears the weight of your upper body. It is also responsible for transmitting forces and movements from the upper limbs to the lower limbs, and vice versa. If something is amiss with your back or your trunk overall, any upper- or lower-body movement can be difficult. Your back and trunk are supported by the bony structures of the spine and by the core trunk muscles.

The Structure of the Spine The spine or *spinal column* (also called the *vertebral column*) is the series of bones called *vertebrae* that connect the upper-body and lower-body skeleton and protect the spinal cord. Figure 6.5 shows the basic structure of the spine. Note that the spine has four distinct regions and curvatures: *cervical, thoracic, lumbar,* and *sacral.* The curvatures are an essential part of the force-absorbing capabilities of the spine.

Intervertebral disks are round, spongy pads of cartilage that act as shock absorbers. The disks have fibrous outer rings that are filled with gel and waterlike substances that will distend slightly when compressed. That distention acts to absorb shock. The disks also ensure that there is adequate space between the vertebra. When a change in body mechanics or posture occurs—or when an acute injury occurs—the resulting change to spinal alignment can damage the disk structures.

disk herniation A permanent bulging of an intervertebral disc out of its normal space

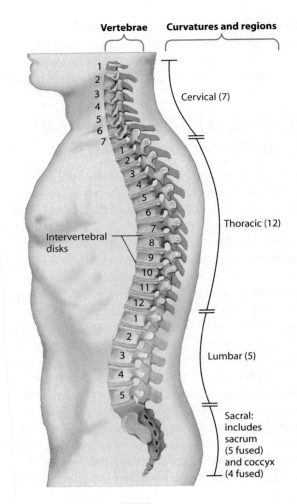

FIGURE 6.5

The spine has four distinct regions and curvatures (cervical, thoracic, lumbar, and sacral) made up of individual or fused vertebrae.

A permanent bulging of the disk out of the normal space is called a **disk herniation.** The disk can bulge toward the spinal column or nerves and cause pain or numbness in the back or other areas of the body. Disk herniations most often occur in the lower lumbar region, where most of the body weight and forces are applied.

Another problem that occurs with trauma or aging is dehydration, hardening, or degeneration of intervertebral disks. Without adequate fluid content and elasticity, disks cannot perform their shock-absorber role very well. The resulting smaller joint space between vertebrae applies pressure to the spinal nerves. This can cause back, hip, or leg pain and muscle weakness. Healthy spinal nerves are essential for sending messages for contraction to your skeletal muscles.

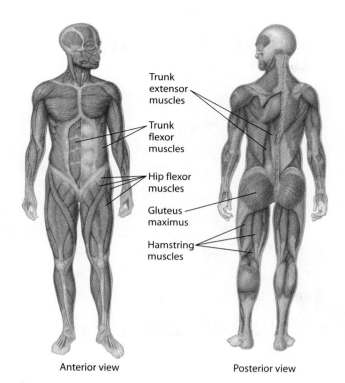

FIGURE 6.6

Strengthening and stretching of the spine-supporting core muscles is essential for a healthy back. The core muscles include extensors of the trunk and hip and flexors of the trunk and hip.

Labels on figure:
- Trunk extensor muscles
- Trunk flexor muscles
- Hip flexor muscles
- Gluteus maximus
- Hamstring muscles
- Anterior view
- Posterior view

The Core Trunk Muscles

The bones of the spinal column could not maintain their healthy curvatures and an upright posture without supporting muscles. Core trunk muscles support the trunk while you are standing, sitting, lying down, or moving. These muscles, located all around your body (Figure 6.6), are essential for supporting the spine and for performing sports, recreation, and everyday activities. **Core muscles** include back, abdominal, hip, gluteal, pelvis, pelvic floor, and lateral trunk muscles. Core muscles work together to effectively transmit forces between your upper and lower body. While weak core muscles can lead to back pain, strong core muscles can lead to increased performance levels in all of your activities.

REDUCE YOUR RISK OF LOWER-BACK PAIN

You can reduce your risk of back pain by improving your body weight, muscle fitness, posture, and movement techniques. Although exercise in general has not been shown to prevent lower-back pain,[16] specific muscle fitness exercises will help stabilize your key spine-supporting muscles.

Lose Weight

The prevalence of lower-back pain rises with increases in body mass index or body weight.[17] An increase in body weight puts extra strain and pressure on all the spinal structures. If the additional weight resides in the abdominal region, the pelvis may get pulled forward and result in a greater curvature of the lower back, causing back pain. Lowering your weight and body fat levels to within recommended ranges will reduce your risk of lower-back pain.

Strengthen and Stretch Key Muscles

Most people's bodies have "weak" muscle areas, "tight" muscle areas, and areas that are both weak *and* tight.

- *Hip flexor muscles* tend to be tight in most people. This stems from extended sitting, resulting in shortened and inactive muscles. If you have tight hip flexor muscles, add hip flexor stretches (see Figure 6.3) to your weekly workout.

- *Hip extensor muscles* also tend to be tight and weak in many people and can benefit from stretching and strengthening.

- *Trunk flexor muscles* (abdominals) are often weak in individuals who are sedentary or overweight. Having a minimal level of strength in your abdominal muscles will help protect your spine and back and improve your exercise performance.

- *Trunk extensor muscles* are responsible for keeping your spine upright while sitting, standing, and moving. If you do a lot of hunched-over sitting, these muscles are probably weak, and you should add safe back extensor strengthening exercises to your program.

The simplest prescription for back health is to maintain a healthy weight and an active lifestyle. If you are predisposed to back pain due to other reasons (e.g., hyperflexibility, sport history, occupation), try to add some specific back health exercises to your current exercise routine. Figure 6.7 illustrates back health exercises that will help you stretch or strengthen these key areas of the trunk and hips.

core muscles Musculature that supports the trunk (back, spine, abdomen, and hips)

FIGURE **6.7** **EXERCISES FOR A HEALTHY BACK***

Refer to Figure 5.7 in Chapter 5 for the muscle diagram. Perform 3 to 10 repetitions of the back health exercises, holding where appropriate for 15 to 30 seconds.

*Videos for many of these exercises are available at www.aw-bc.com/hopson.

1. Cat Stretch

Start on your hands and knees with a flat back. Looking at the ground, align your head with your spine. Drop your head and look back toward your knees while lifting your upper back toward the ceiling.

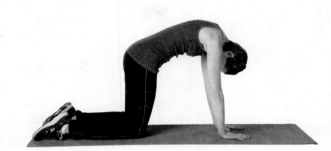

Muscles targeted:

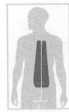 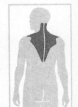

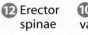 **12** Erector spinae   **10** Trapezius; various neck muscles

2. Arm/Leg Extensions

Start on your hands and knees with a flat back. Looking at the ground, align your head with your spine. Extend your arm straight out in front of you while extending the opposite leg straight out behind you. Keep your arm and leg in a straight line with your spine. Do not lift them too high, because this causes too much arch in your lower back.

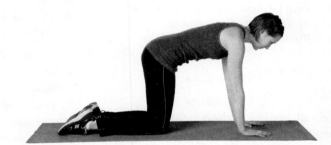

Muscles targeted:

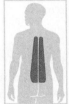 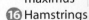

12 Erector spinae   **15** Gluteus maximus
16 Hamstrings

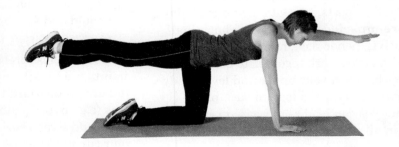

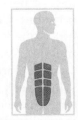

3 Rectus abdominus

3. Pelvic Tilt

Lie on your back with your knees bent and your feet flat on the floor. Relax in a comfortable posture, letting the natural curve of your spine bring your lower back off the mat. Breathe out as you tilt the bottom of your pelvis toward the ceiling, pulling your abdominals in and pressing your lower back flat against the floor.

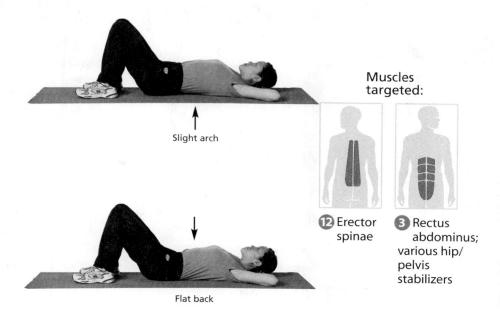

Slight arch

Flat back

Muscles targeted:

12 Erector spinae

3 Rectus abdominus; various hip/ pelvis stabilizers

4. Back Bridge

Lie on your back with your knees bent, your feet flat on the floor, and your arms extended straight along your sides. Lift your hips off the ground and press your pelvis toward the ceiling until your thighs and back are in a straight line. Look at the ceiling and keep your neck extended throughout the exercise (do not tuck your chin to your chest).

Other exercises that can help maintain back health include the plank (p. 139), side bridge (p. 138), knee-to-chest stretch (p. 171), hamstring stretch (p. 173), torso twist and hip stretch (p. 171), hip flexor stretch (p. 172), abdominal curl (p. 137), reverse curl (p. 138), and oblique curl (p. 138).

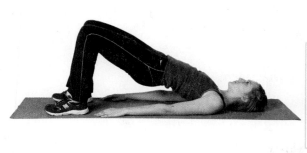

Muscles targeted:

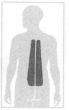

12 Erector spinae

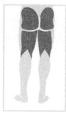

15 Gluteus maximus

16 Hamstrings; various hip muscles

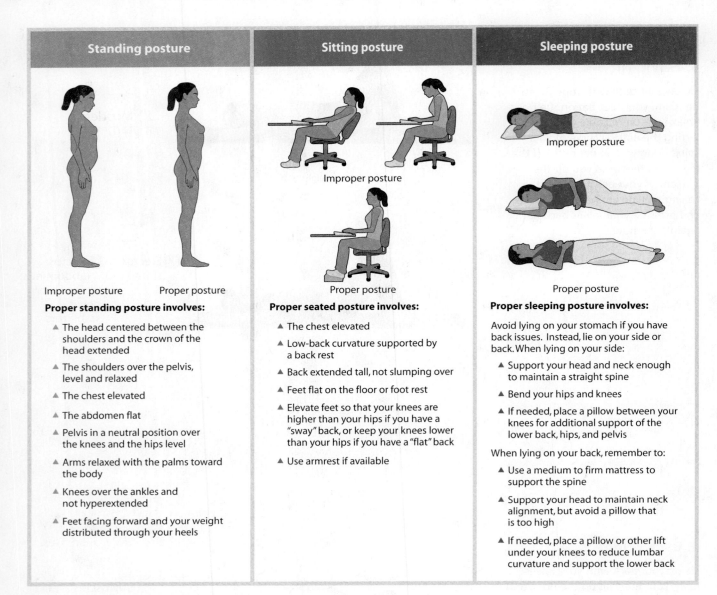

Standing posture	Sitting posture	Sleeping posture

Standing posture

Improper posture   Proper posture

Proper standing posture involves:

▲ The head centered between the shoulders and the crown of the head extended

▲ The shoulders over the pelvis, level and relaxed

▲ The chest elevated

▲ The abdomen flat

▲ Pelvis in a neutral position over the knees and the hips level

▲ Arms relaxed with the palms toward the body

▲ Knees over the ankles and not hyperextended

▲ Feet facing forward and your weight distributed through your heels

Sitting posture

Improper posture

Proper posture

Proper seated posture involves:

▲ The chest elevated

▲ Low-back curvature supported by a back rest

▲ Back extended tall, not slumping over

▲ Feet flat on the floor or foot rest

▲ Elevate feet so that your knees are higher than your hips if you have a "sway" back, or keep your knees lower than your hips if you have a "flat" back

▲ Use armrest if available

Sleeping posture

Improper posture

Proper posture

Proper sleeping posture involves:

Avoid lying on your stomach if you have back issues. Instead, lie on your side or back. When lying on your side:

▲ Support your head and neck enough to maintain a straight spine

▲ Bend your hips and knees

▲ If needed, place a pillow between your knees for additional support of the lower back, hips, and pelvis

When lying on your back, remember to:

▲ Use a medium to firm mattress to support the spine

▲ Support your head to maintain neck alignment, but avoid a pillow that is too high

▲ If needed, place a pillow or other lift under your knees to reduce lumbar curvature and support the lower back

FIGURE 6.8

Proper posture is important for back health.

Maintain Good Posture and Proper Body Mechanics

If you have strong and flexible core trunk muscles, maintaining good posture and body mechanics is easier. The problem is that even with good muscular fitness, poor posture can become a habit. You might always hunch over at the computer and feel unnatural sitting up straight. Maybe you slouch back on the couch when you are watching TV. Over time, poor posture can create back problems.

Poor posture and poor muscle fitness can also lead to improper body mechanics while you perform everyday activities. Poor body mechanics put you at risk of muscle strain and back pain. *Lab6.2* teaches you how to evaluate your posture, and Figure 6.8 illustrates proper postures for standing, sitting, and lying down.

PROPERLY TREAT LOWER-BACK PAIN

If you already experience regular back pain, you can do things to help manage your pain and prevent future recurrences. The box **Tools For Change: Managing Back Pain** lists some strategies.

TOOLS FOR CHANGE

MANAGING BACK PAIN

While experiencing an acute episode of back pain, take the following treatment recommendations into account:[1]

- Limit bed rest to 1 to 2 days at most. Bed rest alone may make back pain worse and may contribute to other problems like muscle weakness and blood clots.

- Ice and heat may help with pain management, inflammation, and mobility. Apply cold treatments for 2 to 3 days after an acute event, and then add heat treatments as needed for increased muscle blood flow and relaxation.

- Engage in low-stress, back-healthy activities such as stretching, swimming, walking, and movement therapy as soon as you can.

- Check with a doctor before taking drugs for pain relief. Common medications include aspirin, ibuprofen, naproxen, topical muscle creams, and prescription muscle relaxers and pain medications.

- Spinal manipulation by a chiropractor or other qualified therapist can help some individuals with pain management and recovery.

- Nonconventional treatments (acupuncture, biofeedback, etc.) are considered by some patients when they are not responding to more traditional methods.

- Seek medical attention if you do not have a noticeable reduction in pain or experience inflammation after 72 hours of self-care.

Source: National Institute of Neurological Disorders and Stroke, *Low Back Pain Fact Sheet* (July 2003) Office of Communications and Public Liaison. National Institutes of Health. Bethesda, MD: NIH Publication No. 03-5161.

CHAPTER IN REVIEW

REVIEW QUESTIONS

1. _____ is a measure of your overall joint stiffness with muscular contraction.
   a. Dynamic flexibility
   b. Static flexibility
   c. Passive flexibility
   d. Anatomical flexibility

2. Which of the following triggers a muscle to relax when there is too much force or tension in the muscle?
   a. Muscle spindle
   b. Baroreceptor
   c. Golgi tendon organ
   d. Reflex receptor

3. The intensity of each stretch should be stretching until you reach
   a. your toes.
   b. slight discomfort but not pain.
   c. moderate burning pain.
   d. your goal.

4. Stretching through smooth, controlled movements that mimic the exercise activity describes
   a. static stretching.
   b. dynamic stretching.
   c. ballistic stretching.
   d. PNF stretching.

5. Which of the following exercise styles uses a slow-moving series of forms to increase coordination, balance, and flexibility?
   a. Dance
   b. Pilates
   c. Yoga
   d. Tai chi

6. Which of the following is the primary underlying cause of low-back pain?
   a. Poor posture
   b. Sedentary living
   c. Muscle weakness
   d. Poor flexibility

7. The fluid of an intervertebral disk bulging outward and pressing on the nervous system structures in the spine is best described as
   a. disk dehydration.
   b. disk degeneration.
   c. disk herniation.
   d. disk hardening.

8. Which of the following sleep postures creates the most tension in your lower back and is not recommended?
   a. lying on your side
   b. lying on your stomach
   c. lying on your back
   d. sleeping in a chair

9. What approximate percentage of people will experience lower-back pain at some point in their lives?
   a. 25 percent
   b. 50 percent
   c. 80 percent
   d. 100 percent

10. Which of the following acute back pain self-care treatments is no longer recommended?
   a. Five days of bed rest
   b. Light exercise
   c. Pain relievers
   d. Cold and hot treatments

CRITICAL THINKING QUESTIONS

1. Explain how stretching can improve your posture and balance.

2. Describe the stretch reflex.

3. List three occupations that are high-risk for low-back pain and explain why.

4. Explain the difference between static stretching and dynamic stretching.

ONLINE RESOURCES

1. **Slide Show: How to Stretch Your Major Muscle Groups**
   www.mayoclinic.com/health/stretching/SM00043

   A slide show of basic stretches for major muscle groups from a leading authority on health, fitness, and wellness.

2. **MedlinePlus—Trusted Health Information for You**
   www.nlm.nih.gov/medlineplus/backpain.html

A U.S. National Library of Medicine and National Institutes of Health service providing information on a variety of health topics, including back pain.

Please visit this book's website at **www.aw-bc .com/hopson** to view videos of flexibility exercises and to access links to additional topics in this chapter.

REFERENCES

1. National Center for Health Statistics, *Health, United States, 2006: With Chartbook on Trends in the Health of Americans.* (Hyattsville, MD: 2006).

2. Mayo Clinic, *Exercising with Arthritis: Improve Your Joint Pain and Stiffness,* Mayo Foundation for Medical Education and Research (MFMER), 2006, www.mayoclinic .com/health/arthritis/AR00009.

3. J. Peeler and J. E. Anderson, "Effectiveness of Static Quadriceps Stretching in Individuals with Patellofemoral Joint Pain," *Clinical Journal of Sport Medicine* 17, no. 4 (2007): 234–41.

4. A. N. Sjolie, "Low-Back Pain in Adolescents Is Associated with Poor Hip Mobility and High Body Mass Index," *Scandinavian Journal of Medicine and Science in Sports* 14, no. 3 (2004): 168–75.

5. M. A. Jones, G. Stratton, T. Reilly, and V. B. Unnithan, "Biological Risk Indicators for Recurrent Non-specific Low Back Pain in Adolescents," *British Journal of Sports Medicine* 39, no. 3 (2005): 137–40.

6. G. Hultman, H. Saraste, and H. Ohlsen, "Anthropometry, Spinal

Canal Width, and Flexibility of the Spine and Hamstring Muscles in 45–55-Year-Old Men With and Without Low Back Pain," *Journal of Spinal Disorders and Techniques* 5, no. 3 (1992): 245–53.

7. N. Kofotolis and M. Sambanis, "The Influence of Exercise on Musculoskeletal Disorders of the Lumbar Spine," *Journal of Sports Medicine and Physical Fitness* 45, no. 1 (2005): 84–92.

8. R. J. Johns, and V. Wright, "Relative Importance of Various Tissues in Joint Stiffness," *Journal of Applied Physiology* 17 (1962): 824–28.

9. I. G. Fatouros, A. Kambas, I. Katrabasas, and others, "Resistance Training and Detraining Effects on Flexibility Performance in the Elderly Are Intensity-Dependent," *Journal of Strength and Conditioning Research* 20, no. 3 (2006): 634–42.

10. T. Yamaguchi, and K. Ishii, "Effects of Static Stretching for 30 Seconds and Dynamic Stretching on Leg Extension Power," *Journal of Strength and Conditioning Research* 19, no. 3 (2005): 677–83.

11. See note 1.

12. J. Reis, M. Flegel, and C. Kennedy, "An Assessment of Lower Back Pain in Young Adults: Implications for College Health Education," *Journal of American College Health* 44, no. 6 (1996): 289–93.

13. National Institute of Neurological Disorders and Stroke, *Low Back Pain Fact Sheet* (July 2003). Office of Communications and Public Liaison. National Institutes of Health. Bethesda, MD: NIH Publication No. 03-5161.

14. M. Iwahashi, H. Matsuzaki, Y. Tokuhashi, K. Wakabayashi, and Y. Uematsu, "Mechanism of Intervertebral Disc Degeneration Caused by Nicotine in Rabbits to Explicate Intervertebral Disc Disorders Caused by Smoking," *Spine* 27, no. 13 (2002): 1396–1401.

15. See note 13.

16. U.S. Preventive Services Task Force, "Primary Care Interventions to Prevent Low Back Pain in Adults: Recommendation Statement," *American Family Physician* 71, no. 12 (2005).

17. R. Orvieto, N. Rand, B. Lev, M. Wiener, and H. Nehama, "Low Back Pain and Body Mass Index," *Military Medicine* 159, no. 1 (1994): 37–38.

Name: _____

Date: _____

Instructor: _____

Section: _____

Materials: Exercise mat and yardstick, a partner

Purpose: To assess your current level of lower-back, hip, and hamstring flexibility and your current level of joint mobility or range of motion.

SECTION I: THE SIT-AND-REACH TEST

This test measures the general flexibility of your lower back, hips, and hamstrings. The results are specific to those regions of your body and do not reflect your flexibility in other body areas.

1. **Warm-up.** Complete 3 to10 minutes of light cardiorespiratory activity to warm up your body and perform light range-of-motion exercises and stretches for the joints and muscles that you will be using.

2. **Get in position for the test.** Sit straight-legged on a mat with your shoes removed and your feet about 10 to 12 inches apart. Have a partner place a yardstick on the mat between your feet with the 15-inch mark at the edge of your heels. You can use a preplaced/taped yardstick, tape the yardstick in place at the heels, or just have your partner hold the yardstick. Place your hands on top of the yardstick's end.

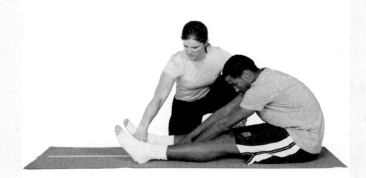

3. **Properly perform the test.** Keep one hand on top of the other. It is important that the fingertips of both hands remain together. Your hands should remain in contact with the yardstick at all times. Reach forward as far as you can by slowly bending forward, reaching with your arms, and sliding your fingertips out along the yardstick. Keep your legs straight, drop your head between your arms, and breathe out as you perform the test. Hold your ending position for at least 2 seconds. Your partner will watch to ensure that you have proper hand position and straight legs during the test.

4. **Find your reach distance.** Your *reach distance* is the most distant point reached with both fingertips. If you cannot keep your hands from separating, the most distant point reached by the fingertips of the <u>hand that is farthest back</u> should be considered the reach distance. Record the reach distance in inches, as measured by the yardstick. Perform the test twice. Have your partner point to your reach distance for each trial on the yardstick. Record the best score of the two trials in the RESULTS section below.

Flexibility RESULTS

Yardstick Sit-and-Reach Test: Reach Distance (in): _____

Rating: _____

5. **Find your flexibility rating by using the chart provided below.** Your rating tells you how you compare to others who have completed this test in the past. Record your results in the RESULTS section above.

Flexibility Ratings

YARDSTICK Sit-and-Reach Test (inches)						
Men	**Superior**	**Excellent**	**Good**	**Fair**	**Poor**	**Very Poor**
18–25 yrs	>27	21–27	18–20	15–17	11–14	<11
26–35 yrs	>27	20–27	17–19	14–16	10–13	<10
36–45 yrs	>27	20–27	16–19	13–15	8–12	<8
46–55 yrs	>25	18–24	14–17	11–13	7–10	<7
56–65 yrs	>23	16–22	12–15	9–11	6–8	<6
>65 yrs	>23	16–22	12–15	8–11	5–7	<5
Women						
18–25 yrs	>28	23–27	20–22	17–19	15–16	<15
26–35 yrs	>27	22–26	19–21	16–18	14–15	<14
36–45 yrs	>27	21–26	18–20	15–17	13–14	<13
46–55 yrs	>26	20–25	17–19	14–16	11–13	<11
56–65 yrs	>25	19–24	16–18	13–15	10–12	<10
>65 yrs	>25	19–24	16–18	13–15	10–12	<10

Source: Reprinted with permission from *YMCA Fitness Testing and Assessment Manual, Fourth Edition.* Copyright © 2000 by YMCA of the USA, Chicago. All rights reserved.

SECTION II: JOINT MOBILITY—RANGE-OF-MOTION TESTS

Range-of-motion tests assess the ability of your joints to move through a normal range of motion. Follow the instructions for each of the tests shown below. Perform each test on both your right and left sides. Stop each movement when you feel resistance. In order to avoid injury, do not try to push past your normal range! Have a partner observe your movements and record your range-of-motion results for each test in the RESULTS section below.

1. **Neck Lateral Flexion**—Sit or stand with your head neutral and looking forward. Tilt your head to the side and drop your ear toward your shoulder.

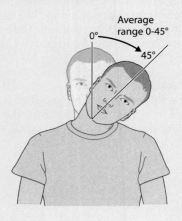

2. **Shoulder Flexion**—Starting with your arms at your sides, reach a straight arm forward and up toward your head.

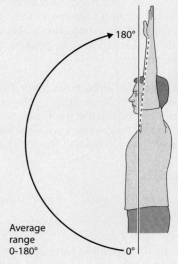

3. Shoulder Extension—With your arms at your sides, reach a straight arm behind you and up.

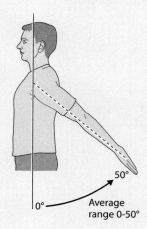

0°
50°
Average range 0-50°

4. Shoulder Abduction—Reach your straight arm out to the side and up to your head.

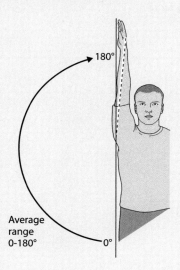

180°
Average range 0-180°
0°

5. Shoulder Adduction—Reach your straight arm down and across your body in front.

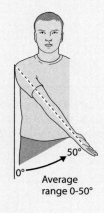

0°
50°
Average range 0-50°

6. Trunk Lateral Flexion—Standing upright with slightly bent knees and your arms at your sides. Bend your torso sideways and reach your arm down your leg for support.

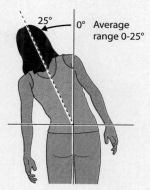

25°
0° Average range 0-25°

7. Hip Flexion—Lying on your back, lift a straight leg up into the air while keeping the other leg bent and your foot flat on the ground.

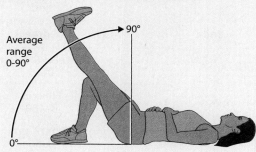

90°
Average range 0-90°
0°

8. Hip Extension—Lying on your stomach with your head on the mat, reach your straight leg up behind you, keeping the other leg flat on the ground.

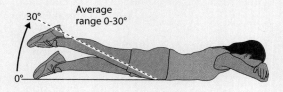

30°
Average range 0-30°
0°

9. Hip Abduction—Standing upright with slightly bent knees, reach your straight leg out to the side.

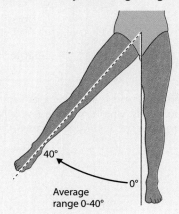

40°
0°
Average range 0-40°

10. **Ankle Dorsiflexion**—Sitting without shoes and your legs extended out in front of you, flex your foot back toward your knee.

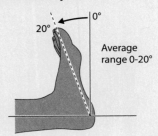

Average range 0-20°

11. **Ankle Plantar Flexion**—Sitting without shoes and your legs extended out in front of you, point your foot toward the floor.

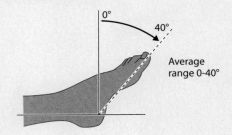

Average range 0-40°

Joint Mobility RESULTS

Joint	Movement and Average Range (degrees)	Full Average Joint Range?	
		Right Side YES or NO?	*Left Side* YES or NO?
1. Neck	Lateral Flexion 0–45		
2. Shoulder	Flexion 0–180		
3. Shoulder	Extension 0–50		
4. Shoulder	Abduction 0–180		
5. Shoulder	Adduction 0–50		
6. Trunk	Lateral Flexion 0–25		
7. Hip	Flexion 0–90		
8. Hip	Extension 0–30		
9. Hip	Abduction 0–40		
10. Ankle	Dorsiflexion 0–20		
11. Ankle	Plantar Flexion 0–40		

Source: Adapted from American College of Sports Medicine, *ACSM's Health-Related Physical Fitness Assessment Manual.* 2nd ed. (Baltimore, MD: Lippincott Williams & Wilkins, 2008); American College of Sports Medicine, *ACSM's Resource Manual for Guidelines for Exercise Testing and Prescription.* 5th ed. (Baltimore, MD: Lippincott Williams & Wilkins, 2006).

Name: _____ **Date:** _____

Instructor: _____ **Section:** _____

Purpose: To evaluate your posture.

Before you begin: Wear clothing that will not interfere with the assessment of your posture. If it is comfortable, men should wear shorts only, and women should wear shorts and a tank top. Remove your shoes. If you have long hair, pull it back into a ponytail for the assessment.

Stand against a wall and have a partner evaluate your posture using the following chart. Your partner should assign you a score of between 1 to 5 for each of the 10 areas of your body shown on the next page.

POSTURE RESULTS

Posture Score	Posture Rating
45 or higher	Excellent
40–44	Good
30–39	Average
20–29	Fair
19 or less	Poor

Source: Adapted from *New York State Physical Fitness Test for Boys and Girls Grades 4–12. A Manual for Teachers of Physical Education,* Division of Physical Education and Research, State University of New York. Albany, NY: New York State Education Dept., 1972.

	Good—5	Fair—3	Poor—1	Score
Head	Head erect, gravity passes directly through center	Head twisted or turned to one side slightly	Head twisted or turned to one side markedly	
Shoulders	Shoulders level horizontally	One shoulder slightly higher	One shoulder markedly higher	
Spine	Spine straight	Spine slightly curved	Spine markedly curved laterally	
Hips	Hips level horizontally	One hip slightly higher	One hip markedly higher	
Knees and Ankles	Feet pointed straight ahead, legs vertical	Feet pointed out, legs deviating outward at the knee	Feet poointed out markedly, legs deviated markedly	
Neck and Upper back	Neck erect, head in line with shoulders, rounded upper back	Neck slightly foward, chin out, slightly more rounded upper back	Neck markedly forward, chin markedly out, markedly rounded upper back	
Trunk	Trunk erect	Trunk inclined to rear slightly	Trunk inclined to rear markedly	
Abdomen	Abdomen flat	Abdomen protruding	Abdomen protruding and sagging	
Lower back	Lower back normally curved	Lower back slightly hollow	Lower back markedly hollow	
Legs	Legs straight	Knees slightly hyperextended	Knees markedly hyperextended	
			Total score	

GET FIT, STAY WELL!

Name: _____   Date: _____

Instructor: _____   Section: _____

Materials: Results from Lab 6.1

Purpose: To learn how to set appropriate flexibility goals and create a personal flexibility program.

SECTION I: SHORT- AND LONG-TERM GOALS

Create short- and long-term goals for flexibility and back health. Be sure to use SMART goal-setting guidelines (specific, measurable, action-oriented, realistic, time-oriented). Select appropriate target dates and rewards for completing your goals.

Short-Term Goal for Flexibility (3 to 6 months)

_____

_____

Target Date: _____

Reward: _____

Long-Term Goal for Flexibility (12+ months)

_____

_____

Target Date: _____

Reward: _____

Optional: Long-Term Goal for Back Health (12+ months)

_____

_____

Target Date: _____

Reward: _____

SECTION II: FLEXIBILITY PROGRAM DESIGN

Complete one line for each exercise you have chosen to do in your program.

Stretching Exercises	Frequency (days/week)	Length (sec)	Reps (number)	Total Time (sec)
LOWER BODY				
1.				
2.				
3.				
4.				
5.				
6.				
7.				
8.				
UPPER BODY				
1.				
2.				
3.				
4.				
5.				
6.				
7.				
8.				

SECTION III: TRACKING YOUR PROGRAM AND FOLLOWING THROUGH

1. **Goal and Program Tracking:** Use the following chart to monitor your progress. Change the frequency, time, sets, and reps frequently to ensure continuing progress toward your goals.

2. **Goal and Program Follow-up:** At the end of the course or at your short-term goal target date, reevaluate your flexibility and answer the following questions:

a. Did you meet your short-term goal or your goal for the course?

b. If so, what positive behavioral changes contributed to your success? If not, which obstacles blocked your success?

c. Was your short-term goal realistic? After evaluating your progress during the course, what would you change about your goals or training plan?

Flexiblity Training Log

DATE	Stretches Completed	COMMENTS (e.g. stretches modified, stretches held longer, how you felt, etc.)

Flexiblity Training Log

DATE	Stretches Completed	COMMENTS (e.g. stretches modified, stretches held longer, how you felt, etc.)

CHAPTER 7

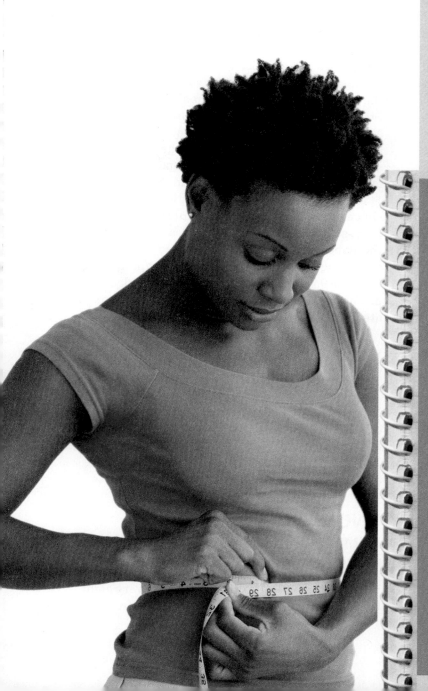

Understanding Body Composition

OBJECTIVES

Define *body composition*.

Explain why the assessment of body size, shape, and composition is useful.

Explain how to perform assessments of body size, shape, and composition.

Evaluate your BMI and body circumferences.

Set goals for a healthy body fat percentage.

CASE STUDY

Jessie

"Hi, I'm Jessie. I started running and resistance training 2 months ago and feel great! I like the new muscle tone in my legs, and I've made a lot of friends from the running group I joined. The ironic thing is, I started working out mainly because I wanted to lose weight, but I actually weigh a little bit more right now than I did when I first started. It doesn't make any sense to me, because my clothes fit better and I look more 'toned.' I've heard that muscle weighs more than fat, but that doesn't make any sense, either—doesn't a pound of muscle weigh the same as a pound of fat?"

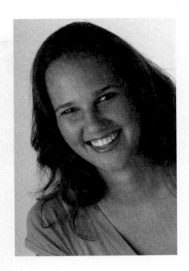

How much of your body is composed of fat? At first, that might seem like an impossible question to answer. But the question can be answered fairly well, and the answer is important to your overall health. **Body composition** refers to the relative amounts of lean tissue and fat tissue in your body. Measuring body composition involves measuring **lean body mass, fat mass,** and **percent body fat.** Your *lean body mass* is your body's total amount of lean or fat-free tissue (muscles, bones, skin, other organs, and body fluids). Your *fat mass* is body mass made up of fat tissue. *Percent body fat* means the percentage of your total weight that is fat tissue—that is, the weight of fat divided by total body weight.

All fat tissue can be labeled as either **essential fat** or **storage fat.** *Essential fat* is necessary for normal body functioning; it includes fats in the brain, muscles, nerves, bones, lungs, heart, and digestive and reproductive systems. Men need a minimum of 3 percent essential body fat. Women need significantly more (12 percent essential body fat) because of reproductive-system-related fat deposits in their breasts, uterus, and elsewhere (see Figure 7.1.) *Storage fat* is nonessential fat stored in tissue near the body's surface and around major body organs. Storage fat provides energy, insulation, and padding. Men and women have similar amounts of storage fat but may differ in the location of larger fat stores. Your individual amount of storage fat depends upon many factors, including your lifestyle and genetics.

In this chapter, you will learn why body size, shape, and composition are useful measurements of fitness and wellness. You'll also learn how each of these measurements are determined and how you can change or maintain your body composition. In Chapter 9, you will combine your knowledge of physical activity, body composition, and diet to create your own weight-management plan.

WHY DO BODY SIZE, SHAPE, AND COMPOSITION MATTER?

You might think of body size, shape, and composition mainly in terms of your physical appearance, but they encompass more than merely how you look. They are important components (as well as measurements) of your overall fitness and wellness.

KNOWING YOUR BODY COMPOSITION CAN HELP YOU ASSESS YOUR HEALTH RISKS

From 1999 to 2004, the proportion of overweight U.S. children and adolescents increased from

body composition The relative amounts of fat and lean tissue in the body

lean body mass Body mass that is fat-free (muscle, skin, bone, organs, and body fluids)

fat mass Body mass that is fat tissue

percent body fat Percentage of total weight that is comprised of fat tissue

essential fat Body fat that is essential for normal physiological functioning

storage fat Body fat that is not essential but does provide energy, insulation, and padding

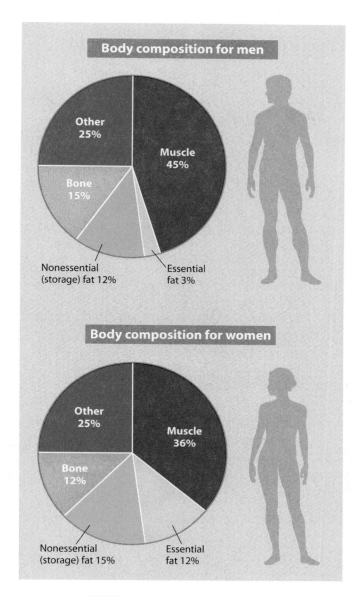

FIGURE 7.1

The body compositions of typical 20- to 24-year-old men and women vary primarily in the amounts of muscle and essential fat.

Data from: McArdle and others, Exercise Physiology: Energy, Nutrition, and Human Performance. *6th ed. (Baltimore, MD: Lippincott Williams & Wilkins, 2007).*

14 percent to 17 percent, significantly increasing their risk for diseases in adulthood.[1,2] Over the same 5 years, the proportion of overweight or obese adults in the United States grew from 64 percent to 66 percent. An alarming 32 percent of American adults are obese.[3]

Studies of obesity, however, often rely on measurements of total body weight rather than measurements of body composition. While measurements of total body weight can be useful in studying large populations, they are less useful in assessing an individual's health risks and body changes. For individuals, estimates of body composition—specifically, of lean and fat mass—provide additional important information. By knowing your percent body fat, you can more effectively determine your risks for chronic disease and decide just how much weight you should try to lose (or gain).

EVALUATING YOUR BODY SIZE AND SHAPE CAN HELP MOTIVATE HEALTHY BEHAVIOR CHANGE

If you are just beginning an exercise program for fitness, it is often more useful to assess changes in body size and shape as a measurement of your progress, rather than weighing yourself daily on a bathroom scale. The reason: healthy increases in muscle tissue (achieved by exercise) may cause you to temporarily gain weight, until the process of body fat loss catches up with muscle tissue gains. This is a *good* thing, but you would not know it if you relied solely on the scale to determine your progress. By monitoring improvements in your body size and shape instead, you can get a more realistic sense of your achievement and stay motivated to stick with an exercise program.

HOW CAN YOU EVALUATE YOUR BODY SIZE AND SHAPE?

How do you determine if your body size and shape are "healthy"? This is a much-debated topic, but there are three common methods of doing so: calculating your body mass index, measuring your *body circumferences,* and identifying the patterns of fat distribution on your body. (Evaluating your body *composition* is a somewhat more complicated process, which we will discuss later in this chapter.)

CALCULATE YOUR BODY MASS INDEX (BMI) BUT UNDERSTAND ITS LIMITATIONS

Body mass index (BMI) is one of the most common measurements that doctors and researchers use to assess risk of weight-related disease, death,

body mass index (BMI) A number calculated from a person's weight and height that is used to assess risk for possible present or future health problems

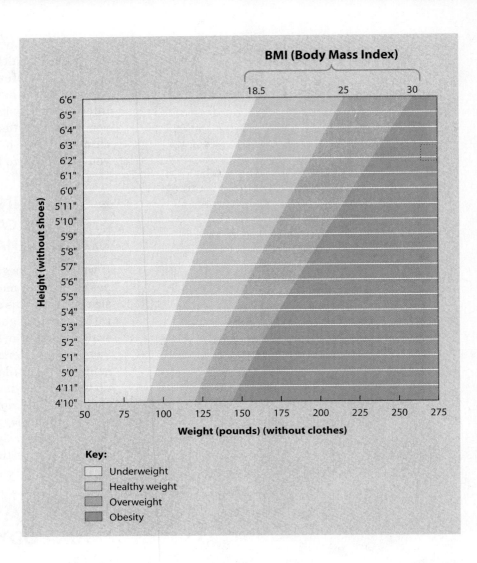

BMI (Body Mass Index)

Key:
☐ Underweight
☐ Healthy weight
☐ Overweight
■ Obesity

FIGURE **7.2**

Estimate your BMI by finding the point at which your weight and height intersect.

and disability. BMI is a measurement based on your weight and height. *Lab7.1* will walk you through how to calculate your BMI. You can also estimate your BMI from the chart in Figure 7.2 or by using an online BMI calculator such as the one described in the following **Try it NOW!** box.

BMI scores place individuals in categories as follows:[4]

Underweight (BMI of < 18.5)

Normal weight (BMI of 18.5 to 24.9)

Try it NOW! **Calculate your BMI online at www.nhlbisupport .com/bmi.**

Overweight (BMI of 25.0 to 29.9)

Obese—Class I (BMI of 30.0 to 34.9)

    Class II (BMI of 35.0 to 39.9)

    Class III (BMI of > 40.0)

Figure 7.3 illustrates how very low and very high BMI scores are correlated with greater risk of death and disability.

The limitation with using BMI scores to assess "fitness" is that they do not differentiate between fat mass and lean mass. BMI is solely determined by height and weight. While BMI measurements can be helpful for individuals of average muscle and bone density, they can be misleading for athletes, bodybuilders, and short or petite individuals. For instance, someone who has an exceptionally heavy skeleton and larger-than-average muscle mass may have a BMI score that classifies him or her as "overweight," even if his or her percent body fat is in the

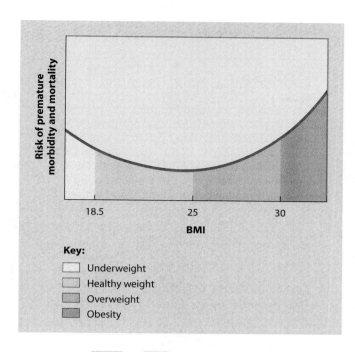

FIGURE 7.3

Extremely low or extremely high BMIs are associated with a greater risk of premature death and disability.

Data from Katherine Flegal and others, "Excess Deaths Associated with Underweight, Overweight, and Obesity," Journal of the American Medical Association *293(2005): 1861–67.*

Key:
- ☐ Underweight
- ☐ Healthy weight
- ☐ Overweight
- ☐ Obesity

"healthy" range. Because of BMI's limitations, it helps to also consider other factors, such as percent body fat, when assessing the overall picture of a person's fitness.

MEASURE YOUR BODY CIRCUMFERENCES

You can measure circumferences of various parts of your body to monitor your body's changes over time and to further assess your risk of disease. If you want to gain or lose weight, you can measure the circumferences of your waist, hips, neck, upper arm, chest, thigh, and calf to monitor changes in your body over time. You can also use waist and hip circumferences to assess disease risk. As shown in Table 7.1, waist circumference (a marker of abdominal fat) can indicate greater risk of diabetes, high blood pressure, and heart disease if it is greater than 102 cm in males or 88 cm in females.[5] As the table also shows, the people at greatest risk are those with high waist circumferences *and* high BMIs.

You can also use waist and hip circumferences to determine your **waist-to-hip ratio (WHR).**

TABLE 7.1

Waist Circumference, BMI, and Disease Risk

Weight Classification	BMI (kg/m²)	Waist Circumference and Disease Risk*	
		Smaller Waist Men 102 cm (40 in) or less Women 88 cm (35 in) or less	Larger Waist Men > 102 cm (40 in) Women > 88 cm (35 in)
Underweight	< 18.5	—	—
Normal Weight	18.5–24.9	—	—
Overweight	25.0–29.9	Increased	High
Obese—I	30.0–34.9	High	Very High
Obese—II	35.0–39.9	Very High	Very High
Obese—III	> 40.0	Extremely High	Extremely High

*Risk for type 2 diabetes, hypertension, and cardiovascular disease, relative to normal weight and waist circumference.

Source: Adapted from National Heart, Lung, and Blood Institute—Expert Panel on the Identification, Evaluation, and Treatment of Overweight in Adults, "Clinical Guidelines on the Identification, Evaluation, and Treatment of Overweight and Obesity in Adults: Executive Summary," *American Journal of Clinical Nutrition* 68 (1998): 899–917. Used with permission.

Waist-to-hip ratio is your waist circumference divided by your hip circumference. A higher WHR is associated with more health risks. Young men with a WHR of 0.94 or more and young women with a WHR of 0.82 or more fall into a high-risk category.[6] *Lab7.2* will walk you through the process of measuring your body circumferences and determining your WHR. Although waist circumference and WHR are both measures of disease risk, waist circumference is generally preferred because it is simpler, because of its relationship with abdominal fat, and because of its strong association to disease risk factors.[7]

IDENTIFY YOUR BODY'S PATTERNS OF FAT DISTRIBUTION

Body fat distribution patterns are mostly genetically determined. You have probably noticed that people take after one parent in the way they "wear their fat." Some individuals tend to accumulate fat around their midsections; others collect it in the lower body or hips. These distributions contribute to an overall body shape that can be correlated to a higher or lower risk of disease.

The two most common body shapes are **android** ("apple-shaped") and **gynoid** ("pear-shaped") (Figure 7.4). A person with *android pattern obesity* has excess body fat on the upper body and trunk and has a greater risk of developing chronic disease than a person with *gynoid pattern obesity,* who carries excess body fat in the lower body. While men tend to store fat in the abdomen and women tend to store it in the lower body, there are exceptions, and fat distribution is strongly influenced by genetics. If you have an "apple-shaped" body, understanding the health risks can help motivate you to keep your "apple" from getting too large and round!

waist-to-hip ratio (WHR) Waist circumference divided by hip circumference

android Body shape described as "apple-shaped," with excess body fat distributed primarily on the upper body and trunk

gynoid Body shape described as "pear-shaped," where excess body fat is distributed primarily on the lower body (hips and thighs)

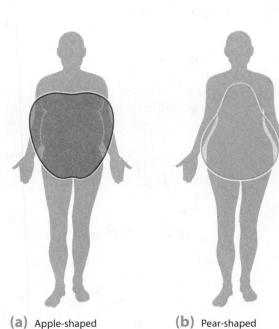

(a) Apple-shaped fat patterning

(b) Pear-shaped fat patterning

FIGURE 7.4

(a) Android ("apple-shaped") fat distribution is associated with greater risk of heart disease and diabetes, more common in men of all ages and postmenopausal women; (b) gynoid ("pear-shaped") fat distribution is more common in premenopausal women.

WHAT METHODS ARE USED TO ASSESS BODY COMPOSITION?

Unlike BMI and body circumference measurements, body composition (lean mass vs. fat mass) can only be estimated indirectly. A true, direct assessment of body composition requires dissection after death; in fact, researchers judge the accuracy of the indirect measures by comparing them with dissection results from cadavers.

Methods of estimating body composition range from assessments that trained fitness instructors can easily administer (such as skinfold measurements and bioelectrical impedance analysis) to sophisticated tests that must be conducted by clinicians in a lab setting (such as dual-energy X-ray absorptiometry, hydrostatic weighing, and air displacement). In the next sections, we examine some of these methods in more detail.

SKINFOLD MEASUREMENTS

Skinfold measurements are an easy, inexpensive way to estimate your percent body fat. **Calipers** (shown in *Lab7.3*) are used to measure the thickness of a fold of skin and subcutaneous adipose tissue. Skinfold measurements at specific sites around the body are recorded and entered into an equation that predicts percent body fat. This prediction of percent body fat has an error range of 3 to 4 percent;[8] for example, if your body fat measurement is 16 percent, the true value could be anywhere from about 12 to 20 percent. Lab 7.3 provides instructions for administering skinfold measurements. Accurate skinfold assessment takes education and practice, so be sure to ask a qualified fitness instructor to help you.

DUAL-ENERGY X-RAY ABSORPTIOMETRY (DXA)

Dual-energy X-ray absorptiometry (DXA) is the "gold standard" for assessing body composition in clinical and research settings (Figure 7.5). It uses low-radiation X rays to distinguish fat, bone mineral, and bone-free lean components of the body. DXA can scan the whole body in a procedure that takes less than 20 minutes, and the range of error is only 1 to 3 percent.[9] However, DXA tests are expensive, require a prescription for a medical X ray, and are not well designed to examine people who are extremely obese.

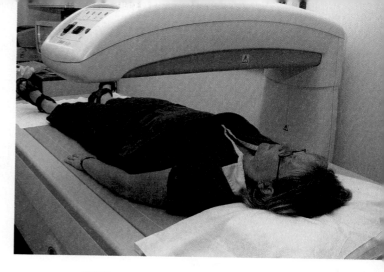

FIGURE 7.5

A DXA machine uses low-radiation X rays to determine body composition.

HYDROSTATIC WEIGHING

Hydrostatic weighing (also called *underwater weighing*) is widely used in research and college settings (Figure 7.6). In this method of body composition assessment, a person is first weighed outside a water tank and then weighed while completely submerged in the tank. Hydrostatic weighing is based on the concept that the more fat a person has, the more he or she will tend to float and the less weight he or she will exert against the bottom of the tank. From this process, a technician can assess total body volume and body density and use them to calculate an estimated percent body fat. The method is valid and reliable (range of error 2 to 3 percent), but access to an equipped facility may be limited, and not everyone is comfortable with being submerged.[10]

skinfold A fold of skin and subcutaneous fat tissue that is measured with calipers to determine the fatness of a specific body area; multiple skinfold measures are combined to estimate total body lean and fat masses

caliper A handheld and spring-loaded instrument with calibrated jaws and a meter that reads skinfold thickness in millimeters

dual-energy X-ray absorptiometry (DXA) A technique using two low-radiation X rays to scan bone and soft tissue (muscle, fat) to determine bone density and to estimate percent body fat

hydrostatic weighing A technique that uses water to determine total body volume, total body density, and percent body fat; a greater difference between out-of-water and in-water weight indicates more body fat

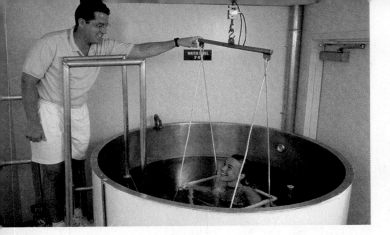

FIGURE 7.6

Hydrostatic (underwater) weighing uses total body water displacement to calculate estimated percent body fat.

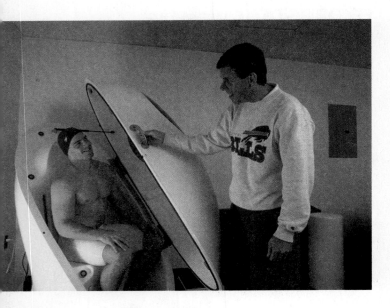

FIGURE 7.7

The Bod Pod uses total body air displacement to calculate estimated percent body fat.

Bod Pod An egg-shaped chamber that uses air displacement to determine total body volume, total body density, and percent body fat

bioelectrical impedance analysis (BIA) A technique that distinguishes lean and fat mass by measuring the resistance of various body tissues to electrical currents

AIR DISPLACEMENT (BOD POD)

While hydrostatic weighing measures total body *water* displacement, the **Bod Pod** is an egg-shaped chamber that measures total body *air* displacement (Figure 7.7). The person being assessed puts on a swimsuit and then sits in the Bod Pod while the air displacement is measured. The measure is used together with other measures (such as weight) to determine total body volume and density and then to estimate percent body fat. Most studies show that the accuracy of Bod Pod measurements is similar to that of hydrostatic weighing; however, the Bod Pod is not yet readily available to the general public.[11]

BIOELECTRICAL IMPEDANCE ANALYSIS (BIA)

Bioelectrical impedance analysis (BIA) works by measuring the resistance of various body tissues to electrical currents. BIA machines send small electrical currents through the body via the hands, feet, or both (Figure 7.8). Fat does not conduct electricity very well, so fat tissues will demonstrate a resistance to the currents. Fat-free tissues, which have more body water, conduct electricity well; thus, fat-free tissues do not offer as much resistance to the currents. These resistance differences are used to estimate percent body fat. Higher resistance indicates higher levels of overall body fat. The error range of BIA is 3 to 4 percent, but accuracy depends upon the quality of the machine and upon the subject's following instructions, especially concerning his/her water intake.[12] Higher or lower levels of body water will significantly alter a BIA machine's results, so it is important to avoid drinking too much or too little prior to assessment.

ESTIMATES FROM CIRCUMFERENCES OR BMI

If you have no other way to assess your body composition, you can roughly estimate your percent body fat from circumference measurements, which you can easily do at home. While not as accurate as the methods described above, circumference measurements can provide a starting point for your weight-management program. The following **Try it NOW!** box provides a website that contains guidelines for taking circumference measurements.

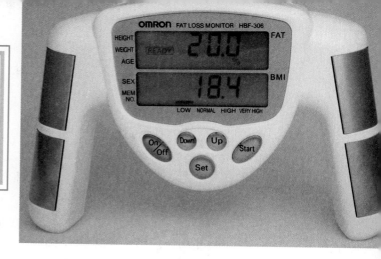

Try it NOW! Estimate your body fat based on weight, height, and circumference measurements in this method developed by the U.S. Navy: www.he.net/~zone/prothd2.html.

You can also use your BMI and Table 7.2 to quickly estimate your percent body fat. The estimate is rough, with an error range of 5 percent, meaning your body fat could be 5 percent higher or lower than the estimate.[13] This method assumes that you have an *average* amount of muscle mass. If you are exceptionally muscular, this method will not yield accurate results.

FIGURE 7.8

Bioelectrical impedance analysis (BIA) machines measure the resistance of different body tissues to electrical currents. These measurements are then used to estimate percent body fat. Shown here is a handheld BIA machine.

TABLE 7.2

Body Fat Prediction from BMI

Age BMI (kg/m²)	Women (% Body Fat)			Men (% Body Fat)		
	African American	Asian	White	African American	Asian	White
20–39 years						
BMI < 18.5	20 or less	25 or less	21 or less	8 or less	13 or less	8 or less
BMI 18.5–24.9	21–31	26–34	22–32	9–19	14–22	9–20
BMI 25.0–29.9	32–37	35–39	33–38	20–25	23–27	21–25
BMI ≥ 30.0	38 or more	40 or more	39 or more	26 or more	28 or more	26 or more
40–59 years						
BMI < 18.5	21 or less	25 or less	23 or less	9 or less	13 or less	11 or less
BMI 18.5–24.9	22–33	26–35	24–34	10–21	14–23	12–22
BMI 25.0–29.9	34–38	36–40	35–40	22–26	24–28	23–28
BMI ≥ 30.0	39 or more	41 or more	41 or more	27 or more	29 or more	29 or more
60–79 years						
BMI < 18.5	23 or less	26 or less	25 or less	11 or less	14 or less	13 or less
BMI 18.5–24.9	24–34	27–35	26–37	12–22	15–23	14–24
BMI 25.0–29.9	35–40	36–40	38–42	23–28	24–28	25–30
BMI ≥ 30.0	41 or more	41 or more	43 or more	29 or more	29 or more	31 or more

Source: Adapted from D. Gallagher, S. B. Heymsfield, M. Heo, and others, "Healthy Percentage Body Fat Ranges: An Approach for Developing Guidelines Based on Body Mass Index," *American Journal of Clinical Nutrition* 72 (2000): 694–701. Copyright © 2000 American Society for Nutrition. Used with permission.

Jessie

"A trainer at my gym gave me a skinfold test, which I thought was really interesting. He told me I have about 36 percent body fat. It is good to know that, because I can retest myself in a few months to see how all of my exercise is paying off!"

1. What other methods could Jessie use to determine her body composition?

2. What methods of assessing body composition are readily available to you? How can you use the results to help you set fitness goals?

HOW CAN YOU EVALUATE AND CHANGE YOUR BODY COMPOSITION?

After you assess your body size, shape, and composition, the next steps are evaluation, goal setting, and (if your results are not within healthy ranges) planning for change.

DETERMINE IF YOUR PERCENT BODY FAT IS WITHIN HEALTHY RANGE

It is difficult to specify the exact level of body fat that is "healthy" or "unhealthy" for an individual, because people accumulate fat very differently, and not all fat is the same. For instance, abdominal fat increases your risk for disease much more than does fat on the calves. Because of these differences, researchers do not agree upon desired body fat percentages for people of all ages, and you will find that research articles, books, and websites differ in their recommendations. That

said, the numbers in Table 7.3 provide a starting point of recommended body fat percentages, especially for someone who is inactive and needs to lose weight. Meanwhile, the box **Facts and Fallacies: Can You Be Overweight and Fit?** explores why the relationships between weight, wellness, and mortality is complicated.

SET REASONABLE BODY COMPOSITION GOALS

You have many choices in setting body composition goals. In this chapter, we have explored methods you can use to assess your overall body size, shape, and composition in your process of self-evaluation. If you are already in the healthy ranges, you can set additional goals for increasing lean mass or decreasing fat mass (within the low limits).

Keep in mind that real body composition changes take time. Losing a lot of weight in 1 week is unhealthy and very hard to do. Quick weight loss is easier for those with more weight to lose, but most

TABLE 7.3

Percent Body Fat Recommendations for Men and Women*

	Recommended	Overfat	Obese
Men	< or = 34 years old: 8–22% 35–55 years old: 10–25% > 55 years old: 10–25%	≤ 34 years old: 23–25% > 35 years old: 26–28%	≤ 34 years old: > 25% > 35 years old: > 28%
Women	< or = 34 years old: 20–35% 35–55 years old: 23–38% > 55 years old: 25–38%	≤ 34 years old: 36–38% > 35 years old: 39–40%	≤ 34 years old: > 38% > 35 years old: > 40%

* Assumes nonathletes. For athletes, recommended body fat is 5 to 15 percent for men and 12 to 22 percent for women.

Source: American College of Sports Medicine, *ACSM's Resource Manual for Guidelines for Exercise Testing and Prescription.* 5th ed. (Baltimore, MD: Lippincott Williams & Wilkins, 2006). Copyright © ACSM. Reprinted by permission of Wolters/Kluwer. Please note that there are no agreed-upon national standards for recommended percent body fat.

FACTS AND FALLACIES

CAN YOU BE OVERWEIGHT AND FIT?

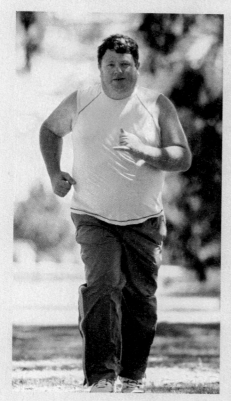

For decades, doctors, researchers, trainers, and even textbooks have discussed the links between fitness, weight, wellness, and mortality. No matter what "facts" you may have heard, however, current research is revealing that the connections are complicated and are still not fully understood.

A recent federal study of 2.3 million American adults analyzed decades of mortality data from people over age 25.[1] The study divided all the subjects into standard BMI groupings: underweight, normal weight, overweight, and obese. It used individuals of normal BMI to establish standard baselines for cancer and cardiovascular-disease-related deaths, as well as for all non-cancer and non-CVD causes of death (such as infections, accidents, lung diseases, and Alzheimer's disease).

The study found that underweight people had higher-than-standard death rates for non-cancer and non-CVD causes. Overweight people had *lower*-than-standard death rates for non-cancer and non-CVD causes but higher rates for cancer, diabetes, and heart disease. Averaging all the various causes of death, overweight people were slightly *less* likely to die in a given period than normal-weight individuals as a group.

Obese people had higher death rates for CVD and slightly higher rates for the cancers associated with body fat: colon, breast, esophagus, uterus, ovary, kidney, and pancreas. They had lower death rates for non-cancer and non-CVD causes, but when combined, their death rates were higher than in normal-weight individuals.

Researchers aren't yet certain why underweight people tend to die in greater percentages from one group of diseases while overweight and obese people tend to succumb to others. In the meantime, other researchers have asked a more direct question: Can you be technically overweight but still fit?

Researchers in one study tested 2,600 subjects over age 60 for fitness levels and for body mass, then followed the subjects' health for 20 years.[2] The study found that having a large waistline or high BMI predicted higher mortality, but not in individuals who tested high for fitness levels. In another study, people who ate the fewest calories but were also the least physically active were more likely to develop and die from heart disease than were those who ate the most calories but also did the most exercise.[3]

The evidence is strong that muscular and cardiovascular fitness helps protect us from illness and disease. It allows us to stay healthier, to maintain mobility, and to experience a higher quality of life. Do you feel energetic, get plenty of exercise, and have a high fitness level? If so, you can probably worry less about current definitions of "overweight" and "high BMI" and instead focus on continuing to maintain or increase your fitness level.

Sources:

1. Katherine M. Flegal, and others, "Excess Deaths Associated with Underweight, Overweight, and Obesity," *Journal of the American Medical Association* 298, no. 17 (2007): 2028–37.
2. X. Sui, and others, "Cardiorespiratory Fitness and Adiposity as Mortality Predictors in Older Adults," *Journal of the American Medical Association* 298, no. 21 (2007): 2507–16.
3. J. Fang, and others, "Exercise, Body Mass Index, Caloric Intake, and Cardiovascular Mortality," *American Journal of Preventative Medicine* 25, no. 4 (2003): 283–89.

weight that is lost quickly consists of water and muscle—the very things you *don't* want to lose. To lose fat only, you have to be committed to exercise and slow, consistent weight loss. Aim for a body composition goal and a target weight that is healthy and that you can maintain for a lifetime. The box **Tools for Change: Losing a Pound of Fat** illustrates some ideas for decreasing fat mass.

FOLLOW A WELL-DESIGNED EXERCISE AND NUTRITION PLAN

Fad diets are just that: fads. Most of the time they do not work or only work for a short period of time. True body changes come from sticking with a carefully planned and executed nutrition and exercise program. Chapters 8 and 9 will help you get started. For additional assistance, seek out qualified medical, nutrition, and fitness experts.

MONITOR YOUR BODY SIZE, SHAPE, AND COMPOSITION REGULARLY

Stay motivated in your body change program by monitoring your progress regularly. Since body fat changes may take time, allow 2 to 4 months between body composition assessments. Other types

TOOLS FOR CHANGE

LOSING A POUND OF FAT

Picture four sticks of butter plus three more thick pats on top. That pile contains 3,500 calories—the same number in a pound of your own body fat. If you 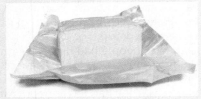 wanted to lose 1 pound of fat by a week from today, you would have to reduce your food intake by 3,500 calories/week, burn off 3,500 calories through exercise, or commit to a calorie-reduction plan coupled with additional exercise.

Consider the following examples of activities that a 150-pound individual could perform in order to lose 1 pound of fat in 1 week:[1]

- Rollerblade or jog for an extra hour each day for a week

- Dance vigorously for an additional 87 minutes daily for a week

- Walk at a moderate speed, on level ground, for 2 extra hours daily for a week

Regardless of your current weight, you can also cut 500 calories/day by eliminating or reducing calorie-rich foods from your diet, such as chips, nuts, cookies, coffee drinks, cheese, cream sauces, gravies, butter, fried meats, and desserts.

Remember that longer duration, moderate cardiovascular activity coupled with weight training is one of the most effective ways to burn fat. Also keep in mind that a realistic exercise-plus-diet routine—one that you feel comfortable sustaining week after week—is the best way to help you reach the healthy body composition you desire.

Source: Frank Katch, Victor Katch, and William McArdle, *Calorie Expenditure Charts for Physical Activity* (Ann Arbor, Michigan: Fitness Technologies Press, 1996).

UNDERSTANDING DIVERSITY

THE FEMALE ATHLETE TRIAD

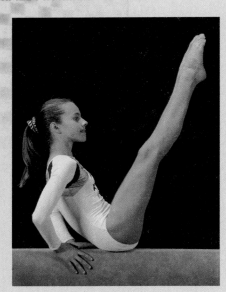

Some female athletes develop a disorder called the *female athlete triad* that requires attention and help from friends, families, and coaches. This condition is characterized by:

- disordered eating (such as skipping meals, starving, or avoiding whole food groups) or true eating disorders (such as anorexia nervosa or bulimia)

- the temporary cessation of menstruation (called *amenorrhea*)

- low bone density (resulting in increased risk of bone breaks and osteoporosis).

The female athlete triad is based on the interrelationships between energy availability, menstrual function, and bone density. Too little caloric intake coupled with too much exercise can lead to hormonal changes and the stopping of menstruation. Improper nutrition, including too little calcium and vitamin D intake, can lead to altered hormones and to bone loss and risk of fractures. What's more, such changes taking place in adolescence or early adulthood can permanently reduce the size of a female's skeleton and increase her lifelong risk for osteoporosis.

Those at especially high risk for the female athlete triad are those in subjectively rated sports (gymnastics, dance, ice skating) or body weight–affected sports (gymnastics, running). Such athletes should carefully monitor their body composition, menstrual health, eating habits, and perhaps bone density. If the triad is suspected, the female should eat more nutritious food and/or exercise less, and may need to seek treatment for an eating disorder.

Sources: A. Nattiv, and others, "American College of Sports Medicine Position Stand. The Female Athlete Triad," *Medical Science in Sports and Exercise* 89, no. 10 (2007): 1867–82; A. Z. Hoch, and others, "The Female Athlete Triad and Cardiovascular Dysfunction," *Physical Medicine and Rehabilitation Clinics, North America* 18, no. 3 (2007): 385–400, vii–viii.

of assessments can be done more frequently. Here is a suggested schedule:

- Body size/shape (mirror and fit of clothes)—assess daily or weekly
- Weight—assess weekly
- Circumferences—measure monthly (or even less frequently)

- BMI—measure monthly (or even less frequently)
- Percent body fat—measure bimonthly (or even less frequently)

Keep a separate log, journal, or notebook of your progress, but do not feel burdened by it. Remember that some people are more motivated by journaling than others—find the monitoring system that works best for you, and use it consistently.

CHAPTER IN REVIEW

REVIEW QUESTIONS

1. The proportion of your total weight comprised of fat is called
   a. body composition.
   b. lean mass.
   c. percent body fat.
   d. BMI.

2. Women have a greater amount of *essential fat* due to
   a. larger calves and thighs.
   b. their eating habits.
   c. less physical activity.
   d. reproduction-related fat deposits.

3. *Storage fat* is
   a. fat that is absolutely essential to normal functioning.
   b. nonessential fat.
   c. completely unaffected by genetics.
   d. fat that cannot be altered in any way.

4. All of the following statements about BMI are true EXCEPT,
   a. BMI is based on height and weight measurements.
   b. BMI differentiates between lean mass and fat mass.
   c. very low and very high BMI scores are associated with greater risk of mortality.
   d. BMI stands for "body mass index."

5. Which of the following BMI ratings is considered "overweight"?
   a. 20
   b. 25
   c. 30
   d. 35

6. Which of the following body circumferences is most strongly associated with risk of heart disease and diabetes?
   a. Hip circumference
   b. Chest circumference
   c. Waist circumference
   d. Thigh circumference

7. Which of the following body shapes or body fat distribution patterns is associated with an increased risk of heart disease and diabetes?
   a. Bell-shaped
   b. Android pattern obesity
   c. Pear-shaped
   d. Gynoid pattern obesity

8. Which of the following body composition methods uses air displacement to estimate total body volume, density, and percent body fat?
   a. Bioelectrical impedance analysis
   b. Hydrostatic weighing
   c. The Bod Pod
   d. Skinfold measurement

9. Which body composition method relies heavily on body water or hydration levels being normal (not too low or too high)?
   a. Bioelectrical impedance analysis
   b. Hydrostatic weighing
   c. The Bod Pod
   d. Skinfold measurement

10. The female athlete triad consists of the following interrelated issues:
    a. disordered eating, low bone density, and menstrual dysfunction.
    b. weak eyesight, poor nutrition, and brittle bones.
    c. low body weight, poor nutrition, diabetes.
    d. excessive exercise, high blood pressure, menstrual issues.

CRITICAL THINKING QUESTIONS

1. Explain the usefulness and limitations of using BMI to determine fitness goals.

2. What factors should you consider when determining a healthy percent body fat range for yourself?

ONLINE RESOURCES

1. **National Heart Lung and Blood Institute Online BMI Calculator**
   www.nhlbisupport.com/bmi
   Calculate your BMI and get healthy tips for changing it.

2. **Centers for Disease Control—Body Mass Index**
   www.cdc.gov/nccdphp/dnpa/bmi

Calculate an adult or child BMI, obtain information about the BMI measure, and get nutrition and weight management information.

Web addresses are subject to change. Please visit this book's website at **www.aw-bc.com/hopson** for updates and additional web resources.

REFERENCES

1. C. L. Ogden, M. D. Carroll, L. R. Curtin, and others, "Prevalence of Overweight and Obesity in the United States, 1999–2004," *Journal of the American Medical Association* 295, no. 13 (2006) 1549–55.

2. J. L. Baker, L. W. Olsen, and T. I. Sorensen, "Childhood Body-Mass Index and the Risk of Coronary Heart Disease in Adulthood," *New England Journal of Medicine* 357, no. 23 (2006) 2329–37.

3. National Center for Health Statistics, "Prevalence of Overweight Among Children and Adolescents: United States, 2003–2004." www.cdc.gov.

4. National Heart, Lung, and Blood Institute—Expert Panel on the Identification, Evaluation, and Treatment of Overweight in Adults, "Clinical Guidelines on the Identification, Evaluation, and Treatment of Overweight and Obesity in Adults: Executive Summary," *American Journal of Clinical Nutrition* 68 (1998): 899–917.

5. Ibid.

6. V. H. Heyward, *Advanced Fitness Assessment and Exercise Prescription.* 5th ed. (Champaign, IL: Human Kinetics, 2006).

7. J. P. Reis, C. A. Macera, D. L. Wingard, and others, "The Relation of Leptin and Insulin with Obesity-Related ardiovascular Risk Factors in U.S. Adults," *Atherosclerosis* (December 24, 2007). [Epub ahead of print].

8–12. See note 6.

13. American College of Sports Medicine, *ACSM's Guidelines for Exercise Testing and Prescription.* 7th ed. (Baltimore, MD: Lippincott Williams & Wilkins, 2006).

Name: _____ **Date:** _____

Instructor: _____ **Section:** _____

Purpose: To learn how to calculate your BMI.

Materials: Weight scale, measuring tape, calculator

SECTION I: CALCULATE YOUR BMI

1. Record your weight and height below:

Weight _____ lb   Height _____ inches

2. Convert your weight and height to metric units:

Weight _____ lb ÷ 2.2 = _____ kg

Height _____ inches × 2.54 = _____ cm ÷ 100 = _____ meters (m)

3. Calculate your BMI:

BMI = _____ ÷ [_____ × _____]
       (weight in kg)   (height in m)   (height in m)

BMI = _____ kg/m²

Note: Square the height (multiply by itself) before dividing into weight.

4. Circle your BMI rating in the table below:

Weight Classification	BMI (kg/m²)
Underweight	< 18.5
Normal Weight	18.5–24.9
Overweight	25.0–29.9
Obese—I	30.0–34.9
Obese—II	35.0–39.9

SECTION II: REFLECTION

1. Is your BMI category what you thought it would be?

_____

2. Remember that BMI categories can be misleading for individuals with above-average muscle mass. Do you fall into this category? _____

3. Monitoring changes to your BMI over time is one way to assess your progress with a fitness program. Two months after you begin a new exercise program, recalculate your BMI. Has it changed?

_____

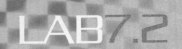

Name: _____ **Date:** _____

Instructor: _____ **Section:** _____

Purpose: To learn how to measure your body circumferences.

Materials: Measuring tape, partner

SECTION I: MEASURING CIRCUMFERENCES

Using a cloth or plastic tape measure, have a partner assist you with the following circumference measures. Be sure to mark your measurements (centimeters or inches) and record them to the nearest 0.5 cm or 0.25 inch.

Site	Description		Measurement
Waist	For those with a visible waist, measure at the narrowest part of the torso or for those with a larger torso, at the navel.		
Hip	Measure with the legs slightly apart. Measure where the hip/buttock circumference is the greatest.		
Upper Arm	Measure midway between the shoulder and elbow.		Right: Left:
Forearm	Measure at the greatest circumference between the wrist and elbow.		Right: Left:
Thigh	Measure with your leg on a bench or chair (knee at 90 degrees). Measure halfway between the crease in your hip and your knee.		Right: Left:
Calf	Measure at the greatest circumference between the knee and ankle.		Right: Left:
Neck	Measure midway between the head and shoulders.		

Source: American College of Sports Medicine, *ACSM's Guidelines for Exercise Testing and Prescription.* 7th ed. (Baltimore, MD: Lippincott Williams & Wilkins, 2006). Copyright © ACSM. Reprinted by permission of Wolters/Kluwer.

SECTION II: EVALUATING CIRCUMFERENCES AND DISEASE RISK

1. Calculate your waist-to-hip ratio (WHR):

WHR = _____ ÷ _____

   (waist circumference)   (hip circumference)

WHR = _____

2. Evaluate your WHR in the table below:

Age (years)	Disease Risk and WHR			
	Low	**Moderate**	**High**	**Very High**
Men: 20–29	< 0.83	0.83–0.88	0.89–0.94	> 0.94
30–39	< 0.84	0.84–0.91	0.92–0.96	> 0.96
40–49	< 0.88	0.88–0.95	0.96–1.00	> 1.00
50–59	< 0.90	0.90–0.96	0.97–1.02	> 1.02
60–69	< 0.91	0.91–0.98	0.99–1.03	> 1.03
Women: 20–29	< 0.71	0.71–0.77	0.78–0.82	> 0.82
30–39	< 0.72	0.72–0.78	0.79–0.84	> 0.84
40–49	< 0.73	0.73–0.79	0.80–0.87	> 0.87
50–59	< 0.74	0.74–0.81	0.82–0.88	> 0.88
60–69	< 0.76	0.76–0.83	0.84–0.90	> 0.90

Source: V. H. Heyward, *Advanced Fitness Assessment and Exercise Prescription.* 5th ed. (Champaign, IL: Human Kinetics, 2006).

Evaluate your waist circumference in the following table:

Disease Risk Category	Waist Circumference (WC)	
	Women	**Men**
Very Low	< 70 cm (< 28.5 in)	< 80 cm (< 31.5 in)
Low	70–89 cm (28.5–35.0 in)	80–99 cm (31.5–39.0 in)
High	90–109 cm (35.5–43.0 in)	100–120 cm (39.5–47.0 in)
Very High	> 110 cm (> 43.5 in)	> 120 cm (> 47.0 in)

Source: G. A. Bray, "Don't Throw the Baby out with the Bath Water," *American Journal of Clinical Nutrition* 70, no. 3 (2004): 347–49. Copyright © 2004 American Society for Nutrition. Used with permission.

3. Record your disease risk from WHR and waist circumference below:

Disease rating for WHR: _____

Disease rating for WC: _____

SECTION III: REFLECTION

1. Do your ratings for disease risk based upon circumferences surprise you? _____

2. Which of your circumference measures are you most interested in changing and why?

_____

Name: _____   Date: _____

Instructor: _____   Section: _____

Materials: Skinfold calipers, appropriate clothing (shorts, tank top, sports bra for women)

Purpose: To assess your current percent body fat.

Directions: Complete the sections below, ideally under the supervision of a trained instructor.

SECTION I: SKINFOLD MEASUREMENT

You will need a partner to help you with your measurements. If you are completing these measurements with an inexperienced partner, be aware that the typical error rate of 3 to 4 percent may be higher. Note the time of day of your measurements and perform any follow-up measurements at the same time of day.

1. Identify the correct skinfold locations. If you are male, locate the chest, abdomen, and thigh locations (see photos below). If you are female, locate the tricep, suprailiac, and thigh locations (see photos).

Chest	A diagonal fold measured midway between the shoulder/armpit crease and the nipple.	
Abdomen	A vertical fold measured 1 inch to the right of the navel.	
Thigh	A vertical fold measured midway between the crease in your hip and the top of your knee.	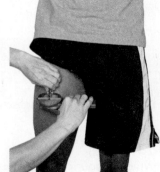

Tricep	A vertical fold on the back of the upper arm midway between the shoulder and elbow.
Suprailiac	A diagonal fold just above the hip bone, on the side of the body at the front edge of your relaxed arm.

Source: American College of Sports Medicine, *ACSM's Guidelines for Exercise Testing and Prescription.* 7th ed. (Baltimore, MD: Lippincott Williams & Wilkins, 2006). Copyright © ACSM. Reprinted by permission of Wolters/Kluwer. Photos owned by Benjamin Cummings.

Have your partner mark these locations with a pen before using the caliper. Mark only the locations on the right side of the body.

2. Your partner will measure each skinfold location and record the results.

Instructions for the partner:
After locating the correct sites, grab a double fold of skin on both sides of the skinfold location. Open your fingers about 3 inches when lifting the fold (> than 3 inches is required for larger individuals). Holding the fold in place, pick up the calipers with your other hand. While still holding the fold, place the caliper jaws on the skinfold location, measuring halfway between the crest and the base of the fold. You should measure perpendicular to the fold and about 1 cm away from your fingers. Read the measurement 2 to 3 seconds after placing the calipers and record the skinfold numbers to the nearest 0.5 mm. For accuracy, measure each site three times and average the two closest numbers. Record the results below and then add up the three skinfold sites to obtain your overall skinfold sum.

MEN			**WOMEN**	
Chest	_____ mm		Tricep	_____ mm
Abdomen	_____ mm		Suprailiac	_____ mm
Thigh	_____ mm		Thigh	_____ mm
Sum of 3 =	_____ mm		Sum of 3 =	_____ mm

3. Find your estimated percent body fat. From the sum of three skinfolds, find your estimated percent body fat in the tables for women and men.

Sum of Skinfolds (mm)	Percent Body Fat Estimates for WOMEN (from tricep, suprailiac, and thigh skinfolds)								
	AGE (years)								
	Under 22	23–27	28–32	33–37	38–42	43–47	48–52	53–57	Over 57
23–25	9.7	9.9	10.2	10.4	10.7	10.9	11.2	11.4	11.7
26–28	11.0	11.2	11.5	11.7	12.0	12.3	12.5	12.7	13.0
29–31	12.3	12.5	12.8	13.0	13.3	13.5	13.8	14.0	14.3
32–34	13.6	13.8	14.0	14.3	14.5	14.8	15.0	15.3	15.5
35–37	14.8	15.0	15.3	15.5	15.8	16.0	16.3	16.5	16.8
38–40	16.0	16.3	16.5	16.7	17.0	17.2	17.5	17.7	18.0
41–43	17.2	17.4	17.7	17.9	18.2	18.4	18.7	18.9	19.2
44–46	18.3	18.6	18.8	19.1	19.3	19.6	19.8	20.1	20.3
47–49	19.5	19.7	20.0	20.2	20.5	20.7	21.0	21.2	21.5
50–52	20.6	20.8	21.1	21.3	21.6	21.8	22.1	22.3	22.6
53–55	21.7	21.9	22.1	22.4	22.6	22.9	23.1	23.4	23.6
56–58	22.7	23.0	23.2	23.4	23.7	23.9	24.2	24.4	24.7
59–61	23.7	24.0	24.2	24.5	24.7	25.0	25.2	25.5	25.7
62–64	24.7	25.0	25.2	25.5	25.7	26.0	26.2	26.4	26.7
65–67	25.7	25.9	26.2	26.4	26.7	26.9	27.2	27.4	27.7
68–70	26.6	26.9	27.1	27.4	27.6	27.9	28.1	28.4	28.6
71–73	27.5	27.8	28.0	28.3	28.5	28.8	29.0	29.3	29.5
74–76	28.4	28.7	28.9	29.2	29.4	29.7	29.9	30.2	30.4
77–79	29.3	29.5	29.8	30.0	30.3	30.5	30.8	31.0	31.3
80–82	30.1	30.4	30.6	30.9	31.1	31.4	31.6	31.9	32.1
83–85	30.9	31.2	31.4	31.7	31.9	32.2	32.4	32.7	32.9
86–88	31.7	32.0	32.2	32.5	32.7	32.9	33.2	33.4	33.7
89–91	32.5	32.7	33.0	33.2	33.5	33.7	33.9	34.2	34.4
92–94	33.2	33.4	33.7	33.9	34.2	34.4	34.7	34.9	35.2
95–97	33.9	34.1	34.4	34.6	34.9	35.1	35.4	35.6	35.9
98–100	34.6	34.8	35.1	35.3	35.5	35.8	36.0	36.3	36.5
101–103	35.3	35.4	35.7	35.9	36.2	36.4	36.7	36.9	37.2
104–106	35.8	36.1	36.3	36.6	36.8	37.1	37.3	37.5	37.8
107–109	36.4	36.7	36.9	37.1	37.4	37.6	37.9	38.1	38.4
110–112	37.0	37.2	37.5	37.7	38.0	38.2	38.5	38.7	38.9
113–115	37.5	37.8	38.0	38.2	38.5	38.7	39.0	39.2	39.5
116–118	38.0	38.3	38.5	38.8	39.0	39.3	39.5	39.7	40.0
119–121	38.5	38.7	39.0	39.2	39.5	39.7	40.0	40.2	40.5
122–124	39.0	39.2	39.4	39.7	39.9	40.2	40.4	40.7	40.9
125–127	39.4	39.6	39.9	40.1	40.4	40.6	40.9	41.1	41.4
128–130	39.8	40.0	40.3	40.5	40.8	41.0	41.3	41.5	41.8

Source: A. S. Jackson, and M. L. Pollock, "Practical Assessment of Body Composition," *The Physician and Sportsmedicine* 13, no. 5 (1985): 76–90.

Sum of Skinfolds (mm)	Percent Body Fat Estimates for WOMEN (from tricep, suprailiac, and thigh skinfolds)								
	AGE (years)								
	Under 22	23–27	28–32	33–37	38–42	43–47	48–52	53–57	Over 57
8–10	1.3	1.8	2.3	2.9	3.4	3.9	4.5	5.0	5.5
11–13	2.2	2.8	3.3	3.9	4.4	4.9	5.5	6.0	6.5
14–16	3.2	3.8	4.3	4.8	5.4	5.9	6.4	7.0	7.5
17–19	4.2	4.7	5.3	5.8	6.3	6.9	7.4	8.0	8.5
20–22	5.1	5.7	6.2	6.8	7.3	7.9	8.4	8.9	9.5
23–25	6.1	6.6	7.2	7.7	8.3	8.8	9.4	9.9	10.5
26–28	7.0	7.6	8.1	8.7	9.2	9.8	10.3	10.9	11.4
29–31	8.0	8.5	9.1	9.6	10.2	10.7	11.3	11.8	12.4
32–34	8.9	9.4	10.0	10.5	11.1	11.6	12.2	12.8	13.3
35–37	9.8	10.4	10.9	11.5	12.0	12.6	13.1	13.7	14.3
38–40	10.7	11.3	11.8	12.4	12.9	13.5	14.1	14.6	15.2
41–43	11.6	12.2	12.7	13.3	13.8	14.4	15.0	15.5	16.1
44–46	12.5	13.1	13.6	14.2	14.7	15.3	15.9	16.4	17.0
47–49	13.4	13.9	14.5	15.1	15.6	16.2	16.8	17.3	17.9
50–52	14.3	14.8	15.4	15.9	16.5	17.1	17.6	18.2	18.8
53–55	15.1	15.7	16.2	16.8	17.4	17.9	18.5	19.1	19.7
56–58	16.0	16.5	17.1	17.7	18.2	18.8	19.4	20.0	20.5
59–61	16.9	17.4	17.9	18.5	19.1	19.7	20.2	20.8	21.4
62–64	17.6	18.2	18.8	19.4	19.9	20.5	21.1	21.7	22.2
65–67	18.5	19.0	19.6	20.2	20.8	21.3	21.9	22.5	23.1
68–70	19.3	19.9	20.4	21.0	21.6	22.2	22.7	23.3	23.9
71–73	20.1	20.7	21.2	21.8	22.4	23.0	23.6	24.1	24.7
74–76	20.9	21.5	22.0	22.6	23.2	23.8	24.4	25.0	25.5
77–79	21.7	22.2	22.8	23.4	24.0	24.6	25.2	25.8	26.3
80–82	22.4	23.0	23.6	24.2	24.8	25.4	25.9	26.5	27.1
83–85	23.2	23.8	24.4	25.0	25.5	26.1	26.7	27.3	27.9
86–88	24.0	24.5	25.1	25.7	26.3	26.9	27.5	28.1	28.7
89–91	24.7	25.3	25.9	26.5	27.1	27.6	28.2	28.8	29.4
92–94	25.4	26.0	26.6	27.2	27.8	28.4	29.0	29.6	30.2
95–97	26.1	26.7	27.3	27.9	28.5	29.1	29.7	30.3	30.9
98–100	26.9	27.4	28.0	28.6	29.2	29.8	30.4	31.0	31.6
101–103	27.5	28.1	28.7	29.3	29.9	30.5	31.1	31.7	32.3
104–106	28.2	28.8	29.4	30.0	30.6	31.2	31.8	32.4	33.0
107–109	28.9	29.5	30.1	30.7	31.3	31.9	32.5	33.1	33.7
110–112	29.6	30.2	30.8	31.4	32.0	32.6	33.2	33.8	34.4
113–115	30.2	30.8	31.4	32.0	32.6	33.2	33.8	34.5	35.1
116–118	30.9	31.5	32.1	32.7	33.3	33.9	34.5	35.1	35.7
119–121	31.5	32.1	32.7	33.3	33.9	34.5	35.1	35.7	36.4
122–124	32.1	32.7	33.3	33.9	34.5	35.1	35.8	36.4	37.0
125–127	32.7	33.3	33.9	34.5	35.1	35.8	36.4	37.0	37.6

Source: A. S. Jackson, and M. L. Pollock, "Practical Assessment of Body Composition," *The Physician and Sportsmedicine* 13, no. 5 (1985): 76–90. Copyright © 1985 JTE Multimedia, LLC. Used with permission.

4. Record your estimated percent body fat and rating.

% body fat = _____

Circle your body fat rating below:

Body Fat Rating	WOMEN	MEN
Athletic/Low	14–20%	6–13%
Fitness	21–24%	14–17%
Acceptable	25–31%	18–25%
Obese	> 32%	> 26%

Source: American Council on Exercise, ACEfitness.org. Reprinted with permission from the American Council on Exercise.

SECTION II: REFLECTION

1. Did your estimated percent body fat or rating surprise you? _____

2. How does your percent body fat rating compare with your other disease risk ratings from Lab 7.2?

_____

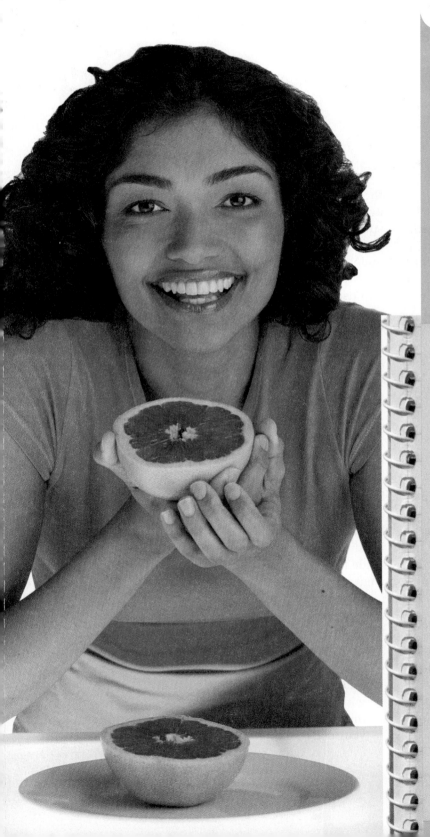

CHAPTER 8

Improving Your Nutrition

CASE STUDY

Chau

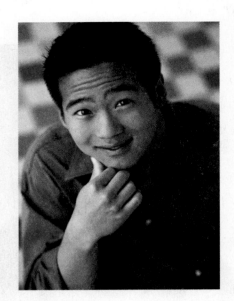

"Hi, I'm Chau. I'm a freshman and live on-campus in a dorm with my roommate, Tom. I moved here to Connecticut from Chicago. Living away from home for the first time has been quite an experience! I've been studying like crazy, taking a full load of classes, and trying to figure out if I want to major in history or poli sci. Plus, I'm in a few clubs and I'm playing a lot of soccer—my favorite sport. I'm not on the team, but I like to play for fun, and I'll join in if I see a pick-up game forming. I'm so busy that I'm always rushing, and then I'll realize I'm starving! When I lived at home, there just always seemed to be food around. Now, I feel like I'm often scrambling at the last minute to find something to eat."

Suppose someone offered to supply you with a perfect diet for life that contained all the nutrients you need, plus the right number of daily calories to keep you at your ideal weight forever. The only catch is that the food in this diet is gray, gummy, tastes like vitamin pills, and squirts out of a large plastic tube. Would you sign up? Probably not! Life would be bleak, indeed, without the pleasure of seeing, smelling, and tasting a variety of foods.

Hunger—the drive to eat—is one of our most basic motivations, compelling us to go out, find, and consume the food that will supply our bodies with energy and raw materials. Our food contains **nutrients,** chemical compounds that supply the energy and raw materials we need to survive. Nutrients include water, proteins, carbohydrates (starches and sugars), lipids (fats and oils), vitamins, and minerals. Proteins, carbohydrates, and lipids contain atoms and molecules arrayed in particular three-dimensional configurations that give them unique shapes and properties. Our cells can break down these food molecules and, in the process, change their shapes and release energy stored in

their chemical bonds. The energy quickly becomes available to drive the activities within our cells, tissues, and organs. The breakdown of nutrients also liberates raw materials that cells can take in, modify, and use in repair and growth.

Nutrition is the study of how people consume and use the nutrients in food. Nutrition researchers explore some of the basic questions about what we should be eating and how food affects our long-term health and disease. Is it better to eat butter or margarine? Should you drink tea, coffee, both, or neither? Should you take a daily vitamin pill? Is red meat okay? How much salt is too much?

Nutritional findings are sometimes contradictory. Since the 1970s, consumers have been advised to throw away butter, and use margarine instead; then to do just the reverse; then to avoid almost all fats; then to avoid almost all carbohydrates, and so on. Some people have grown skeptical about nutritional information. As in every area of science, new studies in nutrition occasionally contain data that appear to invalidate older studies. Nevertheless, the field has made tremendous advances toward understanding what we should be eating, what we should be avoiding, and why. The kinds of healthy diets we discuss in this chapter can help you stay in the optimal zone of the fitness and wellness continuum. Keep in mind:

- A good diet helps sustain desirable body mass and weight and helps keep your fat-to-lean ratios within a recommended range. This, in turn, can improve appearance, enable greater comfort with your body, and reduce the risk of chronic illnesses related to being overweight and obese.

nutrient A chemical in food that is crucial for growth and function; includes proteins, carbohydrates (starches and sugars), lipids (fats and oils), vitamins, and minerals

nutrition The study of how people consume and use the nutrients in food

- A good diet can help alleviate feelings of stress and depression, while a poor diet can contribute to them.

- A good diet can act as preventive medicine, helping you to avoid chronic diseases, frequent colds and infections, and the effects of vitamin deficiency. Conversely, poor diet is one of the biggest contributors to cardiovascular disease, diabetes, obesity, arthritis, osteoporosis, and several types of cancers. If you are young and currently well, such conditions may seem improbable and remote. However, the dietary habits you establish now either diminish or promote your later risk for all types of chronic illness. Optimal fitness and wellness—both now and in your future—requires a good understanding and application of nutrition principles.

WHY ARE THE COLLEGE YEARS A NUTRITIONAL CHALLENGE?

If you are like most college students, you often reach for cheap snacks and fast food to save time and money. You grab something tasty. You eat it quickly. And you move on to the next class, job, study session, or social event. You may worry about calories and weight. But most students don't think much about vitamins, minerals, and other nutrients, or concern themselves much with the challenge of eating well during the college years.

The typical student's diet resembles the typical American diet: nearly one-third of Americans' total calories come from chips, cookies, donuts, desserts, french fries, candy bars, sugary drinks, beer, wine, and other alcoholic beverages.[1] The number-one takeout food is pizza, followed by Chinese food and fast food (burgers, fries, and so on). Other favorite "staples" of the American diet are coffee drinks, tacos, burritos, sandwiches, and salads. The most frequently eaten vegetables in America are iceberg lettuce and potatoes.

MOST STUDENTS HAVE LESS-THAN-OPTIMAL EATING HABITS

College students, in general, have poor eating habits (Figure 8.1). Results of the American College Health Association's 2006 annual survey of nearly 95,000 students from colleges and universities throughout the United States highlighted the dietary deficiencies of today's students.[2] Fewer than 8% consumed the recommended 5 servings of fruits and vegetables each day. Nearly 60% reported eating only 1–2 servings each day, and 31% consumed 3–4 servings. Approximately 60% reported that they did not exercise at all, or only exercised for 30 minutes or more on 1–2 days per week. Less than 35% reported exercising 30 minutes/day on at least 3–5 days per week. In short, like their older counterparts, young adults report that they are interested in improving their health; yet, they fall far short of the mark in meeting national dietary and exercise guidelines. It is no wonder that the term "Freshman 15" has become common language among students to describe their excess weight gain during the first year on campus.

Lack of nutritional knowledge contributes to students' poor eating habits. On the other hand, good information and understanding make a measurable difference in students' nutritional wellness, including the amount of weight they gain. The information throughout this book, especially in this chapter and in our discussion of weight management, can help you in the same ways.

FIGURE 8.1

Students consume more than they need of certain nutrients, which diminishes wellness. They also tend to consume less than they need of the nutrients that can improve wellness.

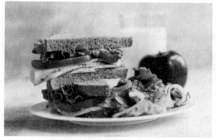

(a) Students do not consume enough fruit, vegetables, whole grains, milk, and fiber

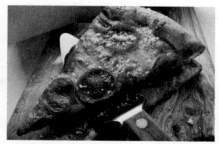

(b) Students consume too much protein, saturated fat, salt, sugar, and too many refined carbohydrates

COLLEGE LIFE PRESENTS OBSTACLES TO GOOD NUTRITION

Food is easy to find in the ever-present vending machines, cafeterias, bars, restaurants, and markets on campus and off. Despite all these food suppliers—and partly because of them, in fact—students face numerous obstacles to good nutrition. These include time and money pressures, lack of home-cooking facilities, personal habits and attitudes, and the emotional stresses college can present.

Fast food and takeout appear to solve both time and money issues, but the food at these restaurants often provides poor nutrition. The box **Tools for Change: Tips for Ordering at Fast-Food Restaurants** lists tips for healthier choices while eating out. Even when students cook for themselves, however, nutritional misconceptions and a tight budget can still impede a good diet. If you do shop and cook, a few simple steps can help you achieve a healthy affordable diet: buy fruits and vegetables that are in season. Watch for sales, use coupons, and/or shop at discount stores. Make a shopping list and stick to it. Buy more plant proteins (e.g., beans and tofu) and less meat, fish, or poultry. And if possible, cook in quantity and freeze portions for later.

Our natural cravings for sweet, fatty, and high-protein foods can lead to poor nutrition. Childhood eating patterns can also be obstacles to good nutrition. Students don't enroll in college and then immediately develop poor food habits. They often come with preexisting preferences based on insufficient nutritional knowledge: for example, eating junk food, skipping breakfast, snacking frequently, and limiting meat and/or vegetable consumption.

Self-perception about body image can be another obstacle to eating well. Three-fifths of female college students and half of males are dissatisfied with their body size and shape.[3] Of these, the vast majority want to lose weight, while a small minority want to gain weight or add muscle. This phenomenon can help explain why some students skip meals; avoid particular classes of foods such as fats or carbohydrates; go on drastic very-low-calorie diets; or take other less-than-successful measures that can cause an imbalance of nutrients, vitamins, and minerals.

Stress and social eating are additional contributors to poor diet. People under stress often eat more, especially high-calorie foods, and get too little sleep, which can lead to using food, caffeine, sugar, and alcohol to alter mood and energy levels. People under stress also tend to seek out the relief of socializing for relaxation, and when people get together, they eat and drink. The box **Tools for Change: Tips for Ordering at Sit-Down Restaurants** on page 222 describes healthy and unhealthy food items on a wide variety of menus.

Choosing foods for the first time without parental guidance leads some to make poor selections. This is particularly true when there are few nutritious options available. Research shows that when nutritious foods are readily available in a cafeteria setting, many students will choose them. Male students, for example, chose more fruits and vegetables and leaner meats in dormitory dining halls than did males eating in apartments, in restaurants, and so on. Female students eating in dining halls chose amounts of fruit closer to USDA recommendations.[4] However, although free choice in cafeteria lines does seem to encourage *better* nutrition for many students, it can still lead to consuming too many calories.

TOOLS FOR CHANGE

TIPS FOR ORDERING AT FAST-FOOD RESTAURANTS

It's not necessary—or even possible, at times—to stop eating at fast-food restaurants. It is important, however, to learn to order healthier alternatives from the menu. Here are some ideas:

- In general, skip high-fat, high-sodium, deep-fried foods such as french fries, onion rings, fried chicken, fish fillets, chicken nuggets, or apple pies.
- Avoid the empty calories of drinks sweetened with sugar or corn syrup and instead choose water, skim or low-fat milk, unsweetened iced tea, diet soft drinks, or fruit juice.
- Use only small amounts of salad dressings, ketchup, and other sauces.
- For sandwiches, avoid extra-large or double-patty servings, added cheese, and white bread buns.
- Try an entrée salad, but use only a small amount of dressing or low-fat dressing on the side.
- For dessert, try fresh fruit and yogurt, or apple slices and low-fat dip.
- At snack bars, avoid white flour bagels; smoothies containing high-fat yogurt and sugar; soft pretzels; coffee drinks; and sweetened granola bars. Instead choose whole fruit, unsweetened fruit juice, veggie sticks, unsalted nuts, or iced coffee with skim milk.

Source: Nutrition: Family Health Guide 2004. Consumers Union of United States, Inc. Yonkers, NY 10703–1057, the nonprofit organization that publishes Consumer Reports®. Reprinted with permission for educational purposes only. No commercial use or reproduction permitted. www.ConsumerReports.org.

CASE STUDY

Chau

"Mostly, I eat in the dorm cafeteria. I have a meal plan that covers 60 meals a month. That means I have to take care of about 30 meals on my own. The idea was that I'd eat two meals a day in the dorm—probably breakfast and dinner—and grab lunch somewhere between classes. So far, though, it's not quite working out that way. On days when I don't have an early class, I tend to sleep through breakfast. Then, I've got to rush to my 11:00, which means grabbing donuts and coffee in the campus store. Sometimes I manage to get back to the dorm for lunch, but if I don't, I usually eat something on the run at the food court. The good thing is that my dorm has a late night café that accepts my meal plan. So if I'm up late studying, I can grab a pizza or bowl of cereal to stay fueled.

I don't pay much attention to my diet or how many calories I'm eating. I'm young and pretty active. I figure at my age, it's more about getting enough calories then eating a 'balanced meal.' After all, doesn't it kind of balance out naturally?"

1. What aspects of college life are influencing Chau's dietary choices?

2. Would you describe Chau's eating habits as excellent, average, or poor? What is he doing right? What should he do differently?

3. How does your living situation and schedule help or hinder your efforts to eat right? What small lifestyle changes could you make to improve your diet?

WHAT ARE THE MAIN NUTRIENTS IN FOOD?

The next time you reach for an apple, an energy bar, or a slice of pizza, don't just think of it as food to satisfy your appetite. Think of it as a refueling stop to input energy compounds and raw materials. We humans share the need to "refuel" with every other kind of animal, from soaring eagles to bloblike sea cucumbers. Our bodies can't originate energy-containing raw materials for activity, growth, and repair. Like all animals, we must obtain these compounds from foods and liquids in sufficient quantities to supply our daily needs, and then modify them into the specific kinds of building blocks our cells require.

Essential nutrients are nutrients we must obtain from food for normal body functioning. Nutritionists classify them into several categories: protein, carbohydrates, fats, vitamins, minerals, and water (Figure 8.2 on page 223). Our bodies chemically modify and use nutrients to build the thousands of components we need to allow our muscles to contract, our nerves to conduct, our cells to divide, and so on. Consuming nutrients keeps our internal "production line" efficiently manufacturing cell parts and usable energy compounds.

Nutritionists measure the nutrients in individual foods, the energy stored in those nutrients, and the way our bodies release and use raw materials and energy during the digestion process. They measure the released energy in **calories.** One calorie (lowercase *c*) is the amount of energy required to raise the temperature of 1 gram of water 1 degree Celsius. When they refer to specific foods, nutritionists usually apply the larger measure **kilocalories** (kcal) or **Calories** (capital *C*). A kilocalorie or Calorie is equivalent to 1,000 calories, as follows:

$$1 \text{ Calorie (Cal)} = 1 \text{ kilocalorie (1 kcal)}$$
$$= 1,000 \text{ calories (cal)}$$

For example, an apple the size of a tennis ball provides 50 Calories or 50,000 calories, enough to raise the temperature of 1 kilogram of water by 50 degrees C. This book uses *calories* when referring to food energy in general and *Calories* for exact energy counts from quantities of specific foods. Active adults need about

essential nutrient A nutrient necessary for normal body functioning that must be obtained from food

calorie A measure of the amount of chemical energy that foods provide. One calorie (lowercase *c*) can raise 1 gram of water 1 degree C.

kilocalorie (kcal) One thousand calories. Also designated Calories (capital *C*). Nutritionists use kcal or C when they refer to specific foods. A medium-sized apple provides 50 Calories.

TIPS FOR ORDERING AT SIT-DOWN RESTAURANTS

Learning to choose healthy items from cafeteria lines and restaurant menus is an important step toward wellness and weight management. Here are the best and worst common items on 5 popular kinds of restaurant menus. "Good Choices" contain fewer than 30 grams of fat, provide more fiber from whole grains, include fruits and vegetables, and have less sodium and fewer calories. "Poor Choices" have 30 to 100 grams of fat and provide less fiber, more sodium, and more calories than the other alternatives.

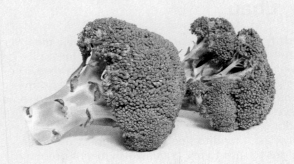

Ordering Italian

Tips: Choose pastas with red sauces, not cream or cheese sauces. Choose smaller portions of pasta. Avoid thick layers of melted cheese.

Good Choices: Large green salad, vinaigrette dressing on the side (hold the salami); spaghetti with marinara or tomato-and-meat sauce; minestrone soup

Poor Choices: Eggplant parmigiana smothered in cheese; fettuccine alfredo with rich cream sauce

Ordering Mexican

Tips: Choose soft tortillas (not fried) with fresh salsa, not guacamole. Order grilled shrimp, fish, or chicken. Ask for black or pinto beans made without lard or fat. Avoid cheeses and sour cream or ask for them on the side.

Good Choices: Bean burrito, no cheese; chicken fajitas, lots of vegetables, no sour cream

Poor Choices: Beef chimichanga, deep fried; chile relleno, battered and fried

Ordering Chinese

Tips: Share a stir-fry. Request brown rice instead of white. Ask for vegetables steamed or stir-fried with less oil. Order moo shu vegetables instead of pork. Avoid fried rice, breaded dishes, egg rolls and spring rolls, and items loaded with peanuts or cashews. Go light on soy sauce, which is high in sodium.

Good Choices: Hot-and-sour soup; stir-fried vegetables; shrimp with garlic sauce; Szechuan shrimp; wonton soup

Poor Choices: Crispy chicken, deep fried; kung pao chicken with lots of peanuts and rich sauce; moo shu pork (high in saturated fat from meat and eggs); sweet-and-sour pork with deep-fried meat in thick sugary sauce

Ordering Japanese

Tips: Avoid soy sauces. Avoid deep-fried dishes like tempura. Eat sashimi and sushi (raw fish) only where the food is freshly made to avoid possible bacteria or parasites.

Good Choices: Steamed rice and vegetables; tofu as a meat substitute; broiled or steamed chicken and fish

Poor Choices: Fried rice dishes (high in saturated fat); miso (high in sodium); tempura

Ordering Thai

Tips: Avoid coconut-based soups and curries. Ask for steamed, not fried, rice. Try for brown rice rather than white. Thai iced tea is filled with sugar and high-fat evaporated milk.

Good Choices: Clear broth soups; stir-fried chicken and vegetables; grilled meats

Poor Choices: Coconut milk soup with chicken (high in saturated fat); peanut sauces for satay; deep-fried or batter-fried meats and vegetables

Source: Frazaos, E. 1999. "America's Eating Habits: Changes and Consequences." Washington, DC: United States Department of Agriculture Economic Research Service Report.

2,000 to 2,500 Calories of food energy per day. Taking in more calories from food than you burn off through activity, exercise, and metabolism results in fat storage and weight gain. One gram of fat delivers 9 Calories; 1 gram of alcohol 7 Calories, and one gram of either proteins or carbohydrates 4 Calories.

PROTEINS ARE BUILDING BLOCKS OF STRUCTURE AND FUNCTION

About 50 to 60 percent of your body weight is water; of the remainder, about half is protein. At 150 pounds, your body would contain about

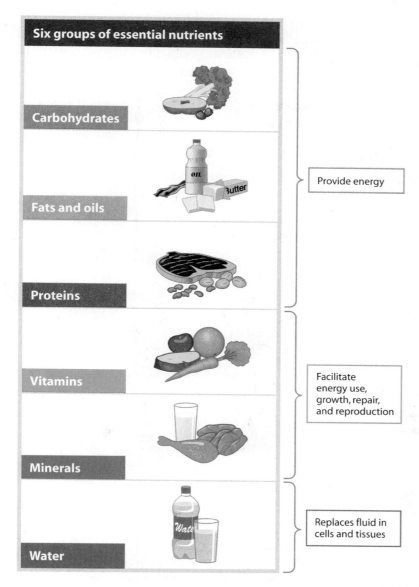

Six groups of essential nutrients

Carbohydrates

Fats and oils

Proteins

Vitamins

Minerals

Water

Provide energy

Facilitate energy use, growth, repair, and reproduction

Replaces fluid in cells and tissues

FIGURE 8.2

The six essential groups of nutrients in our foods provide energy, facilitate vital activities, and supply needed fluid for cells and tissues.

from disease, the enzymes that control all chemical reactions in the body, and many types of hormones that regulate body activities. Proteins also help transport oxygen, carbon dioxide, and various nutrients to body cells. When the body runs low on fats and carbohydrates as sources of ready energy, it can break down its own proteins as well. Protein supplies 4 Calories of energy per gram.

Protein molecules are chains of subunits called *amino acids.* Sometimes called the "building blocks of life," amino acids contain carbon, hydrogen, oxygen, and nitrogen arrayed in particular ways. There are 20 different kinds of amino acids, each with a different three-dimensional shape. Our cells can build 11 of these types, but we must consume the other 9 types in our foods.

Your body uses the 20 types of amino acids to build tens of thousands of kinds of proteins. Many of these are *structural proteins* that make up parts of cells, tissues, and organs. Many kinds of structural proteins enable cells to move, to divide, and to transport materials around internally. Other structural proteins make up your hair strands, your fingernails and toenails, and the lenses of your eyes. A steady supply of amino acids in the diet allows your body to continuously build, repair, and replace its own structural proteins.

Proteins that perform crucial functions (rather than make up physical structures) are called *functional proteins* and include **enzymes.** Enzymes are proteins that enable thousands of kinds of chemical reactions to occur simultaneously within each body cell every second, including the enzyme reactions that break down food, absorb nutrients, and build new cell parts.

75 pounds of water and about 37.5 pounds of protein, depending on your muscle mass. **Proteins** are major structural components of nearly every cell and are especially important to the building and repairing of bone, muscle, skin, and blood cells. Proteins are also critical to cell and body functioning: They make up the antibodies that protect us

protein Biological molecule composed of amino acids. Proteins serve as crucial structural and functional compounds in living organisms.

enzyme Protein that facilitates chemical reactions but is not permanently altered in the process; biological catalyst

Proteins in the Diet Our bodies can manufacture only 11 of the 20 kinds of amino acids. Nutritionists call the other nine, which we must consume in food, the **essential amino acids.** Dietary protein that supplies all the essential amino acids is called *complete protein,* or *high-quality protein.* Typically, protein from animal products is complete. *Incomplete proteins* lack some of the essential amino acids and therefore some of the building blocks we need to produce the full spectrum of proteins for growth, repair, and activity. Proteins from plant sources are often incomplete, lacking one or two of the essential amino acids. Nevertheless, it is relatively easy for a vegetarian to combine plant foods to obtain *complementary proteins* from plant sources (Figure 8.3). Eating peanut butter on whole grain bread is a good example of combining plant foods to get all the essential amino acids. Eating corn and beans on the same day is another example. We'll talk more about plant proteins in our discussion on vegetarian diets (page 255).

Plant sources of proteins fall into three general categories: **legumes** (beans, peas, peanuts, and soy products); grains (whole grains, corn, and pasta products); and nuts and seeds. Certain vegetables such as broccoli and leafy greens like spinach also contribute valuable plant proteins. People who aren't strict vegetarians can combine incomplete plant proteins with complete low-fat animal proteins such as lean chicken, fish, turkey, or red meat or nonfat dairy products.

Daily Protein Needs Nutritionists typically recommend that in a 2,000-Calorie diet, you should get about 10 percent of your calories (or about 200 Calories or more) from protein. Although over a billion of the world's people face daily protein deficiency, few Americans suffer it. In fact, the average American consumes more than 100 grams (400 Calories or more) of protein daily,

Eaten in the right combinations, plant-based foods can provide complementary proteins and all essential amino acids

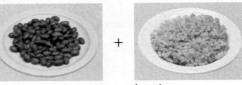

Legumes and grains

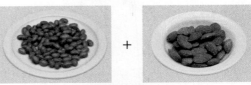

Legumes and nuts and seeds

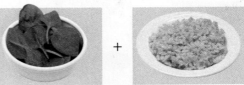

Green leafy vegetables and grains

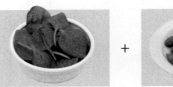 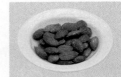

Green leafy vegetables and nuts and seeds

FIGURE 8.3

Combining plant foods from different groups (for example, grains and legumes) on the same day can provide complementary proteins and all the necessary amino acids, even without eating meat or other animal foods.

essential amino acid One of 9 of the 20 types of amino acids, or building blocks, that our bodies cannot manufacture and that we must consume in our foods

legume Fruit or seed of plants of the legume family. Legumes include beans, peas, peanuts, and seeds. Soy products are derived from soy beans, which are legumes.

with as much as 70 percent of it coming from animal parts and products and dairy products high in unhealthy saturated fats. Consuming too much protein, particularly animal protein, can place added stress on the liver and kidneys and can cause *gout,* a painful disease that involves the buildup of certain crystalline compounds in the big toe joint and other areas. An overload of protein may also increase calcium excretion in urine, which can increase your risk of bone loss and bone fractures.[5]

Group	Daily protein requirement (g/kg body weight)		Calculating your daily protein requirement	Example (for average adult)
Most adults	0.8 g/kg		❶ Determine your body weight	❶ Weight = 110 lb
Recreational athletes	1.0 –1.1 g/kg		❷ Convert pounds to kilograms: lb ÷ 2.21 lb/kg = kg	❷ 110 lb ÷ 2.21 lb/kg = about 50 kg
Elite athletes in training	1.2 –1.6 g/kg		❸ Multiply by 0.8 g/kg for average adult to get requirement in grams per day	❸ 50 kg × 0.8 g/kg = 40 g Result: a 110 lb adult would need 40 grams of protein a day

FIGURE 8.4

Use these formulas to determine your daily protein requirements, depending on your activity level.

Here's how you can calculate your own exact daily protein needs (Figure 8.4). A young healthy adult needs about 0.75 to 0.8 gram of protein per kilogram of body weight per day. A woman weighing 132 pounds (60 kg) therefore would need 48 grams (60 × 0.75). One gram is equal to 0.035 ounce; therefore, she would need about 1.68 ounces of protein (0.035 × 48 = 1.68), which she could get, for example, by consuming 1 cup of skim milk, 3 ounces of chicken breast, and 3 ounces of salmon during the course of a day.

In recent years, millions of people have tried the Atkins diet and similar diets that nearly eliminate carbohydrates and prescribe large quantities of protein. While these diets *can* lead to weight loss, the dieter is losing weight due to total calorie reduction, not due to some magical property of dietary protein itself. Diets that are not nutritionally balanced are almost always flawed. People with fluid imbalances, kidney or liver problems, or cardiovascular disease should avoid these diets as they raise risk factors for various chronic diseases.

Protein and Fitness It is fairly common for athletes and fitness buffs to load up on animal protein under the misguided notion that eating more protein will cause them to build bigger muscles. But muscles grow in response to being worked: you must use them to grow them! The

many vegetarian Olympic athletes are proof that training and effort—not mountains of animal protein—are the crucial ingredients. Research has also shown that 1.0 gram/kg of protein is enough for all but the top athletes, most of whom can get all they need for heavy endurance and strength training in 1.5 to 1.6 g/kg/day.[6]

It's true that under some circumstances, you may need extra protein for cellular repair and replacement, such as when you are fighting off a serious infection. Most of us, though, need to be much more concerned with getting low-fat proteins than with meeting our daily protein needs.

Try it NOW! Follow the steps and example illustrated in Figure 8.4 to calculate how much protein you need each day. • Compare this result to how much protein you consume on any given day. • Are you taking in more protein than you really need?

CARBOHYDRATES ARE MAJOR ENERGY SUPPLIERS

Carbohydrates, including the sugars and starches, have ring- and chainlike three-dimensional structures that allow them to store and supply much of the energy we need to sustain normal daily activity. The **simple carbohydrates** or sugars are common in whole, unprocessed foods such as beets, sugarcane, carrots, other vegetables, and fruits. The **complex carbohydrates** include the starches found abundantly in grains (such as rice and wheat); cereals (such as oats); some fruits and vegetables (such as bananas and squash); and many root vegetables (such as potatoes, yams, and turnips).

Our cells can rapidly break down sugar molecules and release energy stored in their chemical bonds. For this reason, sugars such as glucose, sucrose (table sugar), and lactose (milk sugar) are a source of immediate energy for the body. Your muscle cells and your brain and nerve cells are particularly dependent on a steady supply of glucose, whether from fruits and vegetables or from the starches in grains. This dependence is the reason low blood sugar, or *hypoglycemia,* can leave you feeling foggy-headed, weak, and shaky.

Starches and other complex carbohydrates (also called *polysaccharides,* meaning "many sugars") can be a source of "timed release" energy. The body's cells must break starch molecules down into sugar subunits before releasing the chemical bond energy contained in those sugars. This slower breakdown makes most starches important energy-storage compounds and structural building materials in plants and animals.

carbohydrate Member of a class of nutrients containing sugars and starches, which supply most of the energy that sustains normal daily activity

simple carbohydrate Carbohydrate made up of one or two sugar subunits and that delivers energy in a quickly usable form. Glucose, a *monosaccharide,* has one sugar subunit. Table sugar, a *disaccharide,* has two sugar subunits.

complex carbohydrate Important energy-storage compound and structural building material in plants and animals. Also called *polysaccharides,* the complex carbohydrates are made up of long chains of sugar molecules and deliver "timed release" energy.

fiber Indigestible carbohydrates in the diet that speed the passage of partially digested food through the digestive tract. Fiber helps control appetite and body weight by creating a feeling of fullness without adding extra calories.

FIBER

Horses and cows can survive on grass and hay alone because their digestive systems can break down and derive energy from *cellulose* (a structural carbohydrate that makes up the cell walls of plants.) However, we can't accomplish this metabolic trick, so all the cellulose we consume acts as indigestible **fiber** in one of two forms. *Insoluble fiber,* found in bran, whole grain breads and cereals, and in most fruits and vegetables, speeds the passage of foods and reduces bile acids and certain bacterial enzymes. *Soluble fiber,* which is in oat bran, dried beans, and some fruits and vegetables, attaches to water molecules. Soluble fiber appears to help lower blood cholesterol levels and the risk of cardiovascular disease. Both kinds of fiber assist the passage of partially digested food through the digestive tract. They also help control appetite and body weight by creating a feeling of fullness without adding extra calories.

Over 90% of Americans do not consume the recommended daily amount of fiber. The typical American eats about 12 grams of fiber per day, less than half of the daily recommended amount of 25 to 30 grams or more.[7] Some professional groups believe the requirements should be higher, perhaps even double the recommended amount. Food labels must list the fiber contents of foods and often break that number down into insoluble and soluble fiber.

Soluble fiber helps to reduce blood cholesterol, lowering the risk of coronary heart disease. While the links between fiber consumption and reduced cancer risk are weak, eating fiber-rich foods is still recommended because they contain other nutrients that may help reduce cancer risk and have other health benefits.[8] Fiber also helps prevent constipation by absorbing moisture like a sponge and producing softer, bulkier stools that are easily passed. Fiber-induced gas may also initiate bowel movements.

Reducing constipation also helps protect against diverticulosis—the formation of tiny pouches in the

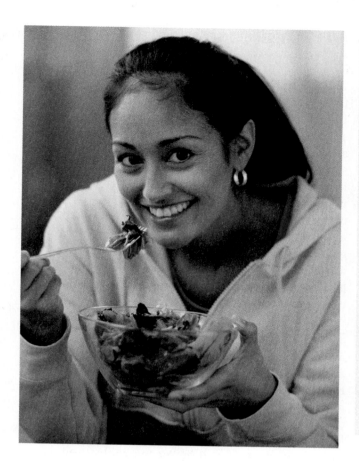

TIPS FOR EATING MORE FIBER

Most Americans need to double their daily fiber intake. To increase yours, think "whole" and "traditional" foods instead of refined foods and choose more of these:

- Whole grains, including stone-ground wheat, bulgur wheat, wheat bran, wheat berries, whole barley, whole millet, whole quinoa, oatmeal, oat bran, popcorn, barley, cornmeal, whole rye, brown rice, and rice bran

- Peas, beans, nuts, and seeds

- Leafy greens such as baby spinach, endive, radicchio, arugula, mizuna, watercress, or dandelion greens

- Bran or flaxseed sprinkled on cereals or salads

- Fresh fruits and vegetables, including, when edible, their cleanly scrubbed skins

- Plenty of liquids each day

At the same time, choose fewer of these:

- White bread, buns, or flour tortillas

- Cereals that list "enriched" flour as the main ingredients

- Cookies, pastries, desserts, candies

colon that bulge out through the intestinal wall like bubbles protruding through holes in a tire. These pouches tend to get inflamed and can cause intestinal pain, bloating, bleeding, blockages, and other symptoms. About 10 percent of Americans over 40, 20 percent over 50, and half over 60 have these little pouches, based on diets too high in refined carbohydrates and too low in whole grains, vegetables, and fruits.[9]

The Glycemic Index of Foods Nutritionists use a tool called the **glycemic index** to measure the rate at which foods raise levels of glucose in the blood. If you eat food with a high glycemic index, your bloodstream becomes flooded with glucose, and this, in turn, leads to an upsurge of the hormone insulin. Over time, this flooding and surging can contribute to being overweight and to type 2 diabetes and heart disease.

Using the glycemic index of foods to control the amount of sugar in your bloodstream requires some practice. The glycemic index is less than straightforward; not all sweet foods have a high index and many starchy or fatty foods do. The index depends on how a starch is cooked, how highly processed a food is, how much indigestible roughage or fiber is left, and how much fat the food contains. The glycemic index of a

medium-sized baked potato is 76; for 1 cup of white spaghetti, it is 44. A slice of pizza has an index almost 10 times higher than a half-cup of ice cream. Dates have an index almost 7 times higher than dried apricots. The glycemic index of foods can help you plan a healthy diet, but it is just one factor to consider because some low–glycemic index foods are poor nutritional choices overall (i.e., premium ice cream, sausages) and some high–glycemic index foods are good choices overall (i.e., bran flakes, watermelon). Keep in mind that, like salt, sugar is often present but hidden in common food products. Ketchup, Russian dressing, and certain types of coffee creamer derive 30 to 65 percent of their calories from sugar. Also, the amount of sugar released into your bloodstream depends on how much of a given food you eat, and in what combination foods are eaten. The combination of glycemic index plus portion size is called *glycemic load*.

glycemic index A measurement of the rate at which foods raise levels of glucose in the blood, and in turn, trigger the release of insulin and other blood-sugar regulators

The best approach to control your sugar intake is to develop a habit of reading food labels before you buy or eat something to discover the amount of dietary sugars in foods. Then, use the glycemic index and glycemic load charts (see this book's website for web links to these charts) to help you get a feel for which foods raise your blood sugar levels quickly and which do not.

"Low-Carb" Foods Because so many Americans are overweight, there is great interest in dietary trends such as cutting fats or loading up on proteins. In recent years, food manufacturers have introduced thousands of "low-carb" foods, influenced, in part, by the popularity of high-protein weight loss diets. As we've seen, however, whole grain foods are packed with healthful nutrients and fiber. The culprit is not the "carbs" themselves but the quantity most people eat and the refining of the carbohydrates. Whole fruits and vegetables, and foods made with whole grains, seeds, and nuts, are nutrient-dense and retain the fibrous cellulose in their skins and husks. Most "low-carb" foods are highly processed and contain substitute sugars like mannitol, sorbitol, and dextrose. There is no solid evidence that these "low-carb" products protect you from diseases, and they cost much more than simple fruits, vegetables, whole grains, nuts, seeds, and beans.

lipid A category of compounds including fats, oils, and waxes that do not dissolve in water

fat A lipid such as butter, lard, and bacon grease, all of which are solids at room temperature

oil A lipid such as corn and olive oil, which is usually a golden liquid at room temperature

fatty acid The most basic unit of triglycerides

triglyceride Lipid molecule made up of three fatty acid chains or "tails" attached to one glycerol "head" containing a three-carbon backbone. Common form of fats in foods and in organisms.

saturated fat A lipid, usually a solid fat like butter, in which most of the chains of carbon atoms are loaded (or "saturated") with as many hydrogen atoms as the chain can carry. Saturated chains are straight, allowing them to pack together and act like a solid.

FATS ARE CONCENTRATED ENERGY STORAGE

The recent "low-carb" craze was preceded by a "low-fat" craze that labeled all fats and oils as harmful. In fact, fats play vital roles in maintaining healthy skin and hair, padding the body organs against shock, insulating us against temperature extremes, storing energy to fuel muscle activity, and promoting healthy cell function. Although they are widely misunderstood nutrients, fats make foods taste better, carry the fat-soluble vitamins A, D, E, and K to cells, and provide certain essential compounds we can't get from other foods or manufacture in our own cells. They also provide a concentrated form of energy and raw materials that can stand in whenever carbohydrates are in short supply.

Types of Fats *Fat* is a common term for **lipids,** a class of molecules that includes fats and oils. **Fats,** such as butter, lard, and bacon grease, are solids at room temperature. **Oils** are usually golden liquids at room temperature; examples are corn and olive oils. Some oils, such as sesame oil, are almost colorless. Lipids also include *waxes,* such as beeswax, and *steroids,* such as steroid hormones, cholesterol, and certain vitamins.

Structurally, fats and oils are made up of long chains of carbon atoms, usually 4 to 14 linked in a line. These chains are called **fatty acids.** The fatty acids in most foods and in the body occur in the form of **triglycerides,** molecules that have a "head," which contains the compound glycerol, and three tails (Figure 8.5a). The "tails" are made up of fatty acid chains of various lengths.

In lipid molecules of all types, the chemical bonding of carbon atoms is the key to whether the chains remain straight and form solid fats, or kink and form liquid oils. Carbon atoms can form four bonds to other atoms. Where carbons are linked to each other in a chain (—C—C—), each carbon has two bonds left over,

$$C-\overset{\displaystyle |}{\underset{\displaystyle |}{C}}-\overset{\displaystyle |}{\underset{\displaystyle |}{C}}-C$$

and these often link to hydrogen atoms:

$$C-\overset{\displaystyle H}{\underset{\displaystyle H}{C}}-\overset{\displaystyle H}{\underset{\displaystyle H}{C}}-C$$

In a fatty acid chain where every available carbon bond is *saturated* or filled with hydrogen atoms, the fat itself is called a **saturated fat.** Saturated

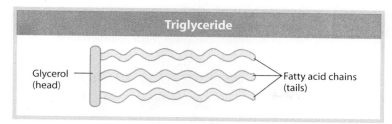

Triglyceride

Glycerol (head) — Fatty acid chains (tails)

(a)

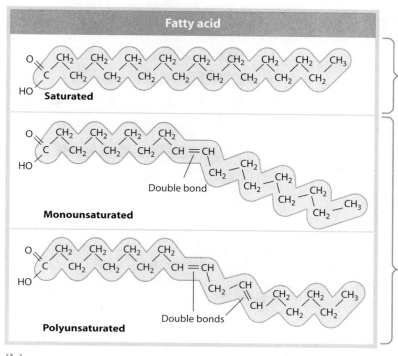

Fatty acid

Saturated

Monounsaturated

Double bond

Double bonds

Polyunsaturated

(b)

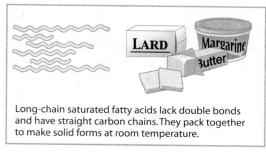

Long-chain saturated fatty acids lack double bonds and have straight carbon chains. They pack together to make solid forms at room temperature.

(c)

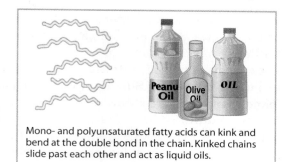

Mono- and polyunsaturated fatty acids can kink and bend at the double bond in the chain. Kinked chains slide past each other and act as liquid oils.

(d)

FIGURE 8.5

(a) Structure of triglyceride. (b) The chemical makeup of fatty acid chains in fats and oils helps explain why saturated fats (c) like lard or butter are usually solid, and why mono- and polyunsaturated fats (d) like olive and corn oil are usually liquids.

chains remain straight and can pack closely against each other and create the properties of a solid. This explains why butter, beef fat, and lard—all saturated fats—occur as solids at room temperature (Figure 8.5c).

In an oil, there are also chains of carbon atoms, but at certain spots, the carbons have two bonds to other carbons (—C=C—). As a result, they have fewer bonds left over and can't be saturated or filled with hydrogen molecules at these points. The chains are said to be **unsaturated.** These double-bonded spots also cause the chains to kink and bend (Figure 8.5d). Because the chains can't pack tightly together, they slide past each other, generating a slippery liquid oil rather than a solid fat.

Fatty acid chains containing just one kinked (unsaturated) region are called **monounsaturated fatty acids** (MUFAs) (*mono* means "one"). Olive oil, canola oil, and cashew oil are all high in monounsaturated

unsaturated fat A lipid, usually a liquid oil, in which most carbon chains lack the maximum load of hydrogen atoms. Unsaturated chains are kinked and can't pack tightly, thus they can slip past each other and act like liquids.

monounsaturated fatty acid (MUFA) Lipid whose fatty acid chains have just one kinked (unsaturated) region. Olive oil, canola oil, and cashew oil are high in mono-unsaturated fatty acids.

fatty acids. Chains containing two or more linked regions are called **polyunsaturated fatty acids** (PUFAs; *poly* means "many"). Corn oil, safflower oil, and cottonseed oil are all high in polyunsaturated fatty acids (Figure 8.5d).

Food manufacturers sometimes alter the properties of oils by adding hydrogen atoms to liquid oils, a process called hydrogenation. This results in partially hydrogenated oils that contain some *trans fatty acids* or **trans fats.** These have cooking properties of solid fats as well as their potentially negative effects on health. Margarines, shortenings, and many processed foods contain *trans* fats. Nutritionists often recommend that you eliminate or decrease foods containing *trans* fats from your diet. The *trans* fat content of foods is now indicated on food labels. We will discuss the health consequences of eating *trans* fats later.

All of our food sources of fats and oils contain *both* saturated and unsaturated fats, in different ratios (Figure 8.6). For example, a tablespoon of safflower oil contains 0.8 gram saturated fat, 10.2 grams of monounsaturated fat, and 2 grams polyunsaturated fat. Sunflower oil, on the other hand, contains more saturated fat (1.4 grams), less monounsaturated fat (2.7 grams), and much more polyunsaturated fat (8.9 grams) than safflower oil. Even butter is a mix of fat types. One tablespoon of butter typically contains 7.2 grams saturated fat, 3.3 grams monounsaturated fat, and a trace of polyunsaturated fat. In general, lipids high in saturated fats are unhealthy for you, especially if you eat them frequently. While animals tend to make saturated fats and plants make unsaturated fats, some plants generate oils that are very high

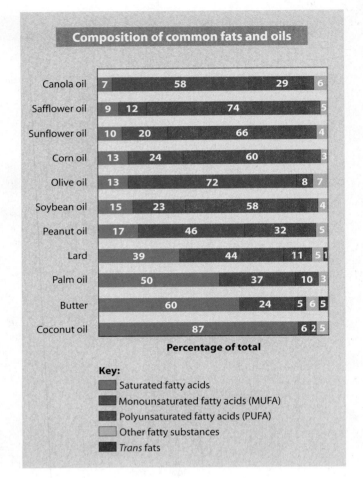

Composition of common fats and oils

	Saturated	MUFA	PUFA	Other	Trans
Canola oil	7	58	29	6	
Safflower oil	9	12	74	5	
Sunflower oil	10	20	66	4	
Corn oil	13	24	60	3	
Olive oil	13	72	8	7	
Soybean oil	15	23	58	4	
Peanut oil	17	46	32	5	
Lard	39	44	11	5	1
Palm oil	50	37	10	3	
Butter	60	24	5	6	5
Coconut oil	87			6 2	5

Percentage of total

Key:
- Saturated fatty acids
- Monounsaturated fatty acids (MUFA)
- Polyunsaturated fatty acids (PUFA)
- Other fatty substances
- *Trans* fats

FIGURE **8.6**

Common fats and oils have varying percentages of saturated and unsaturated fats, making them more or less healthful in the diet.

---

polyunsaturated fatty acid (PUFA) Lipid whose fatty acid chains have two or more kinked (unsaturated) regions. Corn oil, safflower oil, and cottonseed oils are high in polyunsaturated fatty acids.

trans **fat** An unsaturated lipid or oil with hydrogen atoms added to cause more complete saturation and make the oil function as a solid. Margarines and vegetable shortenings are examples of *trans* fats.

essential fatty acid Lipid components, including linolenic acid, EPA, DHA, and linoleic acid, which the body cannot manufacture and which we must obtain in polyunsaturated oils

in saturated fats. Cocoa butter, palm kernel oil, and coconut oil contain more saturated fat per tablespoon than butter, beef fat, or lard! Since lipids high in mono- and polyunsaturated fats are much healthier for you, it pays to learn good sources of them.

Omega-3 and Omega-6 Fatty Acids

There are some types of fatty acids that our cells cannot construct and therefore we must consume in our diet. These fatty acids are called **essential fatty acids.** They include *linoleic acid,* an omega-6 fatty acid, and *linolenic acid,* an omega-3 fatty acid. An **omega-6 fatty acid** is polyunsaturated and has double-bonded carbons at two sites, including one at the sixth carbon along the carbon chain. An **omega-3 fatty acid** has double-bonded carbons at three sites, including one at the third carbon along the chain. Other omega-3 fatty acids include EPA and DHA, which the human body can modify into linolenic acid. Polyunsaturated oils such as canola oil, corn oil, soybean oil, and sunflower oil all contain high levels of omega-6 fatty acids. Polyunsaturated oils such as flaxseed oil, walnuts, and, to a lesser degree, certain fish oils, canola oil, and soybean oil contain relatively high percentages of omega-3 fatty acids. The body can modify both types of essential fatty acids into various fats we need for cell membranes, nerve function, and healthy blood vessel walls.

Dietary Fats and Your Health

As your body breaks down the fats and oils in the food you eat, it packages the lipids into particles called **lipoproteins** that can move along easily in the bloodstream. Lipoproteins contain lipid and protein portions, and carry both triglycerides and **cholesterol,** the most common steroid in the body (recall that steroids are one structural class of fats). Our cells need and make cholesterol to keep membranes pliable and use it as a building block for making steroid hormones and other substances. In common usage, lipoproteins carrying cholesterol are simply called *cholesterol.*

Eating saturated fat and *trans* fat raises the level of **low-density lipoproteins** (also called **LDLs** or "bad cholesterol") in your bloodstream. Over time, elevated levels of LDLs can lead to plaque deposits inside the blood vessels. These plaques can constrict blood flow, raise blood pressure, and lead to heart disease, heart attacks, and strokes. Eating saturated fat also raises the level of **high-density lipoproteins** (**HDLs** or "good cholesterol") in the blood, but to a lesser degree. HDLs prevent and reduce plaque deposits in the blood vessels and therefore help protect against cardiovascular disease, strokes, and heart attacks.

You may be wondering how something the human body makes and needs for its own cell membranes and hormones can be a harmful compound in the diet. When some people consume cholesterol, their body cells make less cholesterol and their overall level stays constant. In other people, however, that "leveling mechanism" works inefficiently, and they tend to accumulate the extra dietary cholesterol in blood-vessel-narrowing plaques.[10] To be safe, the USDA recommends that you consume less cholesterol in the diet by cutting back on red meat, egg yolks, and high-fat dairy products.

Research shows that *trans* fatty acids contained in the solidified oils used to make shortening and some margarines can be even more damaging than saturated fats. *Trans* fats increase LDLs and simultaneously lower HDLs, a doubly negative effect. The USDA recommends choosing products with little or no *trans* fats.[11] *Trans* fats also raise triglyceride levels. After a meal, the liver takes cholesterol and triglycerides that we don't use immediately in our tissues, packages them into HDLs and LDLs, and sends them through the blood to be stored in fat cells.[12] Coincidentally, consuming large quantities of refined starches, sugars, and/or alcohol also raises blood triglycerides. This helps explain why eating big helpings of such starches and sugars, as so many

omega-6 fatty acid A lipid in a class of lipid components that includes linoleic acid; abundant in polyunsaturated oils such as canola oil, corn oil, soybean oil, and sunflower oil. The fatty acids are polyunsaturated and have doubled-bonded carbons at two sites, including one at the sixth carbon along the chain.

omega-3 fatty acid A lipid in a class of lipid components that includes linoleic acid, EPA, and DHA; abundant in polyunsaturated oils from flaxseeds, walnuts, and certain fish. Found in lesser amounts in canola and soybean oils. The fatty acids are double-bonded at three sites, including one at the third carbon along the chain.

lipoprotein A lipid plus protein transport particle that can move along easily in the bloodstream; carries triglycerides or cholesterol

cholesterol A waxy lipid in the steroid class that is an important component of cell membranes and is transported in the blood by carriers called *LDL* and *HDL*. Some cholesterol in the blood comes from the diet; most is made in the liver.

low-density lipoprotein (LDL) A form of lipoprotein sometimes called "bad cholesterol." LDL levels rise in response to saturated fats in the diet and can contribute to plaque deposits inside blood vessels.

high-density lipoprotein (HDL) A form of lipoprotein sometimes called "good cholesterol." HDL levels rise in response to polyunsaturated fats and prevent and reduce plaque deposits in the blood vessels.

Americans do, can lead to obesity, diabetes, and heart disease.

Eating mono- and polyunsaturated fats lowers LDLs and raises HDLs, a doubly positive effect. As Figure 8.6 on page 230 showed, most kinds of cooking oils are high in mono- and polyunsaturated fats and low in saturated fats, but there are exceptions, such as palm kernel oil and coconut oil. That's one reason it is important to read food labels rather than make assumptions about the fats in particular foods.

Some nutritionists encourage people to consume more oils. A popular plan called the Mediterranean diet encourages people to use olive oil liberally in cooking and at the table. Nutritionists from Harvard Medical School also encourage people to eat healthful plant oils at most meals.[13] The new USDA pyramid still recommends limiting fats and oils to 20 to 35 percent of daily calories but does encourage most of those to be mono- and polyunsaturated.

A Healthy Plan for Fats in Your Diet

Most of us need to cut down on saturated fats while getting more heart-healthy fats into our diet. Here are some ideas:

- Always read food labels, looking at both the amount of saturated fat and the percentage it represents of your daily recommended maximum for saturated fat and total fat.

- Don't be fooled into thinking that cookies, crackers, or chips are healthy foods because they are labeled "low-fat." Watch out for high levels of added sugars, refined flour, salt, and *trans* fats (the label may read "vegetable shortening" or "partially hydrogenated vegetable oil").

- For salad dressings, sautéing, and other cooking needs, choose oils like canola, soy, olive, and safflower that contain high levels of mono- and polyunsaturated fats.

- Whenever possible, instead of butter or margarine, use soft, buttery spreads that list "0 *trans* fats" on the label. For topping bread and crackers, alternatives to butter include all-fruit jams (no sugar added), fat-free cream cheese, tomato salsa, olive oil, or low-fat salad dressing.

- Choose lean meats, fish, or poultry instead of fatty meats such as bacon, sausages, hot dogs, bologna, pepperoni, or organ meats. Remove skin. Avoid frying. Drain off fat after cooking.

- Choose dairy products that have 0 or 1 percent fat, such as skim milk, nonfat yogurt, and fat-free cottage cheese. Avoid reduced-fat dairy products (2 percent fat) and whole-milk dairy products (4 percent fat) whenever possible. Choose nonfat or low-fat frozen yogurt or sorbet rather than ice cream.

- Cook with chicken broth, wine, vinegar, low-calorie salad dressings, or unsaturated oils (mono- and polyunsaturated) rather than butter, margarine, sour cream, mayonnaise, and creamy salad dressings.

- Eat fatty fish (i.e., salmon, tuna, bluefish, herring, or sardines) one or two times per week. However, be aware of high mercury levels in some types of fish (see **Facts and Fallacies: Is It Safe to Eat Fish?**).

- Add green, leafy vegetables, walnuts, walnut oil, and milled flaxseed to your diet.

- Limit processed and convenience foods. These often contain refined carbohydrates in addition to *trans* fats.

- Don't demand daily nutritional perfection from yourself. Try to balance your intake of different foods over a few meals and a couple of days at a time. If you have a high-fat breakfast or lunch, balance it with a low-fat dinner. If you forget to eat many fruits and vegetables today, eat extra servings tomorrow and cut back on fats and proteins.

VITAMINS ARE VITAL MICRONUTRIENTS

Vitamins are organic compounds that we need in tiny amounts to promote growth and help maintain life and health. Vitamins take part in the minute-by-minute cellular reactions that help maintain our nerves and skin, contribute to the production of blood cells, help us build bones and teeth, assist in wound healing, and help convert food energy to accessible fuel for cellular activities. Some vitamins are toxic in high doses, and for many vitamins, time

vitamin Organic compound in foods that we need in tiny amounts to promote growth and help maintain life and health

FACTS AND FALLACIES

IS IT SAFE TO EAT FISH?

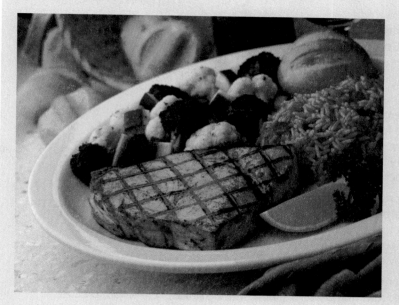

You may have heard that eating too much of certain kinds of fish can pose health hazards, especially to women of childbearing age and to children. At the same time, there are many nutritional benefits to eating fish, including high levels of healthy omega-3 fatty acids. So what's safe and what's not?

The problem is that mercury (either released in the air due to industrial pollution, or naturally occurring) can accumulate in bodies of water, where it becomes methylmercury and contaminates fish. People who eat fish containing high amounts of methylmercury can, in turn, accumulate mercury in their bloodstream. Women of reproductive-age and children need to be careful about their fish consumption because mercury can damage the brain and nervous systems in developing fetuses and young children.

The EPA advises women and children to avoid four types of fish altogether: tilefish, swordfish, shark, and King mackerel (1), as these fish tend to contain exceptionally high levels of mercury. They also advise the two groups to limit consumption of fish containing low-levels of mercury—such as salmon, canned light tuna, and catfish—to 12 ounces (two average meals) per week. Other seafood containing low levels of mercury include anchovies, clams, codfish, crab, herring, lobster, and North Atlantic mackerel (2).

Sources:
1. Environmental Protection Agency. "What You Need to Know about Mercury in Fish and Shellfish." http://www.epa.gov/waterscience/fishadvice/advice.html. Updated July 19, 2007.
2. U.S. Department of Health and Human Services. "Mercury Levels in Commercial Fish and Shellfish." http://www.cfsan.fda.gov/frf/sea-mehg.html. Updated February 2006.

---

spent on the shelf, the heat from cooking, and certain other environmental conditions can diminish their potency in foods.

Some vitamins can dissolve only in water and some only in fat. *Water-soluble vitamins,* including vitamin C and the B vitamins, dissolve easily in water and can be absorbed directly into the bloodstream. Excess water-soluble vitamins are usually excreted in the urine and cause few toxicity problems. Because they are not stored in the liver, body fat, or other tissues, we need to consume water-soluble vitamins on a regular basis in our foods. *Fat-soluble vitamins,* including vitamins A, D, E, and K, must associate with fat molecules in order to be absorbed through the intestinal tract. Excess, unused quantities of the fat-soluble vitamins tend to be stored in the body. High levels can accumulate in the liver and cause damage. Table 8.1 lists 13 vitamins, their food sources, their chief functions in the body, and the symptoms caused by consuming too little or too much of each.

Vitamin vendors often make various claims about the benefits of taking vitamin supplements to augment what we consume in foods. For the most part, a careful diet will provide your vitamin needs, but because many people eat too few fruits and vegetables, they don't get optimal levels. In addition, certain groups of people, and all of us at certain life stages, do have special vitamin needs. People over 50, for example, must be careful to get enough vitamin B_{12} since absorption of certain nutrients,

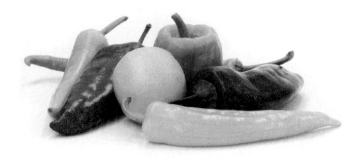

TABLE 8.1

Guide to Vitamins

Vitamin	Best Food Sources	Main Functions in Body	Deficiency Symptoms	Toxicity Symptoms
Water-Soluble Vitamins				
B_1 (Thiamin)	Meat, pork, liver, fish, poultry, whole grain and enriched breads and cereals, pasta, nuts, legumes	Energy harvest and use from nutrients; normal appetite; nervous system function	Poor appetite, heart irregularities, mental confusion, muscle weakness, poor growth	None known
B_2 (Riboflavin)	Dairy products, dark green vegetables, liver, meat, whole grain and enriched breads and cereals	Energy harvest and use from nutrients; healthy skin, normal vision, normal growth	Eye problems, skin cracking around nose and mouth	None known
Niacin	Meat, eggs, poultry, fish, milk, whole grain and enriched breads and cereals, nuts, legumes, yeast, all protein foods	Energy harvest and use from nutrients; healthy skin, nervous system function, digestion	Skin rash, loss of appetite, dizziness, weakness, irritability, fatigue, mental confusion, indigestion	Flushing, blurred vision, glucose intolerance, abnormal liver function
B_6 (Pyridoxine)	Meat, poultry, fish, shellfish, legumes, whole grain foods, leafy greens, bananas	Breakdown of proteins and fats, formation of red blood cells and antibodies, conversion of niacin	Nervous disorders, skin rash, muscle weakness, anemia, convulsions, kidney stones	Sensory nerve damage, skin lesions
Folate	Leafy greens, liver, legumes, seeds	Forming red blood cells, breakdown of proteins, cell division, proper formation of neural tube in embryo	Anemia, heartburn, diarrhea, smooth tongue, poor growth and development	Nerve damage; high levels may mask a vitamin B_{12} deficiency
B_{12}	Meat, fish, poultry, shellfish, milk, cheese, eggs, yeast	Nerve cell maintenance, red blood cell formation, building of new genetic material	Anemia, smooth tongue, fatigue, nerve degeneration progressing to paralysis	None known
Pantothenic acid	Widespread in foods	Crucial factor in energy harvest and use	Rare; sleep disturbances, nausea, fatigue	None known
Biotin	Widespread in foods	Crucial factor in energy harvest and use; building fat molecules; energy storage in muscles	Loss of appetite, nausea, depression, muscle pain, weakness, fatigue, rash	None known

TABLE 8.1 *continued*

Vitamin	Best Food Sources	Main Functions in Body	Deficiency Symptoms	Toxicity Symptoms
C (Ascorbic Acid)	Citrus fruits, cabbage-type vegetables, tomatoes, potatoes, dark green vegetables, peppers, cantaloupe, strawberries, mangos, papayas	Helps heal wounds; maintains connective tissue, bones, and teeth; strengthens blood vessels; antioxidant; boosts immunity, aids absorption of iron	Scurvy, anemia, blood vessel damage, depression, frequent infections, loose teeth, bleeding gums, bleeding, muscle wasting, rough skin, weak bones, poor wound healing	Nausea, abdominal cramps, diarrhea, red blood cell breakdown in some people, kidney stones in people with kidney disease. Upon withdrawing from high doses, deficiency symptoms may appear
Fat-Soluble Vitamins				
A	Milk, cream, cheese, butter, eggs, liver, dark leafy greens, broccoli, deep orange fruits and vegetables	Healthy vision; growth and repair of tissues; formation of bones and teeth; immunity; building hormones; cancer protection	Night blindness; rough skin; frequent infections; impaired growth, especially of bones and teeth; eye problems leading to blindness	Miscarriage, birth defects, red blood cell breakage, nosebleeds, abdominal cramps, nausea, blurred vision, bone pain, dry skin, rashes, hair loss, others
D	Sunlight on skin; fortified milk and margarine, eggs, liver, fish	Healthy bones and teeth; aids absorption of calcium and phosphorus	Rickets in children; weakened bones and bone problems in adults; abnormal growth; joint pain; soft bones	Raised blood calcium, constipation, weight loss, irritability, weakness, nausea, kidney stones, mental and physical retardation, calcium deposits
E	Vegetable oils, leafy greens, wheat germ, whole grains, butter, liver, egg yolk, milk, nuts, seeds, fortified cereals, soybeans, avocado	Healthy red and white blood cells; healthy cell membranes in lungs and elsewhere; antioxidant activity	Muscle wasting, weakness, damage to red blood cells, anemia, bleeding, fibrocystic breast disease	Interference with anticlotting medication, intestinal discomfort, increased risk of stroke
K	Liver, milk, leafy greens, cabbage-type vegetables, vegetable oils	Aids digestion, blood clotting, regulation of calcium in blood, builds bone tissue	Bleeding	None known

UNDERSTANDING DIVERSITY

DO YOU HAVE SPECIAL VITAMIN AND MINERAL NEEDS?

Most nutritionists agree that you should try to get your daily vitamins and minerals from a healthful diet rather than eating carelessly and relying on supplements. People in a number of population groups, however, are at risk for vitamin deficiencies. If you belong to one of these groups, you should pay extra attention to your diet and perhaps also consider taking a multivitamin.

- Women of reproductive age who could become pregnant need 400 micrograms of folate per day to prevent potential neurological defects in a developing fetus. Pregnant women need 600 micrograms per day.

- Premenopausal women, especially those with heavy menstrual bleeding, need to get 18 milligrams of iron per day in foods or in total from foods and a multivitamin. Men and postmenopausal women need 10 milligrams per day and need to be careful not to get too much.

- Everyone needs a good supply of calcium each day from low-fat dairy products, fortified juices, and other sources. The daily value for people under 50 is 1,000 milligrams. Pregnant women, nursing mothers, teens, and older adults need extra calcium (1,200 to 1,500 milligrams per day) for the development and maintenance of bones and to lower the risk of osteoporosis.

- Older adults, dark-skinned individuals, and people who do not get regular exposure to sunlight have a special need for vitamin D (25 micrograms per day or 1,000 International Units per day).

- People over 50 naturally produce less stomach acid and absorb less vitamin B_{12} from foods. Older adults should be careful to get at least 2.4 micrograms per day or more, especially if they take stomach acid blockers.

- Cigarette smoking decreases bone density and interferes with the body's normal use of vitamin C. Smokers therefore need to consume higher levels of calcium (1,200 mg per day) and of vitamin C (110 mg in women, 125 mg per day in men) compared to 90 mg for nonsmoking adults.

- Vegetarians, especially strict vegans, can become deficient for iron, vitamin B_{12}, calcium, and vitamin D.

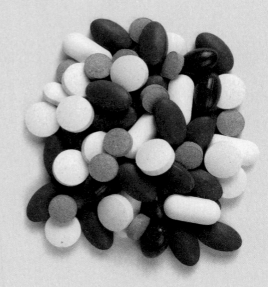

They must be careful to get their daily values from plant foods or take a multivitamin.

- People with diseases that disrupt normal metabolism or nutrient absorption (diabetes and certain cancers, for example) can develop vitamin or mineral deficiencies. Physicians often recommend special diets or multivitamins as part of their treatment.

If you plan to take a multivitamin, apply common sense. There is no need to get more than the RDI for vitamins and minerals. In some cases, high doses exceeding 100 percent can lead to serious side effects. Since fat-soluble vitamins and certain minerals can build up in the body, be sure a multivitamin has less than the RDI for vitamins A, D, E, and K, and for magnesium, chromium, selenium, and zinc. To be safe, people in high-risk groups should consult a doctor before taking supplements regularly.

Sources: Center for Science in the Public Interest. "The Multivitamin Maze" and "How to Read a Multi Label," *Nutrition Action Healthletter* (March 2006): 6–7; National Institutes of Health. "NIH State of the Science Panel Urges More Informed Approach to Multivitamin/Mineral Use for Chronic Disease Prevention." NIH News. National Institutes of Health Internet publication, May, 17, 2006. www.nih.gov; U.S. Department of Health and Human Services. "USDA Dietary Guidelines for Americans," 2005.

including B_{12}, declines naturally with age. The box **Understanding Diversity: Do You Have Special Vitamin and Mineral Needs?** discusses both the vitamin needs of specific groups and the issue of taking vitamin supplements versus getting vitamins from food alone.

Advertisers would have you believe otherwise, but few Americans suffer from true vitamin deficiencies if they eat a fairly balanced diet. Very high levels of certain vitamins can even lead to a toxic condition know as *hypervitaminosis.*

MINERALS ARE ELEMENTAL MICRONUTRIENTS

The micronutrients called **minerals** allow our nerves to transmit impulses, our hearts to beat, oxygen to reach our tissue cells, and our digestive tracts to absorb vitamins from food. They are usually not toxic, and we excrete excess quantities of most minerals from the body. The **major minerals** (also called *macrominerals*) are elements that the body needs in relatively large amounts. The major minerals include sodium, calcium, phosphorous, magnesium, potassium, and chloride. We need smaller amounts of the **trace minerals** (also called *microminerals*), which include iron, zinc, copper, iodine, selenium, fluoride, and chromium. Table 8.2 on page 238 lists most of the major and trace minerals, their functions, food sources, and symptoms of deficiency and/or toxicity. We discuss three minerals—sodium, calcium, and iron—in more detail because of their crucial roles in the body and their excesses or deficiencies in many students' diets.

We need sodium, the Na in sodium chloride (NaCl), or table salt, for regulating the water contents of blood and body fluids; for the transmission of nerve impulses; for muscle contraction, including the heartbeat; and for several metabolic functions inside cells. However, most of us consume much more than we need. The average adult at rest and not sweating profusely needs only 500 mg of sodium (about one-quarter teaspoon) per day. Nutritionists estimate, however, that the average American man consumes 3,100 to 4,700 mg per day and the average woman 2,300 to 3,100 mg per day in salted snacks and processed foods! The Recommended Dietary Allowance (RDA) Subcommittee recommends restricting sodium to no more than 2,400 mg per day; less is better. Pickles, salty snack foods, processed cheeses, many breads and bakery products, and smoked meats and sausages often contain several hundred milligrams of sodium per serving. Many fast-food entrées and convenience entrées pack 500 to 1,000 mg of sodium per serving.

Many experts believe that there is a link between excessive sodium intake and hypertension (high blood pressure). Although this theory is controversial, researchers began recommending several years ago that people with hypertension cut back on sodium to reduce their risk of cardiovascular disorders.[14]

High sodium intake may also increase calcium loss in urine, which increases your risk for debilitating fractures as you age. The issue of calcium

> *Try it NOW!* Shake your salt habit! Take simple steps today to reduce your overall sodium intake: choose low-sodium or salt-free food products. • Order popcorn without salt. Switch to kosher salt—it has 25% less sodium than regular table salt. • Instead of adding salt to food you prepare, try using fresh or prepackaged herb blends to season foods.

consumption has gained national attention as the incidence of weak, porous bones has risen, particularly among older women and, increasingly, among older men. The element calcium (Ca) is crucial for the development and maintenance of bones and teeth, for blood clotting, muscle contraction, nerve transmission, and fluid balance between the cell's interior and its environment. Nevertheless, most Americans consume less than the 1,000 mg to 1,300 mg of calcium per day recommended by government guidelines.

Osteoporosis is a disease of thinning, weakened, porous bones that affects more than 44 million Americans over age 50. The risk for it climbs if you consume too little calcium during childhood and adolescence when bones are developing, if you have a naturally small frame, and/or if you consume too little calcium during adulthood. Bone weakness

mineral An element such as calcium or sodium that allows vital physiological processes, including nerve transmission, heartbeat, oxygen delivery, and absorption of vitamins

major mineral A mineral needed in relatively large amounts, including sodium, calcium, phosphorus, magnesium, potassium, and chloride

trace mineral An element the body needs in very tiny amounts; includes iron, zinc, copper, iodine, selenium, fluoride, and chromium

osteoporosis A disease of thinning, weakened, porous bones during which too little calcium is deposited or retained in the bones

TABLE 8.2

Guide to Selected Minerals

Mineral	Best Food Sources	Main Functions in Body	Deficiency Symptoms	Toxicity Symptoms
Calcium	Milk and dairy products, small fish with bones, tofu, leafy greens, legumes	Building bones and teeth; muscle contraction and relaxation; nerve function; blood clotting; blood pressure	Stunted growth in children; bone weakness and thinning in adults	Mineral imbalances, shock, kidney failure, fatigue, mental confusion
Phosphorus	All animal tissues	Component of every cell; helps regulate pH balance	Unknown	Can unbalance calcium; can lead to calcium deficiency, spasms, convulsions
Magnesium	Nuts, legumes, whole grains, deep leafy greens, seafood, chocolate	Bone hardening; protein synthesis; enzyme activity; normal function of muscles and nerves	Weakness, confusion, poor growth, impaired hormone production, muscle spasms, disturbed behavior	Mega-doses can lead to nausea, cramps, dehydration, death
Sodium	Salt, soy sauce, processed foods, cured, canned, pickled foods	Helps maintain normal fluid balance and pH within body	Muscle cramps, mental apathy, loss of appetite	Hypertension, water retention, increased calcium loss
Chloride	Salt, soy sauce, processed foods, cured, canned, pickled foods	Component of stomach acid and needed for digestion; helps maintain normal fluid balance	Dangerous changes in pH, irregular heartbeat	Vomiting
Potassium	Meats, fruits, milk, vegetables, grains, legumes	Involved in biochemical reactions that help build protein, maintain fluid balance, transmit nerve impulses, contract muscles	Muscle weakness, paralysis, confusion; accompanies dehydration; can cause death	Muscular weakness, vomiting, irregular heartbeat; can stop heart
Iodine	Iodized salt, seafood	Component of thyroid hormone, helps regulate metabolism	Goiter; mental and physical retardation due to thyroid deficiency	Goiter or enlargement of thyroid gland

can lead to pain, stooped posture, and fractures, and can diminish mobility and independence. Half of all American women and one-quarter of all American men will break a bone as a result of osteoporosis.

Dairy products are among the richest dietary sources of calcium, but calcium-fortified orange juice and soy milk are also good sources, as are leafy green vegetables and many other foods (see Table 8.2). Be aware that the added phosphoric acid (phosphate) in carbonated soft drinks can cause you to excrete calcium and thus deplete needed calcium from your bones. Calcium/phosphorus imbalance may lead to kidney stones, bone spurs, and to the deposits or plaques inside blood vessels that contribute to cardiovascular diseases.

TABLE 8.2 *continued*

Mineral	Best Food Sources	Main Functions in Body	Deficiency Symptoms	Toxicity Symptoms
Iron	Beef, fish, poultry, shellfish, eggs, legumes, dried fruits	Crucial component of hemoglobin in red blood cells, myoglobin in muscles; takes part in oxygen transfer, energy use	Anemia: weakness, pallor, headaches, frequent infections, difficulty concentrating	Nausea, vomiting, dizziness, rapid heartbeat, damage to organs, death
Zinc	Meats, fish, poultry, grains, vegetables	Component of insulin and many enzymes; takes part in DNA, protein synthesis, immune response, taste, wound healing, normal development, sperm production, vitamin A transport	Growth failure in children, delayed sexual development, loss of taste, poor wound healing	Fever, nausea, vomiting, diarrhea, headaches, depressed immune function
Copper	Meats, drinking water	Absorption of iron; component of several enzymes	Anemia, bone changes (rare)	Liver damage if toxicity is due to certain diseases; nausea, diarrhea, vomiting
Fluoride	Drinking water (natural or fluoridated), tea, seafood	Formation and maintenance of bones and teeth	Susceptibility to tooth decay and bone loss	Discoloration of teeth, joint pain, stiffness
Selenium	Seafood, meats, grains	Helps protect body compounds from oxidation	Muscle pain and possible deterioration; possible damage to nails and hair	Vomiting, nausea, rash, brittle hair and nails, cirrhosis of liver
Chromium	Meats, whole foods, fats, vegetable oils	Associated with insulin; needed for breakdown and use of glucose	Diabetes-like condition with poor glucose utilization	Unknown. Occupational overexposure damages skin and kidneys

Vitamin D improves absorption of calcium; that's why dairies are required by law to add it to milk. Sunlight shining on your skin also increases the body's own manufacture of vitamin D, so a moderate amount of sunlight helps improve calcium absorption. The best way to obtain calcium, like all nutrients, is to consume it as part of a balanced diet, but certain people do need calcium supplements (see the **Understanding Diversity** box on page 236).

Each of us needs the element iron (Fe) for producing healthy blood, for muscle function, and for normal cell division. Females aged 15 to 50 need about 18 mg/day; males aged 19 to 50 need about 10 mg/day. Worldwide, iron deficiency is the most common nutrient deficiency, affecting more than

CASE STUDY

Chau

"I kind of understand that your body uses different nutrients for different needs. But because I've been growing a lot over the last few years, I've been more concerned with quantity than quality. I've never had a weight problem, though I have gained a little bit of weight over the past few months. I realize I'm eating a lot more carbs than I used to, mostly cereal and white bread. And Tom's girlfriend is always baking him cookies, so I load up on those. I also eat a ton of cheese pizza. Still, I don't worry about fat. Everyone in my family is thin!"

1. Chau often eats meals prepared on campus, where he doesn't have access to nutrition labels.

How could Chau estimate the amount of protein, carbohydrate, and fat in his diet?

2. Given what you know about Chau's diet, which nutrients might he be deficient in? Which nutrients might he be consuming too much of? What can he do to eat a more balanced diet?

3. Think about your own diet. How often do you consume omega-3 fatty acids, and in what foods? How often do you consume fiber? What nutrients, if any, are you deficient in? What changes could you make to achieve more balance in your diet?

---

1 billion people. In developing countries, more than one-third of the children and women of childbearing age suffer from **iron-deficiency anemia,** in which the body fails to produce enough of the red hemoglobin pigment in the blood, leading to unusually low oxygen levels, unusually high carbon dioxide levels, and resulting in mental and physical fatigue. About 5 percent of all Americans get too little iron in their food.[15] Among toddlers, adolescent girls, and women of childbearing age, about 10 percent show iron-deficiency anemia. Table 8.2 lists good dietary sources of iron.

Getting the right amount of iron is important. Researchers have linked iron deficiency to a host of problems, including poor immune system functioning and a propensity toward certain cancers. Some research has also suggested a link between too much iron in the diet and/or stored in the body and a higher risk for cardiovascular disease.

Acute iron toxicity due to ingesting too many iron-containing supplements remains the leading cause of accidental poisoning in small children in the United States. Dozens of children have died from overdoses of as few as five iron tablets.[16]

iron-deficiency anemia A disease in which the body takes in too little iron and makes too little oxygen-carrying hemoglobin

dehydrated Depleted of normal, necessary levels of body fluids

WATER IS OUR MOST FUNDAMENTAL NUTRIENT

Imagine you are stranded on a desert island for a reality TV show and you can take along just one provision. Would you choose food, water, or a cell phone? We hope you said water!

Humans are mostly water—close to 60 percent. Watery fluids bathe each of our internal cells. They help maintain a proper balance of salts within our blood and tissues, help maintain pH balance, and help facilitate the transport of substances throughout the body. Human blood plasma (the fluid portion of blood exclusive of red and white blood cells and other solid components) is approximately 91.5 percent water.[17] This proportion must remain fairly constant for blood to efficiently carry oxygen and nutrients to the cells and carry away carbon dioxide and other wastes.

Even under the most severe conditions, the average person can live for weeks on the energy stored in their body fat. You can also get along without certain vitamins and minerals from foods for an equal amount of time before experiencing serious deficiency symptoms. Without water, however, you would become **dehydrated,** or depleted of normal levels of body fluids, within hours. Within 1 day without drinking water, you would probably begin to feel sluggish, dizzy, and nauseated, and would experience headaches, muscle cramps, or weakness. After a few days without water, your tongue would be parched and swollen, your heart would be racing, and you'd very likely go into shock and die.

A person's need for water varies dramatically based on age, size, diet, exercise, overall health, and environmental temperature and humidity levels. Most of us get enough water through foods and beverages just by satisfying our thirst. People with certain diseases such as diabetes or cystic fibrosis, however, excrete extra fluid and must generally take in a higher volume. On a hot day, especially if exercising, you need to consciously replace fluids lost to sweat and exhalation. It is possible, though, to take in too much water and become ill or even lose consciousness from excess hydration. If your intake is high enough that you gain water weight during an active exercise session, you are probably imbibing too much.

Commercial energy drinks diluted with extra water have become a very popular way for exercisers to replenish water lost through sweat without getting more salt and sugar than they want. However, some energy drinks include ingredients that are ineffectual or that can be harmful in large quantities. Researchers have failed to confirm any health benefit for ingredients such as taurine, bee pollen, and ginkgo biloba.[18] High concentrations of added sugars can boost energy in the short term but can create a rebound of sluggishness later. Added vitamins C and B are unnecessary in a balanced diet. And if overused, energy drinks containing the stimulants caffeine and/or ginseng can speed bone loss, raise blood pressure, and increase the risk of cardiovascular diseases.

HOW CAN YOU ACHIEVE A BALANCED DIET?

The average American adult consumes about 1,000 Calories more per day than the average citizen worldwide and yet still gets unbalanced nutrition with too little of certain nutrients and too much of others. To counter these trends toward overeating and substandard nutrition, the U.S. government sets guidelines, publishes food pyramids, and requires nutrition labels on most packaged and processed foods. The effort is designed to improve our national wellness, and the tools they provide can help you achieve a better diet.

FOLLOW GUIDELINES FOR GOOD NUTRITION

Several government scientific advisory boards serve up an "alphabet soup" of recommended daily intakes for fat, carbohydrates, proteins, vitamins, and minerals. Sorting them out can be challenging. But here's a short introduction to these nutritional guides:

- DRI (Dietary Reference Intake) is a combined listing of 26 nutrients essential to maintaining health. The list identifies recommended and maximum safe intake levels of the nutrients for healthy people, and identifies minimum levels needed to prevent deficiencies and diseases. DRIs are an umbrella category for several older classifications. The National Academy of Sciences Food and Nutrition Board publishes DRIs.

- **RDAs** (Recommended Dietary Allowances) are a listing of the average daily nutrient intake level of vitamins and minerals that meets most people's daily needs. The National Academy of Sciences introduced RDAs in 1941 and updates the list periodically.

- RDIs (Reference Daily Intakes) is a listing of needed daily nutrients based on the National Academy of Science's RDAs. Table 8.3 lists the current RDIs for various vitamins and minerals.

- DRVs (Daily Reference Values). The RDIs left out some nutrients that proved to be important for daily dietary monitoring, so the DRVs cover them. They cover fat (including saturated fat and cholesterol), carbohydrates (including fiber), protein, sodium, and potassium. Table 8.4 lists the current DRVs for these nutrients.

- **DVs** (Daily Values) are the RDIs and the DRVs as printed on food labels. American consumers need to know what's in their food and what they should be eating without sorting through a bunch of confusing acronyms. Therefore, the U.S. Food and Drug Administration (FDA) invented a simpler term, DV, for all the important nutrients from the RDI and DRV lists to include on food labels. If you look on any food label, you will see a column labeled "% Daily Value." We'll return to nutrient labels and how to use them later in this section.

RDAs (Recommended Dietary Allowances) A listing of the average daily nutrient intake level for a list of vitamins and minerals that meets most people's daily needs

DVs (Daily Values) A list of all the important nutrients from two less inclusive government lists—the RDIs (Reference Daily Intakes) and the DRVs (Daily Reference Values). DVs are printed on all nutrition labels.

TABLE 8.3

Reference Daily Intakes (RDIs) for Vitamins and Minerals

Nutrient	Amount
Vitamin A	5,000 IU[1]
Vitamin C	60 mg[2]
Thiamin	1.5 mg
Riboflavin	1.7 mg
Niacin	20 mg
Calcium	1.0 g[3]
Iron	18 mg
Vitamin D	400 IU
Vitamin E	30 IU
Vitamin B_6	2.0 mg
Folic acid	0.4 mg
Vitamin B_{12}	6 mcg[4]
Phosphorus	1.0 g
Iodine	150 mcg
Magnesium	400 mg
Zinc	15 mg
Copper	2 mg
Biotin	0.3 mg
Pantothenic acid	10 mg

[1] international units
[2] milligrams
[3] grams
[4] micrograms; also represented by μg
Source: Adapted from U.S. FDA home page, www.fda.gov/fdac/special/foodlabel/dvs.html; 2006.

You will probably come across the above-mentioned listings the most often. However, when looking into calorie requirements and safe levels of vitamins and minerals you may also see references to a few other daily intakes:

- EAR (Estimated Average Requirement): This is a listing of the intake that meets the requirement of half the healthy people of a certain sex at a certain life stage, such as adolescence, young adulthood, and so on.

- AI (Adequate Intake): Recommendations for daily nutrient intake where actual RDIs aren't known. Some of the values for vitamins and minerals are

TABLE 8.4

Daily Reference Values (DRVs)

Food Component	DRV
Fat	65 g[1]
Saturated fatty acids	20 g
Cholesterol	300 mg[2]
Total carbohydrate	300 g
Fiber	25 g
Sodium	2,400 mg
Potassium	3,500 mg
Protein**	50 g

(Based on 2,000 calories a day for adults and children over 4 only)
[1] grams
[2] milligrams
** DRV for protein does not apply to certain populations; Reference Daily Intake (RDI) for protein has been established for these groups: children 1 to 4 years: 16 g; infants under 1 year: 14 g; pregnant women: 60 g; nursing mothers: 65 g.
Source: Adapted from U.S. FDA home page, www.fda.gov/fdac/special/foodlabel/dvs.html; 2006.

AIs because scientists have yet to discover exact daily requirements for those nutrients.

- TUI (Tolerable Upper Intake Level): Recommendations for the highest levels that pose no risk where too much of a particular vitamin or mineral could be harmful. These are important for establishing the toxicity levels listed in Tables 8.1 and 8.2 on pages 234 and 238, respectively.

- EER (Estimated Energy Requirement): Calorie intake levels based on age, gender, height, weight, and activity level.

- AMDR (Acceptable Macronutrient Distribution Ranges): A range of percentages for carbohydrate, fat, and protein consumption that provides adequate nutrition and reduces the risk of chronic diseases. For example, the AMDR for fat is 20 to 35 percent of total calories. For carbohydrate, it is 45 to 65 percent of total calories. For protein, it is 10 to 35 percent.

There are so many parts to the government's nutritional advice to the public that they published an overview—think of it as a cheat sheet for nutrition—called the Dietary Guidelines for Americans. The latest version came out in 2005 from the USDA and U.S. Department of Health and Human Services. We discuss the government's nutritional guidelines for specific groups later in the chapter.

Determining Your Calorie Needs

If you read the fine print near the bottom of any nutrition label, you will see that the listings of nutrients are based on diets of either 2,000 or 2,500 Calories per day. The U.S. government chose a 2,000 Calorie-per-day diet as the basis for recommending the daily values of 65 grams of fat, 300 grams of carbohydrates, and 50 grams of protein (see Table 8.4). Does that mean you should be eating 2,000 Calories per day even if you are 4'11" and weigh 90 pounds, or 6'8" and weigh 230 pounds? And does it mean that you should adhere to those daily values regardless of your activity level? No on both counts.

A round number like 2,000 Calories makes it easy to extrapolate your actual calorie needs and serving sizes. It is also a maintenance level of energy input for a medium-sized person— about 150 pounds—who expends a medium amount of activity such as 30 minutes of moderate activity a few times per week. Food labels usually also provide a second level, 2,500 Calories, as a calculation base for larger or more active people. Your actual calorie needs depend on your size, age, gender, activity level, cultural factors, medical conditions, and your basal metabolic rate (BMR), which is partly inborn and partly activity-based.

Your BMR, the amount of energy your body uses in a given time period while resting or sleeping, accounts for 50 to 70 percent of your calorie consumption each day and allows you to maintain a steady heartbeat, a temperature of about 98.6 degrees, and so on. You use another 20 percent of your calories moving around and doing physical work such as walking, talking, carrying things, running, or sweeping the floor. Finally, eating and digesting food itself uses up about 5 to 10 percent of the calories you burn each day.

In determining calorie needs, the big variables are body size, BMR, and energy expenditure through physical activity. Larger people, more muscular people, and those who do hard physical work or exercise burn extra calories. You can get a specific calorie estimate using diet analysis tools such as www.mypyramid.gov. Use your own personal calorie estimate to calculate appropriate serving sizes and numbers when reading food labels and planning your diet.

Understanding Portion Sizes

One reason that Americans eat an average of nearly 3,500 Calories per day rather than the world average of 2,400 to 2,600 is the size of our typical food portions. The U.S. government recommends that each of us eat a certain number of servings each day from each food group based on standard serving sizes. Most Americans, however, don't know how to recognize standard portions. It helps to have some visual aids for estimating proper serving sizes and recognizing the right amount of food. Table 8.5 lists various foods, healthy serving sizes in cups and ounces, and visual devices for remembering proper portions. For example, one serving of cooked whole-wheat pasta or brown rice is half a cup, about the size of a woman's fist. This table puts into startling perspective the servings we receive at most restaurants: the mountains of pasta, the big wedges of pie, the stacks of plate-sized pancakes, the bucket-sized soft drinks, and the other servings we accept and expect as normal.

Using Food Pyramids

Perhaps you grew up seeing the USDA's early Food Guide Pyramid on food labels, with their specific daily recommendations for serving numbers of bread, cereal, rice, and pasta; fruits and vegetables; meat, poultry, beans, eggs, and nuts; milk, yogurt, and cheese; and so on. The early pyramids emphasized carbohydrates (with 6 to 11 servings per day) and deemphasized fats and oils (relegating them to the small upper tip of the pyramid along with sweets). It did not, however, distinguish between refined carbohydrates and whole grains, or between artery-clogging saturated fats and healthful unsaturated oils.

In 2005, the USDA issued a new Food Guide Pyramid to accompany its new Dietary Guidelines. While the old pyramids offered serving number ranges for each food group, the new pyramid uses colored bands to symbolize the food groups (Figure 8.7 on page 245) and directs people to retrieve their own

TABLE 8.5

Portion Sizes and Comparisons

Grains: Breads, Cereal, Rice, Pasta	Recommended Portion Sizes
1 slice of bread or medium dinner roll	Roll should be no larger than an egg
1/2 cup cooked rice, pasta, or other grains	Size of a woman's fist
1 ounce ready-to-eat cereal	Small bowl, diameter of a CD
3 cups popped popcorn	Fills a sandwich-sized plastic bag
Fruit	
Whole fruit such as 1 medium apple, banana, or orange	Size of a tennis ball
1/2 cup of raw or cooked fruit	Size of a racquet ball
3/4 cup of fruit juice	Just fills a 6-ounce yogurt container
1/2 cup canned fruit	Less than fills a small yogurt container
1/4 cup dried fruit	Size of a golf ball
Vegetables	
1 cup leafy raw vegetables	Size of a softball
1/2 cup chopped fresh, frozen, or canned vegetables	Size of a tennis ball
Proteins	
2–3 ounces lean baked or roasted meat, fish, or poultry	Size of a deck of cards
2 tablespoons peanut butter or other nut or seed butter	Size of a golf ball
1/4 cup nuts	Size of a golf ball
1/2 cup cooked legumes	Size of a racquetball
3 ounces tofu	Size of a deck of cards
Milk, Yogurt, and Cheese	
1 cup milk or yogurt	Smallest milk carton
1 1/2 ounces natural cheese	Size of six dice
2 ounces processed cheese	Size of eight dice
1/2 cup cottage cheese	Size of a racquetball
1/2 cup ice cream, ice milk, or frozen yogurt	Size of a racquetball

Source: Adapted from Anderson, J. B. *Eat Right! Healthy Eating in College and Beyond,* San Francisco: Benjamin Cummings, 2007: 3.

personalized diet analysis and daily recommendations from the USDA website (www.mypyramid.gov). This site offers 12 personalized pyramids that vary based on your age, sex, and activity.

Nongovernment nutritionists have published several alternative pyramids. One published in 2003 by Harvard Medical School's Department of Nutrition recommends that you minimize all sugars and refined or low-fiber carbohydrates such as white flour, white rice, pasta, and peeled potatoes. It also discourages the consumption of red meat, butter, cheese, and other sources of saturated fat. At the

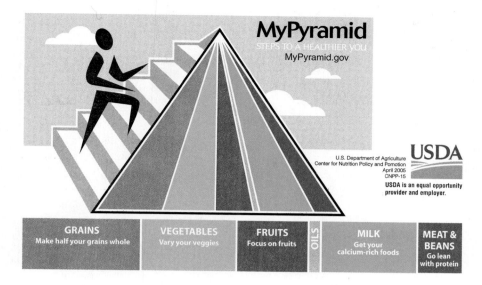

FIGURE 8.7

The 2005 USDA Food Pyramid provides symbolic advice for the proper proportion of each food group in a healthy diet. The stair-stepping figure represents the role of daily exercise in wellness. The USDA website www.mypyramid.gov provides each visitor with an individualized recommendation for daily servings and portion sizes of each food type.

same time, it encourages consumption of vegetables, whole grains, nuts, beans, and unsaturated fats from plant oils (Figure 8.8). There are other pyramids available as well. On the Internet, you can find alternative pyramids for Mediterranean, Asian, Latin American, and vegetarian eating patterns. Visit this book's website for links to other alternative food pyramids.

Try it NOW! Log on to www.mypyramid.gov, find the box called "MyPyramid Plan," and enter your age, sex, and general activity level. The next screen will present you with: the number of daily calories you should consume • the number of servings you should eat from each of the five food groups (grains, vegetables, fruits, milk products, and meat and beans) • pointers for eating enough whole grains and for varying your vegetables each week so you include some dark green ones, some orange ones, some legumes, some starchy vegetables, and others • a reminder to consume enough healthful oils • advice on limiting calories from fats and sugars.

ACQUIRE SKILLS TO IMPROVE YOUR NUTRITION

Do you know the nutritional value of your own daily diet? Do you know how to find out? A few simple skills will help you analyze and improve your diet.

Reading Food Labels The U.S. government requires nutritional labels on the packages of most food products, including the familiar panel entitled "Nutrition Facts" (Figure 8.9). Reading and understanding these labels can help you judge both appropriate portion sizes and the nutritional merits of the foods you eat. By law, every food package must

- prominently identify the product, such as "multigrain cereal" or "low-fat milk";

- state the quantity of food product in the package by weight, volume, or number of pieces so you can judge the value of what you are buying;

- list all the ingredients by common name in order from predominant ingredient to least prominent ingredient by weight;

- give contact information for the food company in case you want more information;

- supply nutritional information in a standardized panel so you can compare and judge the dietary merits of the product before you buy it.

The Nutrition Facts panel provides the greatest concentration of information; it identifies a serving size and how many servings you'll get in a package. For example, one serving of the soup in Figure 8.9 is approximately 1 cup. The panel tells you how many calories each serving provides and how many of

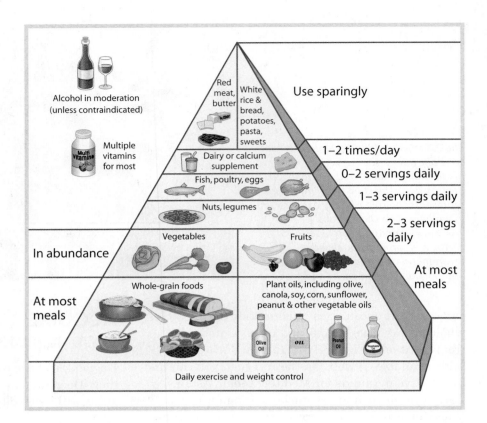

FIGURE **8.8**

Healthy Eating Pyramid

*Source: Eat, Drink, and Be Healthy:
The Harvard Medical School Guide to
Healthy Eating* by Walter C. Willett,
M.D. © 2001 by President and Fellows
of Harvard College (Simon & Schuster)

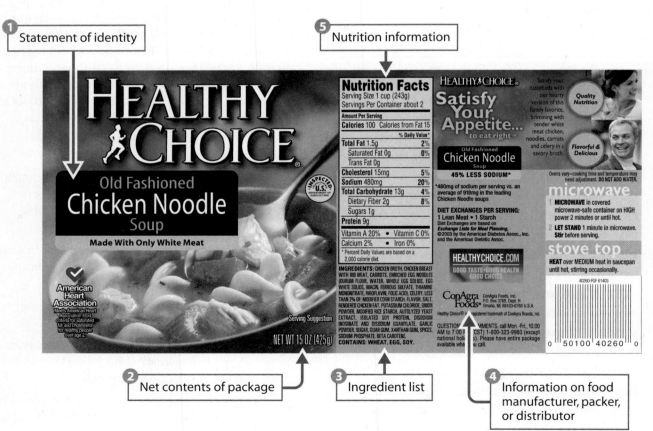

① Statement of identity

⑤ Nutrition information

② Net contents of package

③ Ingredient list

④ Information on food manufacturer, packer, or distributor

FIGURE **8.9**

An important part of improving personal nutrition is reading food labels and understanding the many kinds of information they are required to provide.

those calories come from fat. It lists daily recommended values for nutrients that people should limit in their diets, including total fat, saturated fat, cholesterol, carbohydrates, and sodium. It also lists nutrients that many people should increase in their diets, such as vitamins A and C, calcium, and iron. The label gives the % Daily Value for each nutrient, as discussed earlier and shown in Table 8.4 (on page 242). Finally, each label lists footnotes that show how the percentages of Daily Value are calculated for each nutrient, based on 2,000-Calorie-per-day and 2,500-Calorie-per-day diets.

Without such labels, it would be easy to eat half of a large bag of potato chips and think of that as one serving. Or to pick out a box of sweetened granola with 250 Calories in one-half cup and mistakenly consider a bowl of it to be the nutritional equivalent of high-fiber, low-sugar multigrain flakes with only 100 calories in three-quarters of a cup.

Developing a habit of quickly checking seven items from the typical food label can greatly improve your daily nutrition. *Lab8.1* will encourage this habit. Here are the seven you should look for on a regular basis:

- *What is the normal serving size?* Let's say you bought a bag of corn chips and were planning to eat the whole thing. The label, however, says it contains 8.5 servings. You have just gotten a valuable hint about the calorie density of that food, not to mention the amount of fat and sodium you would get if you ate the whole bag. If you decide to eat just one serving, you can count out your seven or eight pieces and enjoy them—slowly!

- *What is the main ingredient?* If it is water, corn syrup, or enriched (translation, "white") flour, are you getting your money's worth—and good nutrition?

- *How do the total fats and saturated fats compare to the listed daily values?* Just 1 tablespoon of butter, for example, will provide one-third of your DV for saturated fat. Do you really want to consume that much fat in one pat? And what if you were planning to eat something drenched in melted butter like seafood or popcorn, or filled with butterfat, like ice cream or the icing on cake? Those would contain unhealthy levels of dietary fat. Thus, it is best to eat foods like that as one-in-a-great-while treats, if at all.

- *What is the trans fat content?* Reduce or eliminate *trans* fats because of their potentially negative health consequences.

- *How does the sodium compare to % Daily Value?* People diagnosed with high blood pressure, diabetes, kidney disease, and certain other conditions must limit sodium levels. Others should limit sodium to within recommended levels.

- *Does the food provide any fiber?* If not, could you substitute something that does—for example, baby spinach leaves instead of iceberg lettuce in a salad, or a fresh apple instead of canned pineapple, or brown rice instead of white?

- *Finally, what is the % Daily Value of sugars?* Technically, there is no DV for sugars or other sweeteners, but you can see the content in grams listed on food labels. Sugars are common in cereals, sauces, and other processed foods and add empty calories that you could devote to more filling and nutritious foods. Sweeteners come in many forms with many names, including sucrose, brown sugar, honey, corn syrup, corn sweetener, evaporated cane juice, glucose, dextrose, fructose, and maltose. Look for ways to reduce them with more nutritious foods. For example, instead of eating a cup of raisin bran with 19 grams of sugar and 188 Calories of food energy, try choosing one cup of bran flakes with only 5 grams of sugar and 122 Calories, and then adding a cup of sliced, fresh strawberries (high in volume, flavor, vitamin C, and fiber, and containing only 55 Calories).

Keeping a Food Diary Did you have three servings of fruit yesterday or two? Two hundred Calories of fats and sugars or 600? If you are like most people, you can only remember a highlight or two from yesterday's meals, not to mention what you ate the other days of the week. To get an accurate idea of whether your diet is nutrient-rich or poor and provides enough fiber, you will need to record snacks and meals for a few days. This is best done immediately after eating, not hours later when you have discarded wrappers with nutrient labels or lost count of serving sizes.

One way to track your diet is to fill in a food diary like the one packaged with your textbook. Keeping a food diary helps you learn to judge serving sizes. It requires you to read and apply the information on nutrition labels, learn the value of your typical foods, and substitute healthier items for the foods you usually choose.

Using Diet Analysis Software An online program such as www.mypyramid.gov is a powerful tool for keeping track of what you eat, analyzing its nutrient content, and making needed changes in your diet. It is just one of several such programs that can streamline your efforts to achieve better nutrition.

Here are ways you can use this USDA website and its personalized features:

- By clicking on MyPyramid Plan, you can retrieve and then print out a personalized food plan based on your age, sex, and activity level.

- You can use a meal tracking worksheet to keep tabs on each food you ate on a given day, and save this for comparison with additional days.

- You can use the MyPyramid Tracker to assess the nutrients—calories, fats, carbohydrates, vitamins, and so on—in specific foods like a tuna fish sandwich or a slice of pizza (see **Lab8.2**).

- You can make a data bank of nutritional information for foods or meals you eat routinely—say, your typical breakfast of cereal, juice, and toast—so you don't have to enter them individually each time.

- You can do a more detailed analysis of your physical activities to get an estimate of calories burned as you do a particular exercise for a certain period of time.

- Finally, you can keep track of trends in your diet and physical activity over time if you are making changes to benefit your fitness and wellness.

Diet analysis software requires a certain level of comfort with computers and the Internet, and some students will prefer manual methods of keeping food diaries, analyzing nutrient contents, and tabulating calories eaten and expended through exercise.

ADOPT THE WHOLE FOODS HABIT

Analyzing your daily foods for calories and nutrients can help you achieve nutritional wellness. So can a simpler approach: making each bite you take more nutritious by choosing primarily **whole foods,** or dietary items produced with the minimum of refining, addition of preservatives, or processing for quick preparation.

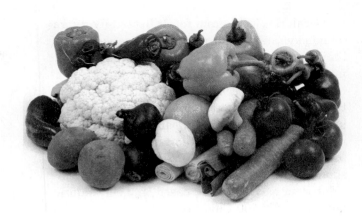

Decades ago, virtually all food was "whole," or real and unchanged. Many packaged foods today, however, have long lists of ingredients and additives that reduce the cost of ingredients, extend shelf life, intensify flavor, and make food preparation easier. People have learned to like the taste and convenience of processed foods, but these products tend to contain hidden fats and sugars, relatively large amounts of sodium, and various additives and preservatives. They also tend to have less naturally occurring fiber and fewer vitamins. A fresh apple, for example, contains more nutrients than a bag of processed, preserved, and dried apple slices. A whole wheat bagel is better for you than a bag of salty "bagel chips." And so on.

Shifting from a diet heavy in processed foods to one rich in whole foods doesn't mean you have to sacrifice good taste or feel hungry or dissatisfied. In fact, you will probably find snacks and meals very filling and delicious if you choose as many foods as possible that are nutrient-dense, high in volume but low in calories, high in fiber, and rich in antioxidants.

Nutrient-Dense Foods You may have heard people talk about foods—sugar, for example—that provide only "empty calories." What they mean is that such foods provide calories for energy without supplying other healthful nutrients. By contrast, **nutrient-dense foods** provide rich sources of vitamins, minerals, antioxidants, and/or fiber, and minimize saturated fat, added sugars, sodium, and refined carbohydrates. Choosing nutrient-dense foods means striving to maximize the food value of each and every meal and snack you consume.

To see what this means in a practical way, compare two small meals—a glass of cola and a hot dog versus a glass of low-fat milk and a small serving

whole foods Dietary items produced and consumed with the minimum of processing, such as refining, adding preservatives, or altering form for quick preparation

nutrient-dense food Food or beverage that provides a high level of nutrients and thus maximizes the nutritional value of each meal and snack consumed

of salmon. The cola provides 105 Calories, all from refined carbohydrates. In about the same number of Calories, the milk provides 8 grams of protein along with vitamin D and calcium. The cola is nutrient-poor; the milk is nutrient-dense.

Now compare the hot dog and salmon. A hot dog on a white-bread bun supplies 420 Calories. It contains more than a whole day's recommended amount of saturated fat, 9 grams of protein, most of a day's allotted sodium, and refined white flour lacking much fiber. In contrast, a serving of salmon provides less than 200 calories, 10 grams of heart-healthy omega-3 fatty acids, twice as much protein, and a small fraction of the sodium. Again, the hot dog has fewer healthful nutrients while the salmon is nutrient-dense.

Learning to reach for nutrient-dense foods every time you get hungry will greatly benefit your life-long fitness and wellness. If your diet consists primarily of processed foods like pastries, coffee drinks, pizza, hamburgers, and cola, you may not even know what wellness feels like! Students often wonder why they should care about the long-term potential consequences of eating too many calories, too much saturated fat, too many refined carbohydrates, and too much sodium. The answer is that dietary excesses can have immediate impacts as well. They can affect your appearance, energy level, athletic performance, social life, ability to fight off infections, and overall sense of well-being. Try shifting toward nutrient-dense foods and away from empty calories, and watch for positive changes in those short-term measures. Focus on establishing habits that keep you looking and feeling vibrantly well today, including the whole foods habit, and your lifelong wellness will improve, too.

High-Volume, Low-Calorie Foods
We eat for many reasons, but the primary one is satiety: a feeling of fullness and the physical and emotional pleasure it brings. Nutrition researchers have discovered that each of us has a characteristic weight of food that we eat in a day. You can eat that weight of food in candy bars, potato chips, steak, and ice cream, but you will be getting too few nutrients and too many calories, and you probably wouldn't feel full for very long between meals. You could eat that same weight of food in celery, iceberg lettuce, and bran and still get too few nutrients, but the volume would help keep you full. The proper goal is somewhere in between: a filling, calorie-appropriate diet that also emphasizes nutrient density. Relatively recent nutritional research showed that

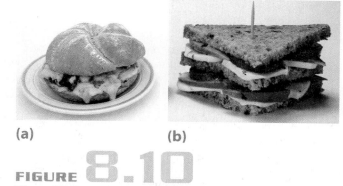

(a)   (b)

FIGURE 8.10

These two sandwiches have approximately the same number of Calories (300), but the one in (a) is small and filled with saturated fat. It contains mayonnaise, butter, cheese, and bacon on a white roll. The sandwich in (b) is large, high-volume, and rich in fiber and vitamins. It contains whole wheat bread, tomato, lettuce, green and red peppers, and cheese.

eating nutritious foods with more volume due to higher air or water content can help people feel full and satisfied longer.[19] This is especially helpful for dieters or for people who want to maintain their weight and not gain more.

Foods with high contents of water, fiber, or protein tend to keep you full and satisfied longer, while those with high contents of fat, sugar, or refined carbohydrates leave you feeling hungry sooner. However, the water must be in the food (as in soups, fruits, and vegetables) and not just in a glass accompanying your meal. Apparently, your brain's satiety center knows the difference and isn't fooled by drinking water. Figure 8.10 compares two sandwiches with approximately the same number of calories, but very different ingredients. Table 8.6 lists familiar foods by calorie density.

High-Fiber Foods
Fiber adds bulk and, often, a chewy quality to food; both help satisfy hunger better and for longer periods. Soluble fiber such as that in oats, barley, and apples, for example, lowers LDL cholesterol. Grains that are intact (like brown rice or bulgur wheat) instead of finely ground (as in whole wheat flour) have a lower glycemic index. High-fiber foods also improve the passage of digested material through the digestive tract.

Antioxidant-Rich Foods
Free radicals are molecules with unpaired electrons that the body produces in excess when it is overly stressed. Free radicals can damage or kill healthy cells, cell

TABLE 8.6

Comparing Calorie Density in Common Foods

Examples of Foods with Low Calorie Density	Examples of Foods with Medium Calorie Density	Examples of Foods with High Calorie Density
Raw celery (1250 grams = 200 Calories)	Brown rice, cooked (179 grams = 200 Calories)	Hot dog, Oscar Meyer beef (61 grams = 200 Calories)
Watermelon (666 grams = 200 Calories)	Enriched spaghetti, cooked (126 grams = 200 Calories)	French fries, McDonald's (59 grams = 200 Calories)
Raw broccoli (588 grams = 200 Calories)	Chicken breast, roasted (121 grams = 200 Calories)	Potato chips, plain salted (37 grams = 200 Calories)
Red or green grapes (290 grams = 200 Calories)	Salmon, cooked, Alaskan wild (110 grams = 200 Calories)	Peanut butter, smooth salted (34 grams = 200 Calories)

Data from U.S. Department of Agriculture, Agricultural Research Service. 2007. USDA National Nutrient Database for Standard Reference, Release 20. Nutrient Data Laboratory Home Page, http://www.ars.usda.gov/ba/bhnrc/ndl

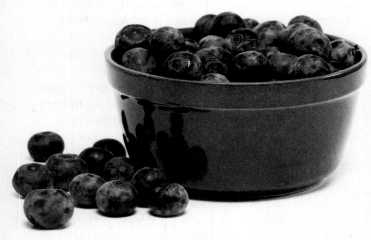

FIGURE 8.11

Fruits and vegetables, such as blueberries and kale, are high in antioxidants.

proteins, or genetic material in cells. **Antioxidants** produce enzymes that scavenge free radicals, slow their formation, and/or actually repair oxidative stress damage. Thus, the theory goes that if you

antioxidant Compound in foods that helps protect the body against the damaging effects of oxygen derivatives called *free-radicals.* Includes vitamins C and E and the yellow, red, orange, and green plant pigments beta-carotene, lycopene, and lutein

consume lots of antioxidants, you will nullify or greatly reduce the negative effects of oxidative stress. Among the more commonly cited nutrients touted as providing a protective effect are vitamin C, vitamin E, beta-carotene, and other carotenoids, and the mineral selenium.

How valid is the theory? To date, many claims about the benefits of antioxidants in reducing the risk of heart disease, improving vision, and slowing the aging process have not been fully investigated, and conclusive statements about their true benefits are difficult to make. Large, longitudinal epidemiological studies support the hypothesis that antioxidants in foods, mostly fruits and vegetables (Figure 8.11), help protect against cognitive decline and risk of Parkinson's disease. However, because of problems with study design and difficulties in isolating dietary effects from supplement effects, it is difficult to assess overall neurological benefits of antioxidants.[20]

Some studies indicate that when people's diets include foods rich in vitamin C, they seem to develop fewer cancers, but other studies detect no effect from dietary vitamin C.[21] Recent studies indicate that high-dose vitamin C given intravenously, rather than orally, may be effective in treating cancer and providing protection from diseases affecting the central nervous system.[22]

Early studies seemed to show that vitamin E had antioxidant effects that could help prevent heart disease and cancer. Large trials involving hundreds of people taking vitamin E supplements, however, have shown very mixed results, with some indicating no benefit.[23] The vitamin E in foods does seem to help protect the cell membranes of red blood cells and the delicate surface lining our lungs.

Foods Containing Folate In 1998, the U.S. Food and Drug Administration (FDA) started requiring food manufacturers to begin fortifying all bread, cereal, rice, and macaroni products sold in the United States with folate (also called *folic acid*). **Folate** is a form of vitamin B that participates in the development of the spinal cord. Folate also helps break down the compound homocysteine, which is produced as the body digests meat and other high-protein foods. By helping break down homocysteine, folate may also protect against cardiovascular disease, heart attacks, and strokes.[24] Vitamin B_6 also participates in breaking down homocysteine.

Phytochemicals Plants make thousands of compounds collectively called *phytochemicals* (meaning literally "plant chemicals"), many of which have antioxidant properties. Fruit, flowers, and plant leaves form a bright palette of colors, in part because plants can generate pigments with antioxidant properties such as *beta-carotene* (yellow and orange pigments), *lycopene* (red pigments), and *lutein,* found in various green, red, yellow, and orange foods.[25]

Most people love the idea of "magic bullets"—pills that will quickly solve their health problems with no other effort. Many people have begun taking antioxidant supplements despite a lack of evidence for their effectiveness in supplement form. Most nutrition researchers recommend getting your antioxidants from nutrient-dense foods or from multivitamin supplements.[26]

DO YOU NEED SPECIAL NUTRITION FOR EXERCISE?

Fitness requires physical activity, but does it also require a special diet? Active people may need some extra nutrients—a little more protein, perhaps, and some extra carbohydrates for fast energy and endurance. But big imbalances in the major nutrients, such as those caused by a high-protein diet or a low-carbohydrate regimen, cannot support improved fitness.

MOST EXERCISERS CAN FOLLOW GENERAL NUTRITIONAL GUIDELINES

Exercisers are often looking for an "edge" and wondering what they can eat, drink, or swallow in pill form that will help them get into shape faster or better. Significantly, sports physiologists and nutritionists have conducted hundreds of studies of recreational, collegiate, and professional athletes, trying to determine optimal energy and nutrient levels for peak performance. Their findings may surprise and disappoint many fitness enthusiasts. But they closely follow general nutritional guidelines with a few minor adjustments.

Carbohydrates The best source of energy before and during exercise is carbohydrates; they should provide up to about 55 to 65 percent of daily calories.[27] Restricting carbohydrates can impede your fitness efforts by leaving you energy-deprived. Sugars can give a little energy boost but can also cause a rise in insulin and a drop in blood sugar that produces fatigue. Many fitness enthusiasts rely on complex carbohydrates during training. Then they consume a sports drink, often diluted with water, to provide hydration and needed energy during a sporting event. Following exercise, they eat complex carbohydrates once again to replace stores of glycogen, a carbohydrate energy-storage compound, in the muscles.

Proteins Most exercisers consume too much protein and fat. As mentioned earlier, for moderate strengthening and endurance exercise, most of us need about 0.75 to 0.8 gram of protein per kilogram of body weight per day. Protein does not in itself help build muscle. Only activity, including weight training, adds new muscle.

ELITE ATHLETES HAVE EXTRA NUTRITIONAL NEEDS

While most exercisers can get complete nutrition from a balanced diet of nutrient-dense foods, some elite athletes do need to modify their eating patterns for better training and performance. Table 8.7 summarizes important recommendations for

---

folate A form of vitamin B that is vital for spinal cord development and helps break down homocysteine as the body digests proteins

TABLE 8.7

Nutrition for Athletes

Nutrient Need for Training	Recommendations
Energy sources in the diet	Carbohydrates should provide 55%–65% of total energy needs
	Fats should provide 25%–30% of total energy needs
	Protein should provide 12%–15% of total energy needs
Consuming sufficient fluids	Drink plenty of fluids before and during strenuous exercise:
	Before exercise, consume 14–22 ounces of fluid (about 2 hours prior)
	During exercise, consume 6–12 ounces every 15–20 minutes
	After exercise, replace fluids lost to sweat and breathing
Meal composition and timing	Consume the maximum carbohydrate calories, then consume dairy and protein foods to make up for energy expenditure
	During heavy training, consume three meals and three snacks per day or more
	Within 1 hour after exercise, replenish glycogen by eating whole-food carbohydrates

Source: Adapted from joint position paper of American College of Sports Medicine, American Dietetic Association, and Dietitians of Canada, January, 2001. www.acsm.org.

athletes from the American College of Sports Medicine and the American Dietetic Association.

Calories People in regular training for competitive sports need extra calories. Athletes often have greater muscle mass than the average person, and muscle tissue consumes more calories than fat tissue, even at rest. A tall young man training with a football or basketball team, for example, could require 5,000 Calories or more daily. High activity levels sustained for long periods—the running during a soccer match, for example—also require extra fuel. About 55 to 65 percent of that extra athletic fuel should come from complex carbohydrates—bread, pasta, cereals, grains, vegetables, and fruits.[28] Some nutritionists recommend up to 70 percent carbohydrates for sustained high-level activities.

Endurance events requiring heavy exertion for more than 90 minutes use two types of internal body fuels, glycogen and fat. Your muscles can store about 90 minutes' worth of glycogen, and additional storage in your liver can fuel a few more minutes of exercise. After that, your body uses its own fat to fuel activity (Figure 8.12). Endurance athletes such as marathon runners, swimmers, and soccer players often consume 60 or 70 percent of their diet in complex carbohydrates starting 2 to 3 days before an athletic event to store sufficient glycogen and fat. Consuming 5 to 7 grams of carbohydrates per kilogram of body weight per day is usually enough for general training, while 7 to 10 grams/kilogram/day will fuel endurance training and strenuous one-time events.

Pre- and Post-event Meals Trainers usually instruct athletes to drink plenty of water, to eat complex carbohydrates 3 or 4 hours before an event, and to avoid proteins, fats, refined sugars, caffeine, and gas-producing foods in the pregame meal. They recommend avoiding protein, because protein takes more time to digest and can lead to increased urination and dehydration. Likewise, fats and oils are slow to digest. Sugar is on the list because it induces a surge of insulin in the blood and later, during the event, can cause an energy dip. Caffeine can lead to increased urination and dehydration and to an accelerated heartbeat. Gas-producing foods can upset digestion.

Most athletes need water and additional carbohydrates during the event, and many choose sports drinks diluted with water to sustain energy and provide sufficient hydration.

Selecting foods for postperformance meals is also important to help restore the muscles' energy supply. After a training or performance session you should eat simple and complex carbohydrates as soon as possible.

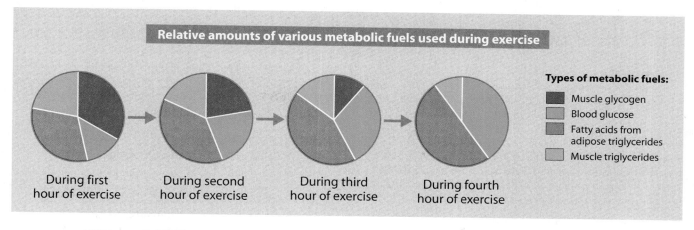

Relative amounts of various metabolic fuels used during exercise

Types of metabolic fuels:
- Muscle glycogen
- Blood glucose
- Fatty acids from adipose triglycerides
- Muscle triglycerides

During first hour of exercise

During second hour of exercise

During third hour of exercise

During fourth hour of exercise

FIGURE 8.12

If you exercise for less than 1 hour, your body uses mostly glycogen and fatty acids (triglycerides) stored in your muscles. If you exercise for 4 hours, the fuel ratios shift dramatically and your activity is mainly powered by blood sugar and the breakdown of fat (adipose) tissue.

Is the popular practice of carbo-loading necessary? If you define *carbo-loading* as eating one huge starch meal the night before an athletic event, then no, it is not necessary or desirable. This kind of consumption can cause the body to retain water, the muscles to feel stiff the next day, and the athlete to feel slow and sluggish when the event starts.

If you define *carbo-loading* as eating 55 to 65 percent of your calories as complex carbohydrates at every meal for 2 to 3 days before an event, then it is desirable because it can load the muscles with glycogen for sustained activity if previous carbohydrate intake was low. Manipulating the pre-exercise diet with more or less sugar, fat, or protein seems to have little effect on most people's performance.[29]

Vitamins and Minerals

The body's energy production and use requires B vitamins; bone- and blood-building require iron and calcium; sweating causes the loss of sodium and potassium that must be replenished during or after events. A balanced diet provides most athletes with enough vitamins and minerals to meet recommended intakes.

Supplements

Optimal muscle growth and strength gain do not require nutritional supplements, however. Most competitive athletes in high school and college do take various kinds of supplements, including megadoses of certain vitamins and minerals as well as purported muscle builders.[30] Where there is no deficiency to start with, these mega-doses provide little or no benefit to performance.[31] The popular creatine monohydrate is chemically related to a natural substance called *creatine phosphate,* which helps fuel muscle contraction. Vendors claim creatine monohydrate helps build muscle, increases energy to improve performance, and delays muscle fatigue. Objective scientific studies suggest that taking creatine orally may cause muscles to temporarily retain more water, and this may boost short-term performance under anerobic conditions. Thus, it may pump up the muscles a bit so they feel bigger (but it is not helpful for endurance events). It does not, however, do what many athletes are hoping for: build permanently bigger muscles. This requires regular physical strength training.

Also popular are individual, concentrated amino acid supplements such as taurine, arginine, glutamine, and leucine. Eating protein-rich foods provides these very same building blocks but in safe concentrations and in naturally occurring mixtures of multiple amino acids. In contrast, supplements provide artificially high concentrations of individual amino acids that may block your body's absorption of the full amino acid spectrum. What's more, amino acid supplements can become contaminated and are far more expensive than eating protein-rich foods. Most importantly, vendors claim that amino acid supplements will help build muscle and sustain contraction, but there is no good evidence of these benefits.

Meal Timing

People use the term *meal timing* in various ways, and some trainers claim that *when* you eat fats, proteins, and carbohydrates will determine how quickly you can build muscles in the gym or how well you can sustain activity during a long bike ride. Carbo-loading and pre- and postevent meals are all forms of meal timing. So are regimens

Chau

"I'm not an 'athlete,' but I do like sports. I've never worried too much about supplementing my diet with extras. I figure as long as I eat enough to feel satisfied, my body's getting what it needs. Some of my friends—like Tom, who's a cross-country runner—are always drinking sports drinks and eating energy bars. I've also noticed Tom often has a pasta dinner two days before a big run, and then he will eat a lighter meal the night before the race. He's also pretty strict about taking a multivitamin every day. It makes me wonder if I should start taking vitamins too."

1. How do Chau's and Tom's nutritional needs differ? Should Chau begin taking vitamin supplements?

2. Explain why Tom plans a pasta dinner two days before a big run, instead of the night before the race.

3. Think about your own level of physical activity. Could you benefit from consuming more calories or adding vitamin supplements to your diet?

---

that instruct you to eat proteins early in the day, carbohydrates at lunch, and so on.

Research shows that the most significant thing about meal timing is the effect on your appetite. Skipping meals, getting ravenously hungry, then "gorging" most of your day's calories at dinner is far more likely to cause fat accumulation than if you "graze" on five or six small meals throughout the day. Japanese sumo wrestlers deliberately apply this principle in order to put on hundreds of pounds of fat. If they spread their daily 6,000 Calories into five or six meals instead of two, they would weigh up to 25 percent less![32]

DO YOU HAVE SPECIAL NUTRITIONAL NEEDS?

In its Dietary Guidelines for Americans, the USDA highlights several groups with special nutritional needs and concerns, including women, children, teens, adults over 50, and vegetarians. We review the groups here, along with diabetic diets and food safety.

WOMEN HAVE EXTRA NEEDS AT CERTAIN AGES

All women must be concerned about calcium, iron, and certain other nutrients, but their recommended values depend on their age and reproductive status. Premenopausal women need to eat enough foods containing iron to replace blood lost through menstruation. They must also get enough vitamin C to help them absorb iron from foods. Any woman who could become pregnant should be careful to get enough folate, because a folate deficiency can lead to neural defects in an embryo even before a woman knows she is pregnant. Finally, all girls and women should get the recommended levels of calcium to build strong bones and prevent osteoporosis.

CHILDREN'S PROPER GROWTH DEPENDS ON NUTRIENTS

The USDA dietary guidelines provide specific pointers for parents and guardians. Adults must ensure that kids and teens get calcium, potassium, fiber, magnesium, and vitamin E in their diets to support their growth and development. Children also need daily intakes of protein, carbohydrates, fats, vitamins, and minerals in nutrient-dense foods, including whole grain products and two to three servings of milk, depending on age. The USDA also recommends that children and teens get at least 1 hour of activity most days of the week to help stem the rapid increase in childhood obesity.

ADULTS OVER 50 HAVE CHANGING NEEDS

To avoid deficiency syndromes, older Americans need to get enough vitamin B_{12}, including from fortified foods and, if necessary, supplements. Review Tables 8.1 and 8.2 on pages 234 and 238, respectively, for amounts and deficiency symptoms for the B vitamins and other nutrients. People over 50 need sufficient calcium to prevent bone-thinning; sufficient potassium for normal muscle contraction and nerve transmission; and sodium within a healthy range to supply cellular needs but lower the risk of high blood pressure.

All adults and children need vitamin D for healthy bones, cell growth, and wound healing. Sunlight hitting the skin helps convert our own natural compounds into vitamin D, but as we age, our skin's ability to absorb sunlight declines. Heavy skin pigmentation and lack of exposure to the sun also limit the conversion of compounds to vitamin D. Older adults must therefore consume extra vitamin D. The same is true for dark-skinned people of all ages, for people who live in far northern latitudes, and for people confined indoors and out of direct sunlight.

The government recommends that older adults stay active by getting moderate to vigorous physical activity most days of the week.

VEGETARIANS MUST MONITOR THEIR NUTRIENT INTAKE

More and more people today are choosing partial or strict vegetarian diets. Between 5 and 15 percent of all Americans claim to be one of the following, arranged in order from the strictest and most exclusive of animal products to the least: Strict *vegetarians* (also called *vegans*) who avoid all foods of animal origin, including dairy products and eggs; *lacto-vegetarians* who avoid animal flesh but eat dairy products; *ovo-vegetarians* who avoid animal flesh but eat eggs; *lacto-ovo-vegetarians* who consume both dairy products and eggs; or *semi-vegetarians,* who consume fish and/or poultry but no red meat. Vegetarians often select organic foods, as do millions of nonvegetarian consumers of both plant and animal products.

Vegetarian diets have certain benefits. Most people who follow a balanced vegetarian diet weigh less than a nonvegetarian of similar height. Most also have healthier cholesterol levels, less constipation and diarrhea, and a lower risk of heart disease. Research indicates that vegetarians may also have a lower risk for colon and breast cancers.[33] It is not clear whether these lower risks are due to their vegetarian diets per se or to some combination of lifestyles such as eating less saturated fat, avoiding smoking, and exercising more.

Despite their benefits, vegetarian diets have certain disadvantages—namely, they can be deficient in protein, vitamin B_2, vitamin D, vitamin B_{12}, or the minerals iron or calcium. With careful food choices, however, vegetarians can avoid these deficiencies:

- Lacto-ovo vegetarians who eat dairy products and small amounts of chicken or fish are seldom nutrient-deficient and consume between 70 and 90 grams per day, which actually exceeds the USDA recommendation for protein. Vegans typically get 50 to 60 grams of protein per day. Through complementary combinations of plant products (review Figure 8.3 on page 224), vegans can get enough essential amino acids.

- Lacto-vegetarians usually get enough vitamins D and B_{12} from dairy products, while strict vegans can develop deficiencies. Fortified products such as soy milk can usually provide enough of these vitamins.

- Vegans are sometimes deficient in vitamin B_2 (riboflavin) since it is found mainly in meat, eggs, and dairy products. They can get enough B_2, however, by eating generous amounts of broccoli, asparagus, almonds, and fortified cereals.

- Because meat is rich in iron and dairy products are rich in calcium, vegans who avoid both can develop deficiencies of these minerals. Solutions include choosing mineral-rich plant foods (see Table 8.2) and/or taking multivitamin/mineral supplements.

In general, vegans can stay in excellent health by eating a wide variety of grains, legumes, fruits, vegetables, and seeds each day. Figure 8.13 shows a vegetarian food pyramid.

THOSE WITH DIABETES MUST REDUCE CARBOHYDRATES

Anyone diagnosed with type 1 or type 2 diabetes will receive specific information from their medical providers about both necessary drug treatments and dietary changes. Because diabetes is a disorder of blood-sugar regulation, patients usually need to cut back on sweets and desserts, both to reduce surges of sugar in the blood and to control obesity, which can both lead to and intensify diabetes. Choosing foods with a lower rather than higher glycemic index (see page 227) is also beneficial, and this usually means less-processed foods and reduced fat content. The American Diabetes Association advises people to eats lots of nonstarchy vegetables and fruits, to choose whole grains over processed grain products, to include beans and lentils in the diet, to eat fish two to three times per week, to choose lean meats and nonfat dairy products, to drink water and diet drinks instead of sugary drinks, to avoid saturated fats and *trans* fats during cooking, and to watch portion sizes.[34]

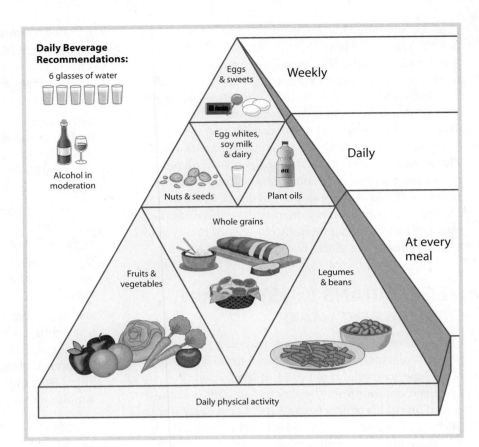

Daily Beverage Recommendations:

6 glasses of water

Alcohol in moderation

Eggs & sweets — Weekly

Egg whites, soy milk & dairy — Daily

Nuts & seeds

Plant oils

Whole grains

Fruits & vegetables

Legumes & beans

At every meal

Daily physical activity

FIGURE 8.13

Vegetarians must be careful to get enough protein, calcium, B vitamins, and other nutrients, and can do so by following this pyramid as a food guide.

Data from the Vegetarian Pyramid, Oldways Preservation and Exchange Trust, www.oldwayspt.org

GOOD FOOD SAFETY PRACTICES ARE FOR EVERYONE

People sometimes think they have the flu when it is actually "food poisoning." Food-borne illnesses usually cause diarrhea, nausea, cramping, and/or vomiting. They usually occur 5 to 8 hours after eating and last only a day or two. For many of us, food poisoning is unpleasant and inconvenient. For the very young, the elderly, or people with cancer, diabetes, AIDS, or other severe illnesses, it can be fatal.

Every year, millions of Americans become sick from unclean or poorly handled foods, sometimes with life-threatening consequences. Since 1994, food-borne pathogens (illness-producing organisms) have sickened more than 76 million Americans annually and have killed more than 9,000.[35]

A rise in the importation of fresh fruits and vegetables from developing countries, as well as increased urbanization, industrialization, travel, and restaurant dining raise the risk of unsafe food handling and resulting illness. To avoid illness, be aware of cleanliness in stores and restaurants. When purchasing food, be aware of the expiration dates on perishable foods. At home, use proper techniques for storing and handling food. This includes several things: Keep hands and cooking surfaces clean. Separate raw foods from cooked foods during storage and cooking. Scrub and thoroughly rinse produce before eating it. Heat foods to high enough temperatures to kill germs. Refrigerate perishable foods. And safely handle the most common sources of food-borne illness: raw eggs, meat, poultry, and fish; unwashed or outdated bean or alfalfa sprouts; and unpasteurized milk and juices.

Some people have concerns about the safety of foods produced with the use of genetically modified organisms or their products, or foods that are irradiated to kill microorganisms and prolong shelf life. You can learn more about these issues by visiting the web links listed on this book's website.

HOW CAN YOU CREATE A BEHAVIOR CHANGE PLAN FOR NUTRITION?

You've no doubt heard the famous phrase, "You are what you eat." But did you know that its origin was a book written in 1825 by Anthelme Brillat-Savain—a French lawyer who loved the pleasures of the table above all else? What he actually wrote was, "Tell me what you eat and I shall tell you what you are." We could modify that slightly to make it perfectly relevant to this book and to you, the reader: tell us what you eat and we'll tell you how fit and well you're likely to be now and in the future!

ASSESS YOUR CURRENT DIET

No matter the details of your current diet, you can probably make significant improvements. The most successful way to change long-ingrained eating habits is to break the task into steps and keep track of your progress.

Recording What You Eat

If you filled in Lab 8.2 using either a manual food diary or the food tracker in www.mypyramid.gov, then you are well on your way to a better diet. Self-awareness is the necessary starting point for change, followed by your own actions for self-improvement.[36]

You should have a pretty clear idea of how many calories you are getting from your daily diet and whether your diet meets, exceeds, or falls short of the daily values for carbohydrates, fats, proteins, fiber, vitamins, and minerals. If there are gaps in your food diary, keep track of your hour-by-hour food consumption for another day or two so you have a clear picture of your typical nutritional profile.

Identifying Your Patterns

Go through your food diary and analyze your reasons for eating each meal and snack. Was it primarily hunger? Primarily socializing? Primarily boredom? If it is hunger, are you satisfying that need with nutrient-dense foods? If it is primarily socializing, are you even hungry at the time? Does peer pressure persuade you to eat an after-dinner snack of pizza and frozen yogurt when you could be happy with a salad, an apple, or a low-cal beverage? If you are eating out of boredom or stress—snacking on chips and cola while studying, for example—could you find a more nutritious alternative like carrot sticks, whole wheat crackers, and

grapes? Or how about an essentially nonnutritive choice such as a diet soft drink or sugar-free gum?

By reflecting on and identifying your own reasons for food preferences and eating habits, you can start to understand your patterns and perhaps change them for the better. It is seldom easy or automatic to improve your diet because it means breaking long-standing habits. But new behaviors become somewhat simpler if you realize when and why you reach for certain foods and that the resistance to change may come from within yourself or your family and friends.

REVIEW YOUR BEHAVIOR CHANGE SKILLS

Examining your current eating patterns is just one part of applying behavior change skills to improve your nutrition. Here are some other ways you can incorporate the behavior change model:

- Look at your motivation. Do you really want a different and better diet? What do you see as the immediate benefits of improved nutrition? What do you expect over the long term? Solidifying your motivation can help you get ready for change.

- Identify barriers to a better diet. What are some of the difficulties you foresee in achieving better nutrition? Time? Money? Eating in less-than-optimal ways with friends and family? Naming some of those barriers and coming up with alternatives can help you on the path to change. If you have trouble brainstorming solutions, the student health service or counseling center may be able to help you.

- Make a commitment to learning about better nutrition. Based on what you learn, list ways in which an improved diet will benefit your life. What could getting more whole grain fiber do for you? How about consuming more fruits and vegetables? Listing these will help you stick with your plan for change.

- Choose a target behavior by identifying your biggest nutritional concern. What is the most pressing issue with your current diet? Review your food diary. If you see that you're getting too much saturated fat every day, outline an approach for getting less saturated fats in your meals and snacks. If you discover that fried meats and cheese (on hamburgers, nachos, pizzas, etc.) are pushing up your daily total, think of lower-fat alternatives from those same menus, or try new places to eat.

- Note where you stand in the typical stages of change. Are you contemplating change? If so, gathering more information or talking more with friends and family might help. Are you planning for change and getting ready to take action?

- Have you noticed any helpful role models? Do you know people with good eating habits and a nutritious diet? Observing their food choices and talking to them about your nutritional issues may help you learn to counter your current habits with others based on better food choices, more successful eating patterns, and solid nutritional information.

GET SET TO APPLY NUTRITIONAL SKILLS

With this chapter, you've already begun to learn and apply nutritional skills. Review your use of them and look for ways to improve those skills and call upon them daily.

- Examine food pyramids to compare your daily servings of various food groups with the amounts that nutritionists recommend from governmental agencies or from academic institutions.

- Read food labels more often and watch for those nutrients you've identified as problematic in your own diet. For example, watch for hidden fats and sugars and look for opportunities to increase fiber.

- Recognize proper portion sizes and note when the helping you are served in a restaurant or cafeteria is way too big (3 cups of pasta instead of half a cup, for example) or way too small (a side salad the size of a golf ball, for example, instead of a softball).

- Use www.mypyramid.gov or other kinds of diet software to get an individual analysis of the daily calories and nutrients you consume and how they compare with the recommended daily intakes of each.

You will use both behavior-change skills and nutritional tools to plan your own program for improved nutrition. Working this plan will give you practice at recognizing nutrient-dense foods. You will begin to choose high-volume, low-density alternatives to high-density, high-calorie foods. You will learn to prefer whole grains to refined ones. And you will start to savor the colors, flavors, and textures of fruits and/or vegetables with every snack and meal.

Your plan may be your first deliberate application of nutritional tools and behavioral-change skills for nutrition. In time, however, it should become a continual and automatic part of each day. The goal is to balance nutrients and control calories naturally as part of your long-term efforts for fitness and wellness and your ongoing management of body mass and weight.

CREATE A NUTRITION PLAN

Begin planning your own program using *Lab8.3.* As you work through the lab, write down your own notes and observations and swap them with others in your class, perhaps during a class discussion or in a small discussion group.

Keep track of calories for your new plan. Are you on track? Where could you cut or add without increasing saturated fats or sugars?

After 2 weeks, discuss the plan and your results with your fitness/health instructor, and revise if necessary. Again, if possible, discuss your experiences with others in your class to exchange successful ideas and get support for your efforts.

For several weeks, continue tracking your daily diet, either manually or using www.mypyramid.gov— at least for the number of servings of the main food groups. This helps you eat sufficient amounts of the foods you needed to increase (for example, whole grains, fruits, vegetables, beans, nuts) and helps you cut back on those that are already overrepresented (for example, saturated fat or refined carbohydrates). Be sure to continue applying nutritional skills such as reading labels and comparing serving sizes to the portions in Table 8.5 (on page 244).

Don't try for perfection! Approach your diet in sets of 2 or 3 days at a time. When you have a day with too few fruits and vegetables, increase them the next day. When you have a day with too little protein, have more the next day. If you get too much protein one day, eat less the next or eat less-concentrated protein foods like tofu, beans, or skim milk.

REVIEW QUESTIONS

1. Essential amino acids are
   a. found only in animal proteins.
   b. found only in plant proteins.
   c. best taken as supplements.
   d. protein building blocks your body can't produce.

2. All are true statements for complex carbohydrates except
   a. they are important energy storage compounds.
   b. they can act as structural compounds in plants.
   c. they can provide fiber in the diet.
   d. they are the best sources of quick energy.

3. Using the glycemic index, one can determine
   a. the percentage of glucose in a food.
   b. the percentage of glycine in a food.
   c. how quickly a food will boost your blood sugar levels.
   d. the caloric content of a food.

4. What do nutritionists sometimes call "bad cholesterol"?
   a. Saturated fat
   b. Butter
   c. HDLs
   d. LDLs

5. Which of these is a poor source of essential fatty acids?
   a. Omega-3 fatty acids
   b. Omega-6 fatty acids
   c. Polyunsaturated oils
   d. Saturated oils such as palm kernel or coconut

6. Vitamins can do all of the following except
   a. help us build bones and teeth.
   b. act as hormones that help regulate the body's use of glucose.
   c. help us convert food molecules into cellular fuel.
   d. take part in wound healing.

7. Calcium can do all of the following except
   a. cause osteoporosis (brittle bones).
   b. facilitate blood clotting.
   c. participate in nerve impulse transmission.
   d. play an important role in muscle contraction.

8. Antioxidants include all of the following except
   a. vitamin C.
   b. beta-carotene.
   c. selenium.
   d. iron.

9. For proper food handling and safety, do all of the following except
   a. scrub and rinse all produce.
   b. avoid pasteurized milk and juices.
   c. observe expiration dates on food packaging.
   d. keep raw foods separated from cooked foods.

10. By law, a food label must
    a. tell the number of sticks in a box of fish sticks.
    b. give the manufacturer's business address on a can of soup.
    c. calculate the percentage of calories from fat.
    d. provide a recommended serving size based on your body weight.

CRITICAL THINKING QUESTIONS

1. Write out a healthy menu for yourself for one breakfast, one lunch, and one dinner, including portion sizes for each type of food you select.

2. Excluding water, what are the major types of nutrients in food? What are the main roles of each?

3. Name several protective functions of dietary fiber.

4. Differentiate *trans* fat and saturated fat. Name two dietary sources of each. Which is worse, and why?

5. How do antioxidants protect the body against the damaging effects of free radicals?

ONLINE RESOURCES

Please visit this book's website at **www.aw-bc.com/hopson** for a list of websites containing information on topics related to this chapter.

REFERENCES

1. U.S. Department of Agriculture, Agriculture Research Service, "What We Eat in America, NHANES 2003–2004," 2006.

2. American College Health Association, "ACHA National College Health Assessment Survey 2006 Reference Group Data Report," *Journal of American College Health,* Vol. 55, No. 4 (January 2007.)

3. W. D. Hoyt, S. B. Hamilton, and K. M. Rickard, "The Effects of Dietary Fat and Caloric Content on the Body-Size Estimates of Anorexic Profile and Normal College Students," *Journal of Clinical Psychology* 59, no. 1 (January 2003): 85–91.

4. L. B. Brown, R. K. Dresen, and D. L. Eggett, "College Students Can Benefit by Participating in a Prepaid Meal Plan," *Journal of the American Dietetic Association* 105, no. 3 (March 2005): 445–8.

5. P. W. Lemon, "Is Increased Dietary Protein Necessary or Beneficial for Individuals with a Physically Active Lifestyle?," *Nutrition Review* 54, no. 4 pt. 2 (April 1996): S 169–75.

6. S. M. Phillips, "Protein Requirements and Supplementation in Strength Sports," *Nutrition* 20, nos. 7–8 (July–August 2004): 689–95.

7. U.S. Department of Agriculture, MyPyramid, 2005.

8. American Cancer Society, "Common Questions About Diet and Cancer," http://www.cancer.org, revised 9/28/2006 (accessed July 27, 2007.)

9. National Institutes of Health, "Diverticulosis and Diverticulitis," *National Digestive Disease Information Clearinghouse* (August 2004): NIH publication no. 04-1163.

10. Janice Thompson and Melinda Manore, *Nutrition: An Applied Approach* (San Francisco: Benjamin Cummings, 2005).

11. United States Food and Drug Administration, "Daily Values Encourage Healthy Diet," FDA internet publication, www.fda.gov/fdac/special/foodlabel/dvs.html.

12. American Heart Association, "What are Triglycerides?," American Heart Association internet publication, www.americanheart.org.

13. Frank B. Hu and Walter C. Willett, "Optimal Diets for Prevention of Coronary Heart Disease," *Journal of the American Medical Association* 288, no. 20 (November 2002): 2569–78.

14. J. Midgley and others, "Effects of Reduced Dietary Sodium on Blood Pressure: A Meta-Analysis of Randomized Controlled Trials," *The Journal of the American Medical Association* 275 (1996): 1590–98.

15. See note 11.

16. Rebecca Donatelle, *Health, The Basics.* 7th ed. (San Francisco: Benjamin Cummings, 2007), 257.

17. John Postlethwait and Janet Hopson, *Explore Life* (Pacific Grove, CA: Brooks/Cole, 2003) p. 400–01.

18. Consumers Union, "A Guide to the Best and Worst Drinks," *Consumer Reports on Health* (July 2006): 8–9.

19. Barbara J. Rolls, Elizabeth A. Bell, and Bethany A. Waugh, "Increasing the Volume of a Food by Incorporating Air Affects Satiety in Men," *American Journal of Clinical Nutrition* 72, no. 2 (August 2000): 361–68.

20. A. Asherio, "Dietary Antioxidant Intakes and Neurological Disease Risks," Paper presented at the Linus Pauling Diet and Optimum Health Annual Conference, Portland, OR: May 2007.

21. See note 10.

22. J. May, "Ascorbic Acid Transporters in Health and Disease," Paper presented at the Linus Pauling Diet and Optimum Health Annual Conference, Portland, OR: May 2007.

23. Gina Kolata, "Large Doses of Vitamin E May be Harmful, Study Says," *New York Times,* November 11, 2004.

24. B. Frei, "Closing Remarks Summary, 2001," Paper presented at the Linus Pauling Institute International Conference on Diet and Optimum Health (Portland, OR: May, 2001).

25. Walter Willett, *Eat, Drink, and Be Healthy. The Harvard Medical School Guide to Healthy Eating* (New York: Free Press, 2003).

26. See note 24.

27. M. Gonzalez-Gross and others, "Nutrition in the Sport Practice: Adaptation of the Food Guide Pyramid to the Characteristics of Athletes Diet," *Archives of Latino American Nutrition* 51, no. 4 (December 2001): 321–31.

28. L. M. Burke and others, "Carbohydrates and Fat for Training and Recovery," *Journal of Sports Science* 22, no. 1 (January 2004): 15–30.

29. W. H. Saris and L. J. van Loon, "Nutrition and Health: Nutrition and Performance in Sports," *Ned Tijdschr Geneeskd* 148, no. 15 (April 10, 2004): 708–12.

30. J. J. Crowley and C. Wall, "The Use of Dietary Supplements in a Group of Potentially Elite Secondary School Athletes," *Asia-Pacific Journal of Clinical Nutrition* 13, suppl. (2004): S39.

31. R. Maughan, "The Athlete's Diet: Nutritional Goals and Dietary Strategies," *Proceedings of the Nutritional Society* 61, no. 1 (February 2002): 87–96.

32. J. B. Anderson and others, *Eat Right! Healthy Eating in College and Beyond* (San Francisco: Benjamin Cummings, 2007).

33. S. Loft, "Diet, Oxidative DNA Damage and Cancer," Paper presented at the Linus Pauling Institute International Conference on Diet and Optimum Health (Portland, OR: May, 2001).

34. American Diabetes Association, "Making Healthy Food Choices," American Diabetes Association, www.diabetes.org/nutrition-and-recipes/nutrition/ healthyfood-choices.jsp (accessed 2006).

35. Centers for Disease Control and Prevention, Center for Infectious Diseases, "Food Borne Illnesses," CDC internet publication, www.cdc.gov (accessed 2002).

36. J. Kurman, "Self-Enhancement, Self-Regulation, and Self-Improvement Following Failures," *British Journal of Social Psychology* 45, pt 2. (June 2006): 339–56.

Name: _____ Date: _____

Instructor: _____ Section: _____

Purpose: To learn how to read food labels and analyze the nutritional content of a packaged food.

Directions: Select any packaged food item from your kitchen or from a grocery store (for example, a box of cereal, a bag of chips, a jar of pasta sauce, or a boxed frozen meal). Find the "Nutrition Facts" panel on the package and answer the following questions.

1. What is the name of the packaged food you are examining?

_____

2. What is the "serving size" stated on the Nutrition Facts panel?

_____

Does this "serving size" match the portion you typically consume of this food in one sitting? Is it bigger or smaller than the amount that you typically consume?

_____

3. Examine the ingredients. What are the main ingredients? (i.e., Which items are listed first?)

_____

Does this list of main ingredients surprise you? How nutritious are the main ingredients?

_____

4. Complete the following table for your chosen food:

Calories (per serving)	Total Fat	Saturated Fat	*Trans Fat*	Sodium	Dietary Fiber	Sugars	Vitamins/ Minerals
	Amount: % Daily Value:	Amount: % Daily Value:	Amount: % Daily Value:	Amount: % Daily Value:	Amount: % Daily Value:	Amount: % Daily Value:	Amount: % Daily Value:

Examine your data. Is this food excessively high in fat, saturated fat, *trans fat*, or sodium? Does it provide any dietary fiber? How much sugar is in this food? Does this food supply any vitamins and minerals?

_____

_____

_____

5. What is your overall assessment of the nutritional value of the packaged food you have examined?

_____

_____

_____

_____

Name: _____ **Date:** _____

Instructor: _____ **Section:** _____

Purpose: To get an initial assessment of your current nutrition and identify areas that need improvement.

Directions: Follow the instructions below. You will need Internet access to complete this lab.*

1. Log on to **www.mypyramidtracker.gov.**

2. Click "Assess Your Food Intake."

3. If you are accessing this site for the first time, click the link for New Users to set up your personalized login and password. When prompted, enter your age, gender, height, and weight. When you're done, click "Proceed to Food Intake."

4. Enter all of the food items you have eaten today. (It's best to complete this at the end of the day, when you are done with all of your meals.) Enter each food individually by entering the name of the food in the search field, clicking "Search," and then clicking "Add," If you cannot find the exact food you are looking for, select the food that is the most similar. After you have "added" a food, it should pop up on the right side of the screen. Click "Select Quantity" and select a serving size from the drop-down menu. Enter the number of servings you consumed. Click "Enter Foods" to enter additional foods. Repeat until you have entered all of the foods you consumed today. (Don't forget to include any snacks and beverages!)

5. When your list of foods consumed is complete, click "Save and Analyze" or "Analyze Your Food Intake."

6. You will see a screen with several links to analyzed data. Click on "Calculate Nutrient Intakes from Foods." This screen will illustrate how your nutrient intake compares to the "recommended or acceptable range." Print this page out.

   a. Does your intake of any nutrient fall short of the "recommended or acceptable" range? If so, which nutrient(s)?

   _____

   _____

   b. Does your intake of any nutrient exceed the "recommended or acceptable" range? If so, which nutrient(s)?

   _____

   _____

7. Click "Analyze Your Food Intake" to return to the main screen containing links to analyzed data. This time, click on "MyPyramid Recommendation." Print this page out.

   How does your food intake compare to the MyPyramid recommendations?

   _____

   _____

Note: For more accurate results, record your intake for at least 3 consecutive days, and then analyze your data again.

* If you do not have Internet access, use the *Behavior Change Log Book and Wellness Journal* that came packaged with your textbook to manually fill out a food diary and analyze your diet.

Name: _____ **Date:** _____

Instructor: _____ **Section:** _____

Purpose: To create a detailed plan for improving your personal nutrition.

Materials: Results from Lab 8.2.

SECTION I: PLANNING CHANGES TO YOUR DIET

1. Look back at your results for Lab 8.2. Which nutrients do you consume too little of?

_____

_____

List at least three foods you could add to your diet in order to increase your consumption of these nutrients:

Food: _____   Rich in: _____

Food: _____   Rich in: _____

Food: _____   Rich in: _____

2. Do you consume too much protein, fat, saturated fat, cholesterol, or sodium? If so, what foods high in these substances could you reduce or eliminate from your diet? List at least 3:

Food: _____   High in: _____

Food: _____   High in: _____

Food: _____   High in: _____

3. How closely did your diet match up with the MyPyramid recommendations? Fill out the chart below.

Current Milk Intake: _____ cups	Recommended Milk Intake: _____ cups
Current Meat and Beans Intake: _____ oz.	Recommended Meat and Beans Intake: _____ oz.
Current Vegetables Intake: _____ cups	Recommended Vegetables Intake: _____ cups
Current Fruits Intake: _____ cups	Recommended Fruits Intake: _____ cups
Current Grains Intake: _____ oz.	Recommended Grains Intake: _____ oz.

How can you adjust your diet to more closely meet the recommended intake levels for each group of foods?

- I would like to increase/decrease my milk intake by _____ cups
- I would like to increase/decrease my meat and beans intake by _____ oz.
- I would like to increase/decrease my vegetables intake by _____ oz.
- I would like to increase/decrease my fruits intake by _____ cups
- I would like to increase/decrease my grains intake by _____ oz.

SECTION II: SHORT- AND LONG-TERM GOALS

Create short- and long-term goals for your healthy eating plan. Be sure to use SMART (specific, measurable, action-oriented, realistic, time-limited) goal-setting guidelines and the information obtained from Section I of this lab and all of your Lab 8.2 materials. Choose appropriate target dates and rewards for completing your goals.

1. Short-Term Goal (3–6 Months)

    a. Goal: _____

    _____

    _____

    _____

    b. Target Date: _____

    c. Reward: _____

    _____

2. Long-Term Goal (12+ Months)

    a. Goal: _____

    _____

    _____

    _____

    b. Target Date: _____

    c. Reward: _____

    _____

SECTION III: BARRIERS TO GOOD NUTRITION; STRATEGIES FOR OVERCOMING THEM

1. What **barriers** or obstacles might hinder your plan for nutrition changes? Indicate your top three nutritional barriers here:

    a.

    b.

    c.

2. Overcoming these barriers to change will be an important step in reaching your goals. Write out three **strategies** for overcoming the obstacles listed:

    a.

    b.

    c.

SECTION IV: GETTING SUPPORT

List **resources** you will use to help you change your nutritional behavior and how each of these resources will support your goals:

    Friend/partner/relative: _____

    School-based resource: _____

    Community-based resource: _____

    Other: _____

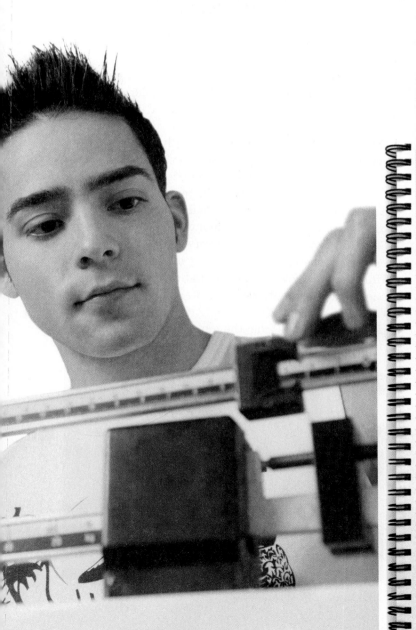

CHAPTER 9

Managing Your Weight

OBJECTIVES

Explain why obesity is both a worldwide trend and a serious concern in America.

Discuss the effects of body weight on wellness.

Acquire effective tools for successful weight management.

List reasons why some diets work but most fail.

Describe the major eating disorders.

Choose a realistic target weight based on your metabolic rate, activity level, eating habits, and environment.

Create a behavior change plan for long-term weight management.

CASE STUDY

Maria

"My name is Maria. I'm 25 and am a full-time student in southern Florida, finishing a BA in child development. I was halfway through college when my daughter, Anna, was born. Now that she's in school, I'm back to taking a full load of classes and hope to finish college in two more years. Overall, I am pretty happy with my life—the only thing I'd really like to change is my weight! Ever since Anna was born, I've been trying to get back my old figure. I'm 5'3"and used to weigh 120 pounds; now I weigh 155. I've tried lots of ways to lose the extra pounds—diet pills, liquid diets, Atkins, South Beach—you name it, I've tried it! Sometimes it works for a while, but eventually the weight always comes back. I'm willing to try again, but how do I find a plan that will stick?"

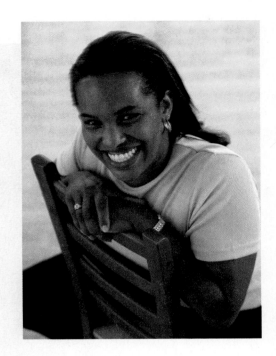

Weight has become a serious issue in America. About two-thirds of American adults are **overweight,** meaning that their body weight is more than 10 percent over the recommended range (see Figure 9.1) and their body mass index, or BMI, is over 25 (see Chapter 6 for a detailed explanation of BMI). Nearly one-third of adults are **obese,** with a BMI of 30 or above, or a body weight more than 20 percent above recommended range. Only about 2 percent of American adults are **underweight,** with a BMI below 18.5 or a weight 10 percent below recommended range.

College students have historically been in better shape than other adult populations. Until fairly recently, only about 25 percent of college students were overweight or obese, a much smaller percentage

than the 66 percent of overweight and obese people in the population as a whole.[1, 2] Because college students tend to be younger, more educated, more likely to exercise, and more socioeconomically advantaged (and thus more likely to have better health coverage), they typically experience fewer health problems than the general population. However, there is evidence that excess weight is becoming an increasing problem for college populations. A recent study of nearly 10,000 college students in Minnesota indicated that over 39 percent of students were overweight, obese, or extremely obese.[3] A similar study of students at the University of New Hampshire indicated that over one-third of students were overweight or obese, and nearly 60 percent of male students had high blood pressure.[4] Results from the most recent national

overweight In an adult, having a BMI of 25 to 29. Also defined as having a body weight more than 10 percent above recommended levels

obese In an adult, having a BMI of 30 or more, or a body weight more than 20 percent above recommended levels

underweight In an adult, having a BMI below 18.5, or a body weight more than 10 percent below recommended levels

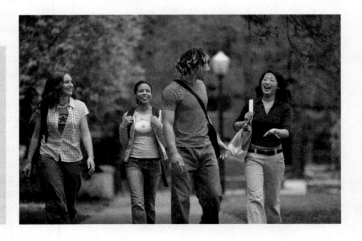

BMI	19	20	21	22	23	24	25	26	27	28	29	30	31	32	33	34	35
Height							**Weight in pounds**										
4'10"	91	96	100	105	110	115	119	124	129	134	138	143	148	153	158	162	167
4'11"	94	99	104	109	114	119	124	128	133	138	143	148	153	158	163	168	173
5'	97	102	107	112	118	123	128	133	138	143	148	153	158	163	158	174	179
5'1"	100	106	111	116	122	127	132	137	143	148	153	158	164	169	174	180	185
5'2"	104	109	115	120	126	131	136	142	147	153	158	164	169	175	180	186	191
5'3"	107	113	118	124	130	135	141	146	152	158	163	169	175	180	186	191	197
5'4"	110	116	122	128	134	140	145	151	157	163	169	174	180	186	192	197	204
5'5"	114	120	126	132	138	144	150	156	162	168	174	180	186	192	198	204	210
5'6"	118	124	130	136	142	148	155	161	167	173	179	186	192	198	204	210	216
5'7"	121	127	134	140	146	153	159	166	172	178	185	191	198	204	211	217	223
5'8"	125	131	138	144	151	158	164	171	177	184	190	197	203	210	216	223	230
5'9"	128	135	142	149	155	162	169	176	182	189	196	203	209	216	223	230	236
5'10"	132	139	146	153	160	167	174	181	188	195	202	209	216	222	229	236	243
5'11"	136	143	150	157	165	172	179	186	193	200	208	215	222	229	236	243	250
6'	140	147	154	162	169	177	184	191	199	206	213	221	228	235	242	250	258
6'1"	144	151	159	166	174	182	189	197	204	212	219	227	235	242	250	257	265
6'2"	148	155	163	171	179	186	194	202	210	218	225	233	241	249	256	264	272
6'3"	152	160	168	176	184	193	200	208	216	224	232	240	248	256	264	272	279
	Healthy weight						**Overweight**					**Obese**					

FIGURE 9.1

Locate your height. Read across to find your weight. Then read up to determine your BMI.

Source: NIH/National Heart, Lung, and Blood Institute (NHLBI). *Evidence Report of Clinical Guidelines on the Identification, Evaluation, and Treatment of Overweight and Obesity in Adults,* 1998.

survey by the National College Health Association also indicate increasing trends of overweight and obesity, as well as increasing indicators of disordered eating.[5]

Regardless of your age and stage of life, several key principles are important to consider as you assess your own dietary, exercise, and weight management strategies:

- Recognize that no diet program, product, or service will magically make weight melt away. Successful weight loss takes time, effort, and motivation. The changes you make in your diet and exercise habits need to become a new way of life, rather than be regarded as short-term fixes.

- Recognize that weight loss, per se, is far less important than your overall percentage of body fat. A high body fat percentage is correlated with numerous health risks. Reducing body fat through resistance exercise, aerobic exercise, and sound nutrition can help lower your risk, improve energy levels, and make you feel better. "Healthy weight loss" means the slow, sustained loss of fat, coupled with increases in muscle mass and the preservation and maintenance of lean body mass.

- Learn how long-term weight management balances calories consumed in foods with calories expended through metabolism, activity, and exercise—an equation called **energy balance.** If you expend more calories than you consume over time, you'll lose weight due to a **negative caloric balance** (Figure 9.2). Consume more calories than you expend and you'll gain weight due to a **positive caloric balance.** Consume and expend approximately the same number of calories over a period of time and you'll reach an **isocaloric balance**—and with it, be able to maintain your weight.

This chapter presents the tools and techniques you need to determine a healthy target weight and create a sound plan for reaching and maintaining it. Incorporating **weight management** into your

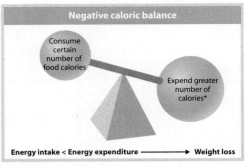

(a)

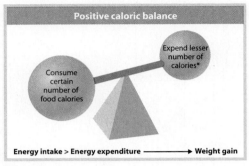

(b)

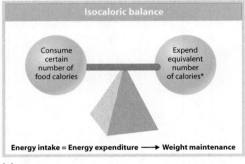

(c)

* Calories are expended through metabolism, activity and exercise

FIGURE 9.2

On any given day, each of us has a personal energy equation with either a negative caloric balance, a positive caloric balance, or an isocaloric balance. Over time, this equation helps determine our body weight.

ongoing wellness program will allow you to realize the significant benefits—physiological, social, and emotional—of sustaining your body mass and body composition within recommended ranges throughout adult life.

WHY IS OBESITY ON THE RISE?

In recent decades, people all over the world have been getting heavier and heavier. What's behind this trend? And why does it matter?

energy balance The relationship between the amount of calories consumed in food with the amount of calories expended through metabolism and physical activity

negative caloric balance A state in which the amount of calories consumed in food falls short of the amount of calories expended through metabolism and physical activity

positive caloric balance A state in which the amount of calories consumed in food exceeds the amount of calories expended through metabolism and physical activity

isocaloric balance A state in which the amount of calories consumed in food is approximately the same as the amount of calories expended through metabolism and physical activity

weight management A lifelong balancing of calories consumed and calories expended through exercise and activity to control body fat and weight

"GLOBESITY" IS A WORLDWIDE TREND

In 2006, the World Health Organization (WHO) estimated that 1.6 billion of the world's people are overweight and that the number could increase to 2.3 billion by 2015. Obese adults number over 400 million worldwide and are a problem in high-income industrialized countries as well as in low- and middle-income developing countries.[6]

Epidemic rates of obesity in the global population, or "globesity," results from energy imbalance. Diets high in processed fats, meats, sugars, and refined starches provide excess calories while labor-saving devices and sedentary lifestyles reduce energy expenditure. In developing countries, entire cultures are moving away from traditional diets—rich in fruits, vegetables, grains, and low-fat proteins—as well as from manual labor. As a result, residents in developing countries are experiencing the same upward shift in body fat percentages and weight that Americans began to show three decades ago. Only the poorest countries of sub-Saharan Africa do not reflect this worldwide trend.[7]

ENERGY IMBALANCE IS COMMON IN AMERICA

In the last quarter century, the percentage of overweight Americans rose 40 percent while the percentage of obese adults more than doubled. The maps in Figure 9.3 reveal that the rapid increase is distributed unevenly, with the southern and upper Midwestern states now showing the highest rates of obesity in the nation.

American children are getting heavier, too. More than 37 percent of American children are overweight or obese. That represents twice as many heavy preschoolers and teens today as in the 1970s, and three times as many children aged 6 to 11.[8] What's behind this widespread energy imbalance?

Overconsumption Americans consume 250 to 500 calories more per day now than they did 30 years ago. Without additional exercise, this imbalance in energy input can lead to considerable yearly weight gain. Many societal factors encourage overeating: portion distortion, the constant availability of food, advertising, and price.

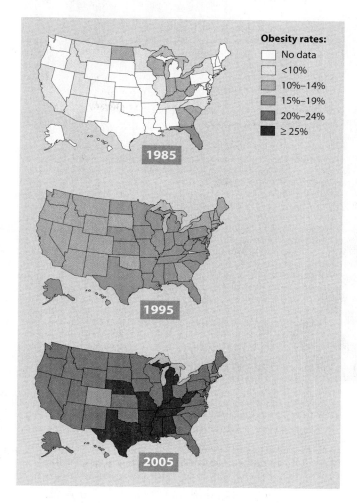

FIGURE 9.3

Obesity rates have risen dramatically over recent decades. Rates are highest in the upper Midwest and in the South.

Source: Centers for Disease Control, 2006.

Food portions in restaurants and supermarkets have grown steadily over the past half-century, along with consumers' preferences and expectations. In 1954, a Burger King hamburger weighed 3.9 ounces. Today, it weighs 4.4 ounces—a 13 percent increase. Most people, however, don't order the regular-sized hamburger, choosing instead the much larger Whopper with 9.9 ounces of meat, or the Double Whopper with 12.6 ounces.[9] In addition, researchers have found that people don't read their own "fullness signals," or feelings of *satiety,* very well. As a result, the bigger the portions (and the more food available), the more they will eat overall.[10]

Easy access to food also encourages overeating. Today, most drugstores, gas stations, schools, and public buildings have vending machines and

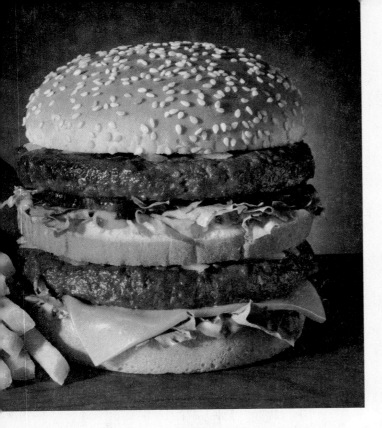

Hand-deliver letters to people when you want to communicate? Probably not! The ease of our modern life is an improvement over the hard physical labor of past generations. The exertion we are spared, however, amounts to hundreds of calories per day that we *don't* burn off as we sit at our desks, drive our cars, and change channels with a remote control.

Even the layout of modern towns and cities contributes to reduced energy expenditure. The majority of Americans live in suburbs—an environment designed and built around automotive transportation. Suburban living is strongly linked to decreased activity, and this, in turn, contributes to a number of medical conditions. The greater the sprawl, the less people walk, the more they weigh, and the more likely they are to have high blood pressure,[14] heart disease, cancer, diabetes, and other diseases.

Biological Factors Our modern food supply, culture, and environment clearly encourage overconsumption and underexercise. But why, then, isn't *everyone* overweight or obese? The answer lies mostly in heredity, demographics, and personal choice.

If most of your relatives—parents, siblings, and others—are overweight or obese, you will be more likely to gain weight during adulthood yourself. Researchers have learned that dozens—perhaps hundreds—of genes help determine your weight.[15] Genes control whether our metabolism is fast and tends to burn off most of our excess calories, or is slow and tends to conserve food energy. Genes also control appetite, fullness, fat storage, fat utilization, and activity levels.

Our natural tendencies to conserve or use energy during rest and activity also influence our weight. Some people tend to save energy by sitting quietly for long stretches and being generally less active all day. Others tend to use energy by being fidgety, jiggling their head, hands, and feet, and getting up to walk around every few minutes. James Levine and colleagues at the Mayo Clinic have demonstrated that lean people burn 279 to 477 more calories per day than obese people through this type of **non-exercise activity**—an expenditure that can significantly affect fat storage and body weight.[16]

The box **Understanding Diversity: Race/Ethnicity, Gender, and Weight** examines how ethnicity and gender can also be factors in an individual's propensity toward weight gain.

minimarts selling packaged food. People eat more candy, cookies, and other treats if they are available in plain sight than if the same food is less accessible.[11] Choice affects eating as well. The more food people have to choose from, the more they tend to eat. People will eat more total food at a four-course meal than at a two-course meal—and even more at a buffet.

The persuasiveness of product advertising also contributes to overeating. An amazing one-third of our daily calories come from just a few categories of highly advertised foods that contribute little more than empty calories: sweets, sodas and fruit drinks, alcoholic beverages, and salty snacks.[12]

The relatively low price of food in America is yet another environmental influence on overconsumption. When experimenters lowered the price of snacks in vending machines, the discount stimulated sales immediately—regardless of whether a snack food had any nutritional value.[13]

Too Little Exercise Do you plant and harvest your own food? Carry your own water from a well?

non-exercise activity Routine daily activities like standing up and walking around that use energy but are not part of deliberate exercise

UNDERSTANDING DIVERSITY

RACE/ETHNICITY, GENDER, AND WEIGHT

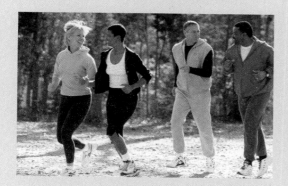

Body weight varies by racial/ethnic groups to some degree, based on genes as well as on cultural preferences for food and exercise. Hispanic males, African American males and females, and white males have the highest percentages of overweight (60 and 70 percent of adults in these groups). Hispanic females and white females have somewhat lower rates of overweight (45 to 55 percent). Asian Americans have the lowest percentages of overweight (men 35 percent, women 25 percent).[1]

Some ethnic groups appear to have "thrifty genes" that helped their ancestors survive during extended periods of famine by slowing down metabolism to conserve food energy. In a modern environment of plentiful food, widespread mechanization, and diminished activity, however, "thrifty genes" can lead to easy weight gain. This helps explain, for example, why 90 percent of Pima Indians are overweight and 75 percent are obese.[2]

Women have a tendency to burn fewer calories than men due to their higher level of essential body fat and lower ratio of lean body mass to fat mass. Because muscle cells burn more energy, and because men usually have more muscle tissue than women, men burn 10 to 20 percent more calories than women do, even at rest. Monthly hormonal cycles and pregnancy also increase the likelihood of weight fluctuation and gain. Significantly, though, adult men are more likely to be overweight than adult women.

Sources:
1. Charlotte. A. Schoenborn and others, "Body Weight Status of Adults: United States, 1997–1998." Advance Data from *Vital and Health Statistics*, no. 330 (September 6, 2002). U.S. Centers for Disease Control and Prevention.
2. P. Jaret, "The Way to Lose Weight," *Health* (January-February 1995): 52–59.

Lifestyle Factors For most people, exercise, activity, nutrition, and other personal choices impact body weight as much or more than do inherited tendencies. For example, 25 percent of Americans do not engage in exercise, sports, or other physical activity during their leisure time.[17] Education is also a factor in both weight and exercise. The more education a person attains, and the more money he or she makes, the less likely he or she is to be overweight or obese. And the higher a person's educational attainment, the more likely he or she is to be physically active.

CASE STUDY

Maria

"I was never overweight as a kid, and I gained a normal amount of weight during my pregnancy, but now I'm considered overweight. My parents, grandparents, and two older sisters are all kind of on the heavy side, so I wonder if my "heavy" gene just decided to kick in! While I was pregnant, I got used to eating more food than I used to, and after giving birth to Anna, I guess I just didn't cut back. I spend a lot of time running around after Anna, but otherwise, I drive everywhere and don't set aside special time to exercise. Meanwhile, it seems like Anna will eat only three things—macaroni and cheese, chicken strips, and pizza—so that's what we eat

most nights. My husband and I joke that all three of us eat like stereotypical college students."

1. **List three factors that probably contributed to Maria's becoming overweight.**

2. **Do you share any of Maria's habits? Is she like any of your friends?**

3. **Are you satisfied with your current weight? If not, are there aspects of your lifestyle that may have led to your current dissatisfaction?**

HOW DOES BODY WEIGHT AFFECT YOUR WELLNESS?

A leading nutritionist has written that "weight sits like a spider at the center of an intricate, tangled web of health and disease."[18] Indeed, research shows that three weight-related factors impact your long-term health: your BMI, increases in BMI over time, and body fat stored in the abdominal regions. You are more likely to remain healthy throughout life if (1) your BMI is between 21 and 23 for women and 22 and 24 for men; (2) you maintain approximately the same BMI and the same waist size throughout your adult life; and (3) your body's fat deposits tend to occur around the hips and thighs rather than the abdomen. High BMIs and abdominal fat (indicated by a large waist size) are associated with higher risk for several chronic diseases.[19]

Being underweight is an important but far less common problem. Fewer than 5 percent of Americans have a BMI under 18.5. Underweight carries its own significant health risks and can be the result of an unusually fast metabolism, excessive dieting, extreme levels of exercise, eating disorders, smoking, or illness.

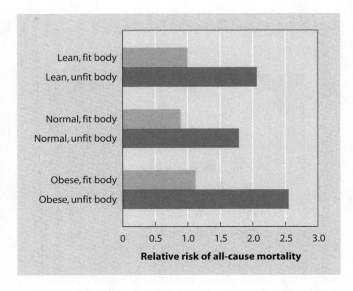

FIGURE 9.4

Being fit significantly reduces your mortality risk in any given year, regardless of your degree of body fat.

Source: Chong Do Lee, Steven N. Blair, and Andrew S. Jackson, "Cardiorespiratory Fitness, Body Composition, and All-Cause and Cardiovascular Disease Mortality in Men," *American Journal of Clinical Nutrition* 69, no. 3 (March 1999): 373–80.

BODY WEIGHT CAN AFFECT LIFE EXPECTANCY

People who maintain a weight and BMI within recommended ranges generally have longer life expectancies than people who are obese or underweight. As Figure 9.4 shows, being fit significantly reduces mortality risk, especially when combined with healthy weight. Being obese (having a BMI of 30 or above) cuts an average of 6 to 7 years from the life of a nonsmoker and 13 to 14 years from a smoker.[20] Research indicates that America's 200-year rise in life expectancy may begin to decline because obesity is so prevalent and can shorten life so dramatically.[21]

Underweight people have a higher death rate than normal-weight or overweight people.[22] In fact, some studies indicate that underweight people may have more than 18 times the risk of dying of cancer, and four times the risk of CVD death.[23] Only obese people have a shorter life expectancy. The statistics for early deaths among the underweight reflect the fact that a low BMI is characteristic of patients with illnesses such as cancer, uncontrolled diabetes, and disordered eating. People who are underweight but

not ill and who are careful to get complete daily nutrition may actually realize greater longevity.[24] Underweight associated with poor nutrition, however, can lead to life-shortening conditions such as anemia, susceptibility to disease and infection, slower recovery from illness, muscle wasting and weakness, and osteoporosis and bone fractures.

BODY WEIGHT CAN PROMOTE OR DIMINISH FITNESS

A stable, healthy-range BMI goes hand in hand with regular exercise. Maintaining weight and BMI within recommended ranges leads to increased energy and reduced likelihood of injury during fitness activities. Safety and comfort, in turn, encourage continued exercise and the many wellness benefits it produces.

Over- and underweight can contribute to poor fitness. The reverse is also true: Low fitness can contribute to unhealthy weight levels. Overweight can lead to a downward fitness spiral: An over-accumulation of body fat leads to strain on the bones, joints, and muscles that makes exercising harder and injury more likely. Stiffness and pain in

CASE STUDY

Maria

"Here's the funny thing: My husband, Tim, is extremely skinny. He's 5'9" and weighs only 130 pounds. We eat the same foods, but he has the metabolism of a humming-bird. I don't know where it all goes. His whole family is thin, so I guess that is part of it. He's just as out of shape as I am, though. We moved to a new apartment recently and need to walk up one flight of stairs—both of us get so out of breath by the time we make it to the door. Just because he's skinnier doesn't mean he's any more fit! What a pair: I want to lose weight, while he wants to gain weight."

1. What chronic health problems is Maria at risk for if she remains overweight?

2. Maria must now walk up and down a flight of stairs every day to leave/return to her apartment. Do you see this as a good or bad thing? Explain your answer.

3. Do you think Tim faces fewer chronic health risks than Maria? What else would you want to know about Tim's and Maria's habits that would help you answer this question?

4. Which of the benefits of maintaining a healthy weight are most important to you?

---

the hands, feet, knees, and back, in turn, make exercising more difficult. They also make work, employment, and activities of daily living—walking up stairs, carrying books or grocery bags, shoveling snow, getting in and out of automobiles, and so on—harder. With lower levels of exercise, fitness and wellness decline.

Below-normal body weight can lead to muscle wasting as the body breaks down muscle tissue for energy when fat stores are low. Muscle wasting, in turn, can lead to weakness and declining ability to exercise and accomplish daily tasks. These inevitably reduce both fitness and wellness unless the underweight individual works hard to maintain strength and endurance.

BODY WEIGHT CAN INFLUENCE THE RISKS FOR CHRONIC DISEASES

Researchers have confirmed that people with excess body fat have higher levels of several serious chronic diseases, including high blood pressure, stroke, heart disease, certain cancers, type 2 diabetes, and metabolic syndrome.[25] Specific cancers linked to high BMI include prostate, colon, rectum, esophagus, pancreas, kidney, gallbladder, ovary, cervix, liver, breast, uterus, and stomach.[26]

Fat accumulation around the waist (a 40-inch waistline or higher for a man, or a 35-inch waistline or higher for a woman) increases the risk for developing **metabolic syndrome.** This serious medical condition is a combination of high blood cholesterol, high blood pressure, abdominal fat

deposits, and insulin resistance or full-fledged type 2 diabetes.

Gaining weight may increase the risk for cardio-vascular disease, diabetes, and other chronic diseases because of *inflammation,* a primitive immune reaction. Fat tissue may be giving off chemicals that trigger inflammation, and inflammation may aggravate heart disease, diabetes, and other conditions.[27] Losing weight, on the other hand, may diminish inflammation and is known to decrease levels of blood cholesterol and triglycerides, and lower blood pressure and diabetes risk.[28] A weight loss of just 10 to 15 pounds can bring measurable health benefits, even to an obese individual.[29]

WHAT ARE EFFECTIVE TOOLS FOR WEIGHT MANAGEMENT?

Understanding role of metabolic rates, setting realistic goals, recognizing your body's set point, and taking lessons from successful weight maintainers will help you achieve your weight goals.

---

metabolic syndrome A medical condition characterized by a combination of high blood cholesterol, high blood pressure, abdominal fat deposits and large waist circumference, and insulin resistance or type 2 diabetes

FACTS AND FALLACIES

DO DIET DRUGS WORK?

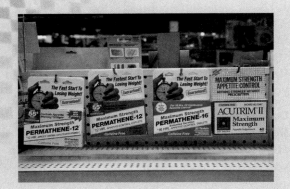

Millions of people think to themselves, "I hate diets and exercise, and they don't work for me, anyway. Why can't I just take a pill to get thin?" Unfortunately, prescription diet drugs can cost over $100 per month and have significant side effects, and even the most effective among them don't bring about much weight loss. What's more, without modified diet and increased exercise, any lost weight comes right back as soon as a person stops taking the pills.[1]

Currently on the market is Meridia (sibutramine), a drug that keeps levels of the neurotransmitter serotonin high and helps to cut hunger. Users average a 10- to 14-pound weight loss over 6 months, or about one-half pound per week. However, the drug can cause headaches, insomnia, high blood pressure, and other symptoms, and can interfere with antidepressant drugs.

Another currently prescribed drug called Xenical (orlistat) partially blocks digestion of fats. Users lose an average of 13 pounds in a year (about 4 ounces per week) with side effects that include oily stools and spotting, gas with fecal discharge, and urgent elimination. A lower-dose over-the-counter version called Alli is being marketed now.

Several prescription drugs suppress appetite, including Phentride (phentermine), and Tenuate (diethylpropion). These drugs are addictive, cause tolerance, and can only be used in the short-term. A French drug called Acomplia (rimonabant) blocks appetites and helps users lose an average of 19 pounds per year (a little over one-third pound per week), but it has undergone limited human testing and is currently unavailable in the United States.

The FDA has banned many other drugs and supplements (for example, drugs containing ephedra or phenylpropanolamine, also called *fen-phen*) because of elevated blood pressure, stroke risk, and other harmful side effects.[2]

You will also find many supplements in the vitamin section of drug and food stores, despite a lack of proof that they are effective or safe. One such product, bitter orange, contains a stimulant similar to ephedra. There have been no conclusive human studies proving either the safety or effectiveness of bitter orange. Claims for several other supplements await supporting evidence. These include herbal laxatives; the heavy metals chromium and vanadium; ginseng and ginkgo; green tea extracts; and an extract from shrimp and crab shells called *chitosan*. Until someone invents a truly effective, low-risk weight-loss drug, the best options are improved diet and increased exercise, perhaps in conjunction with a prescription.

Sources:
1. S. B. Moyers, "Medications as an Adjunct Therapy for Weight Loss: Approved and Off-Label Agents in Use," *Journal of the American Dietetic Association* 10, no. 6 (June 2005): 948–59.
2. B. F. McBride and others, "Electrocardiographic and Hemodynamic Effects of a Multicomponent Dietary Supplement Containing Ephedra and Caffeine: A Randomized Controlled Trial," *Journal of the American Medical Association* 291, no. 2 (January 14, 2004): 216–21.

RECOGNIZE THE ROLE
OF METABOLIC RATE

Lifelong weight maintenance requires deliberately balancing calories consumed and calories expended. Just to stay at roughly the same weight as the years pass and metabolism slows bit by bit, most people must gradually decrease their food intake as they gradually increase their physical activity. Fully 60 to 70 percent of your daily calorie intake—typically between 900 and 1,800 food Calories per day—is consumed as your body sustains functions like heartbeat, breathing, and maintaining body temperature. The rate at which your body consumes food energy to sustain these basic functions is your **basal metabolic rate** (BMR). Your **resting metabolic rate** (RMR) is slightly higher, because it also includes the energy expended as you digest food. BMR has genetic underpinnings but can be influenced by your activity level and your body composition. Since muscle tissue is highly active, the more lean tissue you have, the greater your basal metabolic rate; the more fat tissue you have, the lower your BMR. This explains

basal metabolic rate Your baseline rate of energy use, dictated by your body's collective metabolic activities

resting metabolic rate Basal metabolic rate plus the energy expended in digesting food

why both your activity level and your fitness influence your BMR; the higher your fitness level, the greater your ratio of lean tissue to fat mass is likely to be, and the more energy you will burn while exercising and at rest. Cardiovascular and strength-building exercises contribute most directly to speeding up BMR.

ASSESS YOUR CURRENT WEIGHT AND CHOOSE A REALISTIC GOAL

Figure 9.1 shows healthy weight and BMI ranges based on height. In using weight and BMI charts, people often wonder if their ideal weight should be on the high or low end of the range. If your body fat percentage is low and your muscle development is high, your healthy weight (including your BMI) will be on the higher end of the range. The same is also true if your frame size is large (as judged by a measure such as wrist circumference). If your body fat percentage is high and your muscle development is low, your healthy weight will be in the middle-to-low end of the range. This is also true if your frame size is medium or small. Knowing these factors will help you calculate a realistic weight goal.

RECOGNIZE YOUR BODY'S SET POINT

Perhaps you've noticed that your body is programmed around a certain weight or **set point** that it returns to fairly easily when you gain or lose a few pounds. Many dieters reach a plateau after a certain amount of weight loss and can't seem to trim off more pounds. This plateau is due, in part, to a downshifted metabolism balancing out lower calorie intake: the person's energy balance is now at a weight-maintenance, not a weight-loss, level.

To "outsmart" and reset one's set point, a dieter must lose weight slowly and increase exercise.

Physiologists have known for some time that exercise both speeds resting metabolism and preserves lean body mass so more muscle tissue remains to continue burning extra calories.[31]

TAKE LESSONS FROM *SUCCESSFUL* WEIGHT MAINTAINERS

People who sustain a normal, healthy weight over years or decades tend to do some of the same kinds of things. Successful weight maintainers engage in a physically active lifestyle, averaging an hour per day of moderate to vigorous physical activity.[32]

Successful weight maintainers also tend to have a regular eating pattern. They don't skip meals, they eat breakfast every day, and they don't "cheat" over the weekends by indulging in junk food. They eat a nutritious diet that is low in fats, high in complex carbohydrates, has moderate levels of protein, and has a high volume but a low calorie density. They avoid sodas and juice drinks sweetened with sugar or corn syrup.

Successful weight maintainers also stay conscious of situations that trigger overeating, and they apply strategies to prevent overeating. They are motivated to stay at a healthy weight, and they respond quickly by cutting back calories and increasing activity as soon as their weight starts to creep up.[33]

People who are successful at maintaining a healthy weight typically have tools for coping with problems and handling life stresses. They assume responsibility for their lifestyle behaviors, know where to seek help, and tend to be self-reliant. They have a good social support system, both for their weight maintenance and their lives in general. They are more likely to maintain weight loss if they are satisfied with their new weight.[34]

BALANCE YOUR ENERGY EQUATION

Long-term weight management relies on balancing your energy equation—that is, attaining an isocaloric balance so that the calories you consume are equivalent over time to the calories you burn.

set point A preprogrammed weight that your body returns to easily when you gain or lose a few pounds

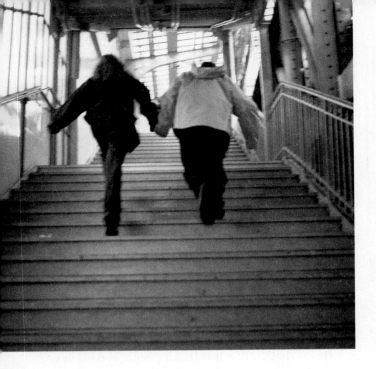

To lose or gain weight, you must deliberately "unbalance" that equation for a while: negative caloric balance for loss, positive caloric balance for gain.

There are several ways to determine your approximate daily calorie consumption and expenditure. *Lab9.1* allows you to calculate your current energy balance and set goals for a better balance. Another approach is logging on to the MyPyramid.gov website to get a target number for calorie consumption based on your age, sex, and level of daily moderate or vigorous activity.

Websites like MyPyramid.gov also provide calorie counts for specific foods and portions so you can keep track of how many calories you consume each day. You can get calorie-counting programs for small handheld computer devices, or find them online at websites like www.caloriecontrol.org. MyPyramid.gov

also supplies calorie expenditure information from various activities, as does Table 9.1.

If you follow good nutritional and eating habits and establish and stick with a regular exercise program, weight maintenance can become second nature to you and a habit you keep throughout adult life.

ESTABLISH A REGULAR EXERCISE PROGRAM

Along with monitored and controlled eating, exercise is essential both to weight change (loss or gain) and to weight maintenance. Exercise burns calories directly, pumps up your metabolic rate to burn additional calories, and builds muscle tissue that burns still more energy. Many people find that in addition to a healthy diet, they need to be active for more than an hour per day in order to lose weight, while 60 minutes per day will sustain weight at current levels. These figures are cumulative: Add 7 minutes of stair-climbing here, plus 11 minutes of brisk walking across campus there, plus 20 minutes of stationary biking, and so on. Aerobic exercise, of course, is the best calorie burner.

The greater the frequency, intensity, and time spent on an activity, the more energy you use and the more calories you burn. There are other considerations for choosing types of fitness exercise as well. The larger the muscle groups you use, for example, the more you boost your metabolism, and in turn, your calorie expenditure. Your baseline physiological activities—heartbeat, breathing, generating body heat, and so on—also consume calories while you are contracting arm, leg, abdomen, and other body muscles. Table 9.1 lists the caloric expenditures for several popular activities, sports, and exercises for adults of three different weight levels.

MODIFY YOUR BEHAVIOR FOR LONG-TERM WEIGHT CHANGE

Weight loss is hard work, but in some ways, it's the easy part of weight management. Most people can lose some weight, but relatively few—perhaps 20 percent—can maintain that lower weight for more than a few months. In one study, more than half of successful dieters thought dieting was easier than weight maintenance. Nevertheless, with the right basic approach, weight loss or gain can simply be phases of lifelong weight stabilization that use very similar tools and techniques.

Try it NOW! **Log on to www.MyPyramid.gov and click on "MyPyramid Tracker." • Set up your own user login and password. • Enter your daily activity level. • Then click "Energy Balance"—how many calories do you need, given your activity level?**

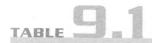

TABLE 9.1

Calories Burned through Activity

Activity, Sport, or Exercise	Calories Expended/Min in 110 lb Person	Calories Expended/Min in 150 lb Person	Calories Expended/Min in 190 lb Person
Aerobics, 10" step	7.0	9.5	12.0
Basketball, pick-up	7.0	9.5	12.0
Biking, slow	5.3	7.1	9.0
Bowling	2.6	3.6	4.5
Dancing, moderate pace	4.2	5.7	9.0
Downhill skiing, moderate pace	5.5	7.5	9.5
Driving	1.8	2.4	3.0
Frisbee, casual	2.6	3.6	4.5
Golf, walking, and pulling clubs	4.4	6.0	7.5
Grocery shopping	3.1	4.2	5.3
Hiking, hills	5.3	7.1	9.0
Jogging, moderate pace	5.3	7.1	9.0
Kickboxing	8.8	12.0	14.7
Office work	1.3	1.8	2.3
Ping-Pong	3.5	4.8	6.0
Reading	0.9	1.2	1.5
Soccer, noncompetitive	6.1	8.3	10.5
Softball	4.4	6.0	7.5
StairMaster: 40 stairs/minute	6.1	8.3	10.2
Stretching	3.5	4.8	5.8
Swimming	~8	~10	~13
Tennis, singles, recreational	7.0	9.5	12.0
Watching TV	1.0	1.4	1.8

Source: Adapted from *Calorie Expenditure Charts*, by Frank I. Katch, Victor L. Katch, and William D. McArdle (Ann Arbor, Michigan: Fitness Technologies Press, 1996).

Readiness requires motivation, commitment, goals, and attitudes. *Lab9.2* at the end of this chapter helps you assess your motivations for weight change and your readiness—your diet IQ.

You must be motivated to change your long-term eating and exercise habits, and you must be willing to work to accomplish those changes. Talking with friends, learning about the benefits of healthy BMI, and writing in a journal about your current eating and exercise habits can all help motivate you to set and reach body goals. Work on your attitude, too. Accept the fact that only through permanently controlled eating and a long-term commitment to activity and exercise can you maintain desired weight, BMI, and body composition over the long-term.

You also need realistic goals in order to change your weight and then maintain the new desired level. Weight and nutrition experts recommend that

CASE STUDY

Maria

"After living in our new apartment for a month, I've noticed something interesting: It's gotten easier to climb up and down the flight of stairs. I guess I'm getting used to it! Of course, that alone is not going to make me lose weight, but it's become the unofficial kickoff to my plan to get more active. One of the things I'm realizing is that I need to stop this idea of 'going on a diet' and instead try to figure out how to change my habits in a way that feels manageable to me. If I just 'go on a diet,' I'll regain everything I lose as soon as I go *off* of it, right? So what I need to do is figure out how to get more active and change my habits in a way that feels natural.

"I weigh 155 right now. I need to lose 35 pounds to get back to my old prepregnancy weight of 120. For now, I'm just going to try losing 10 pounds, at least to start off with. I've heard about weight-loss groups that help you

with meal planning, portion control, and regular exercise. I think that might be a good approach for me."

1. Just by climbing a flight of stairs every day, Maria has increased her daily activity level and is expending more calories than she used to. What other small things could she do to increase her daily physical activity?

2. You've just learned about several tools for effective weight management. Which tools do you see Maria using?

3. Do you have a regular exercise program? If not, what are some steps you can take to begin establishing one?

people set a goal of losing no more than 10 percent of their body weight at a rate of one-half to 2 pounds per week. This requires expending 300 to 500 more calories per day than you consume. Once you have lost 10 percent of your body weight, you should maintain that level for a few months. Then you can set a new weight-loss goal of 10 percent of this new, lower body weight, and so on.

WHY DON'T MOST DIETS SUCCEED?

Many people are convinced that dieting success depends on simply finding the right diet. They bounce from one highly publicized diet to another: low-fat, high carbohydrate; low carbohydrate, high protein and so on. Most experts tend to agree that any calorie-cutting diet can produce weight loss in the short-term, often through water-weight loss. But without improved nutrition and sustained exercise

---

weight cycling The pattern of repeatedly losing and gaining weight, from illness or dieting

rigid diets Weight-loss regimens that specify strict rules on calorie consumption, types of foods, and eating patterns

and activity, lost weight will return and the overall dieting process will have failed. Let's look more closely at the reasons why.

DIETS OFTEN LEAD TO WEIGHT CYCLING

Nearly three-quarters of dieters regain their weight within 2 years (or sooner) after a major diet. Most begin a process called **weight cycling**—a pattern of repeatedly losing and regaining weight.

Marketers of diet plans and foods often promise quick weight loss with no hunger and very little effort, but these usually backfire. People on rigid diets tend to have higher fat-to-lean ratios than people on more flexible plans based on energy balancing of calories eaten and burned.[35] The followers of rigid diets tend to exhibit more depression, anxiety, and binge eating as well. Taken alone, even prescription diet drugs don't work very well unless the patient also makes long-term changes in diet and exercise that produce a favorable energy balance.[36] Research reveals that four-fifths of dieters fail to both cut calories *and* increase exercise.[37] Three-quarters also eat too few fruits and vegetables despite their appetite-satisfying volume.

Rigid and flexible diets are distinctly different. **Rigid diets** specify rules like "eat only 1,200 Calories per day," or "eat only cabbage soup and grapefruit," or "never eat after 6:00 PM." Because rigid diets are unpleasant and restrictive, people seldom stick with them. **Flexible diets** focus on portion size and make allowances for variations in daily routine, appetite, and food availability. For example, if you go to a party and overeat, a flexible diet allows you to cut extra calories tomorrow and increase your exercise regimen to compensate. As a result, people tend to stay on flexible diets longer and in the process, learn better long-term eating habits.

Weight experts refer to a series of diets, each followed by eventual weight gain, as **yo-yo dieting.** Yo-yo dieting can have significant health consequences. As a person regains lost body fat and weight, blood lipids, blood pressure, and diabetes risk rise once again, and with them, the risk of heart disease and other serious illnesses.[38]

MANY DIET PRODUCTS AND PLANS ARE INEFFECTIVE

Dieting is a $30 billion annual industry. Most of the over-the-counter products—"fat burners," "starch blockers," muscle stimulators, diet supplements, weight-loss program memberships, meal replacements, and other diet aids—are ineffective, and some are even dangerous. For example, in 2004, the U.S. Food and Drug Administration banned the popular supplement ephedra (also called *ma huang*) after it caused heart attacks, seizures, and strokes in over 16,000 people and precipitated more than 100 deaths.

What about commercial diet plans and programs? One comprehensive study revealed that most of the best-known diet programs are only minimally effective. A 2005 study revealed that none of the nationally known programs—Weight Watchers, Jenny Craig, Optifast, eDiets.com, and Overeaters Anonymous—really deliver.[39] After 2 years, people who joined Weight Watchers had lost an average of just 6.4 pounds. Nearly half of those who took Optifast dropped out within 6 months, and those who continued did no better than people dieting at home on their own. Those on eDiets.com lost only about 1 percent of their body weight after a year.

Of the many consumer diet products and approaches, low-cost support groups are probably the best alternative for most people and do succeed in providing one very important component of every diet: encouragement and support, either in person, through weekly groups, or online. Campus health centers can usually help students find group support for dieting. It's also important to enlist the personal encouragement of friends, roommates, and family members. If people try tempting you with fattening

foods or undermine your diet efforts in other ways, tell them firmly that you need a different approach.

WHAT ARE EATING DISORDERS?

Skipping meals, going on diet after diet, and binging on junk food are all forms of **disordered eating:** atypical, abnormal food consumption that is very common in the general public and diminishes your wellness but is usually neither long-lived nor

flexible diets Weight-loss regimens that focus on portion size and make allowances for variations in daily routine, appetite, and food availability

yo-yo dieting A series of diets followed by eventual weight gain. Yo-yo dieting can lead to weight cycling.

disordered eating Atypical, abnormal food consumption that diminishes your wellness but is usually neither long-lived nor disruptive to everyday life

Eating disordered	Disruptive eating patterns	Food preoccupied/obsessed	Concerned well	Food is not an issue
• I regularly stuff myself and then exercise, vomit, use diet pills or laxatives to get rid of the food or calories. • My friends/family tell me I am too thin. • I am terrified of eating fat. • When I let myself eat, I have a hard time controlling the amount of food I eat. • I am afraid to eat in front of others.	• I have tried diet pills, laxatives, vomiting or extra time exercising in order to lose or maintain my weight. • I have fasted or avoided eating for long periods of time in order to lose or maintain my weight. • I feel strong when I can restrict how much I eat. • Eating more than I wanted to makes me feel out of control.	• I think about food a lot. • I feel I don't eat well most of the time. • It's hard for me to enjoy eating with others. • I feel ashamed when I eat more than others or more than what I feel I should be eating. • I am afraid of getting fat. • I wish I could change how much I want to eat and what I am hungry for.	• I pay attention to what I eat in order to maintain a healthy body. • I may weigh more than what I like, but I enjoy eating and balance my pleasure with eating with my concern for a healthy body. • I am moderate and flexible in goals for eating well. • I try to follow Dietary Guidelines for healthy eating.	• I am not concerned about what others think regarding what and how much I eat. • When I am upset or depressed I eat whatever I am hungry for without any guilt or shame. • Food is an important part of my life but only occupies a small part of my time.

Body hate/dissociation	Distorted body image	Body preoccupied/obsessed	Body Acceptance	Body ownership
• I often feel separated and distant from my body—as if it belongs to someone else. • I don't see anything positive or even neutral about my body shape and size. • I don't believe others when they tell me I look OK. • I hate the way I look in the mirror and often isolate myself from others.	• I spend a significant amount of time exercising and dieting to change my body. • My body shape and size keeps me from dating or finding someone who will treat me the way I want to be treated. • I have considered changing or have changed my body shape and size through surgical means so I can accept myself.	• I spend a significant time viewing my body in the mirror. • I spend a significant time comparing my body to others. • I have days when I feel fat. • I am preoccupied with my body. • I accept society's ideal body shape and size as the best body shape and size.	• I base my body image equally on social norms and my own self-concept. • I pay attention to my body and my appearance because it is important to me, but it only occupies a small part of my day. • I nourish my body so it has the strength and energy to achieve my physical goals.	• My body is beautiful to me. • My feelings about my body are not influenced by society's concept of an ideal body shape. • I know that the significant others in my life will always find me attractive.

FIGURE 9.5

The continuums of thought associated with healthy eating and positive body image to thoughts associated with disordered eating and poor body image. Adapted from Smiley/King/Avery: Campus Health Service. Original continuum, C. Schislak: *Preventive Medicine and Public Health.* Copyright 1997 Arizona Board of Regents. Used with permission.

disruptive to everyday life. Less common but still disturbingly prevalent are **eating disorders,** which are long-lasting, disturbed patterns of eating, dieting, and perceptions of body image that have psychological, environmental, and possibly genetic underpinnings. Eating disorders can disrupt relationships, emotions, and concentration, and can lead to physical injury, hospitalization, and even death. They require diagnosis and treatment from a psychiatrist or other physician.

Recognizing an eating disorder in yourself or a loved one can lead to treatment that improves or stops the spiral. The statements in Figure 9.5 can help you recognize when thoughts about food and body image verge from normal to abnormal and disordered. People with eating disorders often believe they look fat even when they are rail thin. This unrealistic and negative self-perception can be part of a

eating disorders Disturbed patterns of eating, dieting, and perceptions of body image that have psychological, environmental, and possibly genetic underpinnings, and that lead to consequent medical issues

related syndrome called **body dysmorphic disorder** (BDD), in which a person becomes obsessed with a physical "defect" such as nose size or body shape. It often requires a professional to sort out the symptoms of an eating disorder from BDD since a person can have either or both conditions.

The three common types of eating disorders are anorexia nervosa, bulimia nervosa, and binge eating disorder. About 10 million Americans—9 million of whom are young women—meet the criteria for one of these disorders.[40]

EATING DISORDERS HAVE DISTINCTIVE SYMPTOMS

Anorexia nervosa is a persistent, chronic eating disorder characterized by deliberate food restriction and severe, life-threatening weight loss. People with anorexia first restrict their intake of high-calorie foods, then of almost all foods and purge what they do eat through vomiting or using laxatives. They sometimes fast or exercise compulsively as well. The symptoms of anorexia include refusal to maintain a BMI of 18.5 or more; intense fear of gaining weight; disturbed body perception; and in teenage girls and women, amenorrhea (cessation of menstruation) for 3 months or more. Five to 20 percent of anorexics eventually die from medical conditions brought on by vitamin or mineral deficiencies or physiological results of starvation.

Bulimia nervosa is characterized by frequent bouts of binge eating, followed by purging (self-induced vomiting), laxative abuse, or excessive exercise. Bulimics tend to consume much more food than

most people would during a given time period and feel a loss of control over it. Binging and purging are often done secretly. A medical diagnosis includes binging and purging at least twice a week for 3 months. People with bulimia are also obsessed with their bodies, weight gain, and how they appear to others. Unlike those with anorexia, however, people with bulimia are often normal weight. Also, treatment appears to be more effective for bulimia than for anorexia.

Binge eating disorder (BED), a variation of bulimia, involves binge eating but usually no purging, laxatives, exercise, or fasting. Individuals with BED often wind up significantly overweight or obese but tend to binge much more often than does the typical obese person.

EATING DISORDERS CAN BE TREATED

Because eating disorders have complex physical, psychological, and social causes that unfold over many years, there are no quick or simple solutions for them. That said, eating disorders *are* treatable. The primary goal of treatment is usually to reduce the threat to the patient's life posed by his or her eating behaviors and the physical damage they can cause to the bones, teeth, throat, esophagus, stomach, intestines, heart, and other organs. Once the patient is stabilized medically, long-term therapy can begin. Oftentimes, the affected individual comes from a family that places undue emphasis on achievement, body weight, and appearance. Genetic susceptibility can also play a role.[41] Therapy involves family, friends, and other significant people in the individual's life and focuses on the psychological, social, environmental, and physiological factors that have contributed. Therapy is aimed at helping

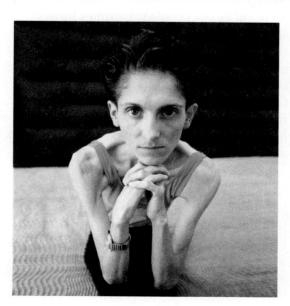

body dysmorphic disorder A psychological syndrome characterized by unrealistic and negative self-perception focusing on a physical defect such as nose size

anorexia nervosa A persistent, chronic eating disorder characterized by deliberate food restriction and severe, life-threatening weight loss

bulimia nervosa An eating disorder characterized by frequent bouts of binge eating followed by purging (self-induced vomiting), laxative abuse, or excessive exercise

binge eating disorder A variation of bulimia that involves binge eating but usually no purging, laxatives, exercise, or fasting

the patient develop new eating behaviors, build self-confidence, deal with depression, and find constructive ways of dealing with life's problems. Eating disorder support groups can be pivotal as well.

HOW CAN YOU CREATE A BEHAVIOR CHANGE PLAN FOR WEIGHT MANAGEMENT?

Let's look at the kinds of attitudes, decisions, and activities you can apply to creating a behavioral change plan for weight management.

CONTEMPLATE WEIGHT MANAGEMENT

The tools and tips in this chapter are designed for direct application in a personal plan. If you are part of the minority of students who are satisfied with your current weight, you can simply pursue and refine your application of good nutritional principles and regular exercise. If you are in the dissatisfied majority, you will need to assess your current weight and BMI using Figure 9.1 to determine whether you truly need to lose or gain weight. You will also need to choose a realistic weight goal based on no more than a 10 percent initial loss or gain. Even if you don't need weight change now, keep in mind that most normal-weight students will become overweight during the postcollege years. The specifics in this section are useful for weight change now or in the future, as well as for stabilizing your current weight and maintaining it for the next few decades.

PREPARE FOR BETTER WEIGHT MANAGEMENT

The steps of the behavioral change model we've discussed in every chapter apply equally well to weight change and weight management.

- **Beliefs and Attitudes** The concepts of self-efficacy and locus of control are central to successful weight management. Do you see yourself as a hopeless victim of "bad genes," overwork, and low budget, or perhaps as too young to worry about nutrition, exercise programs, or deliberate weight management? Or do you believe that you can take effective control of your body composition and weight largely through eating intelligently, limiting your calorie intake, and establishing a program of regular exercise? Talk with others to

CASE STUDY

Maria

"I've never had an eating disorder, but I admit that at times, I've been desperate enough to be tempted to binge and purge. There's so much pressure from all sides. You go to a family party and everyone tells you to eat, eat, eat. At the same time, all you see on TV are super-thin people. How can you please everyone—and yourself?

"Meanwhile, my daughter, Anna, is still very young, but I worry about the pressures she'll feel when she gets older. I hear so many stories about adolescents and high school students with eating disorders. Although I want to lose weight, I don't want Anna to get the message that being thin matters above everything else. There's a big difference between wanting to lose excess weight to become healthier, and feeling a need to lose weight when you are already at a healthy weight."

1. **What signs of eating disorders or disordered eating should Maria watch for as Anna gets older?**

2. **If you recognize symptoms of an eating disorder in yourself or a friend, how should you address the problem?**

clarify your own attitudes in preparation for making an effective weight management plan.

- **Consider Your Motivations** What is motivating you to change or maintain your weight? *Lab9.3* directs you to list and analyze your motivations. The best motivations are usually personal and extended, such as looking good, feeling fit and capable, and staying well over a period of years. People sometimes have very short-term goals that can lead to little more than weight cycling and yo-yo dieting. If one of your reasons is a specific upcoming event (spring break in Florida or a sports match, for example) try identifying some additional reasons with long time frames. Long-term goals help you see beyond poorly designed quick-fix diet remedies.

- **Barriers to Change** What keeps you from changing or maintaining your weight? Do you lack information about good weight management techniques? Do you have poor nutrition and eating habits? Eating triggers that set you off into overconsumption? Lack of social or emotional support? Lack of exercise? Preparing for weight change and management requires that you identify your own particular barriers and brainstorm solutions to them.

- **Visualizing New Behaviors** What specific new behaviors can you adopt that will allow you to change your BMI and body composition to within the recommended ranges? Here are some positive ones:

  Choosing only nutritious foods

  Avoiding foods filled with saturated fats, sweeteners, or sodium

  Tracking the numbers of servings you eat from each food group

  Tracking the calories you consume

  Planning for exercise most days of the week

  Keeping a log of your daily and weekly exercise

  Asking friends for support

  From this list, target one or a few behaviors, concentrate on them first, then move on to other behaviors later. Make a short priority list of the two or three most important behaviors.

- **Write Out Your Specific Goals** Lab 9.3 provides spaces for recording your body fat and body weight goals and the time frame for reaching them.

- **Commit to Your Goals** Behavior change requires commitment. Thinking and talking about your commitment with friends is helpful; so is writing it down and showing it to someone.

- **Set up Support** Solicit the help of people you can trust to support your efforts. Let's say it is 9:30 PM, you've finished studying, you're hungry, but you've already eaten the 1,800 calories on your day's food plan. You call a supportive friend and he or she might say, "Well, you can always have a diet soda and some raw vegetables to fill up. You'll be glad you stuck with your program. Just think, once you've lost weight, you can add back some extra calories each day—and that won't be so long from now!"

TAKE ACTION

Now that you have calculated your target weight and goals for daily calorie consumption and energy expenditure, set your plan in motion and keep track of the results. The box **Tools for Change: Tips for Weight Loss** provides some tips.

ACHIEVE WEIGHT MAINTENANCE

Weight management and weight change are very similar in principle. The tools are the same; your daily calorie goal for weight management will simply be isocaloric while your daily goal for weight loss or gain will have a negative or positive caloric balance. Some degree of calorie-tracking is usually involved in both maintenance and change, and a weekly weigh-in is important. If you have lost or gained 10 percent of your body weight, you will need to maintain that level for a few months before resuming more weight change. The skills you employ during an interim phase of weight maintenance will be excellent practice for the indefinite postchange period: translation, for the rest of your life. Once weight management skills become second nature and you've mastered good nutrition and daily exercise and activity, both change and maintenance become relatively easy for most people.

As for the termination stage, there *is* none for weight management. Maintaining recommended weight and BMI confer so many benefits upon your appearance, energy level, and overall wellness that once you master the needed skill set, you'll rarely miss the junk food you used to eat, nor will you miss the few minutes it will take each day to track energy consumed and expended. The rewards in lifelong wellness are fully worth the trade-off!

Try it NOW! Healthy substitutions at mealtime are the key to weight maintenance success! The next time you make dinner, look at the proportions on your plate. • Veggies and whole grains should take up most of the space; if not, substitute 1 cup of the meat, pasta, or cheese on your plate with 1 cup of legumes, salad greens, or a favorite vegetable. • You'll reduce the number of calories in your meal while eating the same amount of food!

TOOLS FOR CHANGE

TIPS FOR WEIGHT LOSS

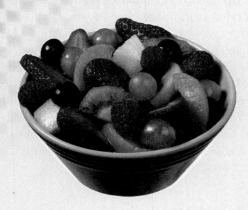

Try these ideas for reframing weight loss in your mind, rather than jumping right in to a diet regimen unprepared:

- Think substitution. Instead of cookies, pie, candy, cake, or ice cream at snack time, substitute fresh fruit. Instead of tortilla chips or French fries, substitute unbuttered popcorn, nuts, or vegetable sticks and low-fat dip.

- Consider yourself successful if you lose 1/2 to 1 pound per week. Faster weight loss stimulates too much hunger, slows metabolism, and loses lean tissue.

- Avoid feeling famished by choosing high-volume, nutrient-dense foods. Items such as clear soups, light salads, whole grains, fruits, vegetables, and beans fill you more quickly and control hunger, at least for a while.

- Avoid rigid dieting. Strictly limiting calorie counts or forbidding yourself certain foods can trigger binging and weight gain, not loss. Flexible dieting works better and emphasizes portion control and lower-calorie, higher-volume foods.

- Don't drink "empty" calories. Drinks sweetened with sugar or corn syrup contribute disproportionately to weight gain.[1] Alcoholic drinks pack a lot of calories and stimulate the appetite.

- Sleep well. Get 7 to 9 hours of sleep each night. Sleep deprivation triggers greater levels of hunger and eating.

- Join a support group. Support groups help most people lose at least a small amount of weight and keep it off.[2]

Sources:
1. G. A. Bray, S. J. Nielsen, and B. M. Popkin, "Consumption of High-Fructose Corn Syrup in Beverages May Play a Role in the Epidemic of Obesity," *American Journal of Clinical Nutrition* 79, no. 4 (April 2004): 537–43.
2. A. G. Tsai and T. A. Wadden, "Systematic Review: An Evaluation of Major Commercial Weight Loss Programs in the United States," *Annals of Internal Medicine* 142, no. 1 (January 2005): 56–66.

CHAPTER IN REVIEW

REVIEW QUESTIONS

1. At more than 20 percent above the recommended weight range for 5′8″ tall, a person is
   a. overweight.
   b. obese.
   c. ideal weight.
   d. at his/her set point.

2. A BMI of 16 in a woman indicates
   a. overweight.
   b. underweight.
   c. normal weight.
   d. obesity.

3. Getting up, walking around, and jiggling your feet when seated are all examples of
   a. energy conservation.
   b. appetite control.
   c. non-exercise activity.
   d. depression.

4. To lose weight, you must establish a(n)
   a. negative caloric balance.
   b. isocaloric balance.
   c. positive caloric balance.
   d. set point.

5. Which of these is not considered an eating disorder?
   a. Anorexia nervosa
   b. Bulimia nervosa
   c. Amenorrhea
   d. Binge eating disorder

6. Metabolic syndrome is characterized by all of the following except
   a. high blood cholesterol.
   b. high blood pressure.
   c. insulin resistance.
   d. small waist circumference.

7. The rate at which your body consumes food energy to sustain basic functions is your
   a. basal metabolic rate.
   b. resting metabolic rate.
   c. BMI.
   d. set point.

8. Successful weight maintainers are most likely to do which of the following?
   a. Indulge in junk food on weekends
   b. Skip meals
   c. Drink diet sodas
   d. Eat a nutritious diet that is low in fats, with high volume but low calorie density

9. Weight cycling is
   a. a pattern of repeatedly losing and regaining weight.
   b. characterized by rigid diets.
   c. characterized by flexible diets.
   d. uncommon.

10. Anorexia nervosa is characterized by
   a. frequent bouts of binge eating followed by self-induced vomiting.
   b. deliberate food restriction and severe, life-threatening weight loss.
   c. the use of laxatives.
   d. obesity.

CRITICAL THINKING QUESTIONS

1. How do height, physical build, and musculature affect recommended weight and BMI?

2. Discuss the chronic disease risks of obesity.

3. What do you see as the greatest contributor to "globesity"? Defend your answer.

ONLINE RESOURCES

Please visit this book's website at **www.aw-bc.com/hopson** to access links related to topics in this chapter.

REFERENCES

1. American College Health Association, "National College Health Assessment. Reference Group Executive Summary Fall 2006" (Baltimore: American College Health Association, 2007).

2. Charlotte A. Schoenborn and others, "Body Weight Status of Adults: United States, 1997–1998." Advance Data from *Vital and Health Statistics* no. 330 (September. 6, 2002).

3. University of Minnesota, Boynton Health Service, "First Ever Comprehensive Report on the Health of Minnesota College Students Looks at Mental Health, Obesity, Financial Health, Sexual Health and More," November 15, 2007.

4. University of New Hampshire, "College Students Face Obesity, High Blood Pressure, Metabolic Syndrome." *ScienceDaily* (June 18, 2007), www.sciencedaily.com.

5. See note 1.

6. World Health Organization, "Obesity and Overweight Factsheet," September 2006.

7. International Union of Nutritional Sciences, "The Global Challenge of Obesity and the International Obesity Task Force," September 2002, www.iuns.org/features/obesity/obesity.htm (accessed August 12, 2007).

8. "Preventing Childhood Obesity: Health in the Balance," Institute of Medicine, National Academies of Science, Washington, D.C., 2005.

9. Erica Goode, "The Gorge Yourself Environment," *New York Times* (July 3, 2003): D1.

10. B. Wamsink, J. E. Painter, and J. North, "Bottomless Bowls: Why Visual Cues of Portion Size May Influence Intake," *Obesity Research* 13, no. 1 (January 2005): 93–100.

11. G. Wamsink, "Environmental Factors that Increase the Food Intake and Consumption Volume of Unknowing Customers," *Annual Review of Nutrition* 24 (2004): 455–79.

12. G. Block and others, "Foods Contributing to Energy Intake in the U.S.: Data from NHANES III and NHANES 1999–2000," *Journal of Food Chemistry and Analysis* 17 (June 2004): 439–47.

13. S. A. French, "Public Health Strategies for Dietary Change: Schools and Workplaces," *Journal of Nutrition* 135, no. 4 (April 2005): 91–92.

14. M. Papas and others, "The Built Environment and Obesity," *Epidemiological Reviews* 29, no. 1 (2007): 129–43. Also M. Rao and others, "The Built Environment and Health," *The Lancet* 370, no, 9593 (2007): 1111–13; and E. M. Berke and others, "Association of the Built Environment with Physical Activity and Obesity in Older Persons," *American Journal of Public Health* (2007).

15. I. S. Farooqi and S. O'Rahilly, "Genetic Factors in Human Obesity," *Obesity Reviews* 8, Suppl 1 (2007): 37–40. Also University of Cambridge, "New Insight into the Link Between Genetics and Obesity," *Science Daily*, www.sciencedaily.com.

16. James A. Levine and others, "Interindividual Variation in Posture Allocation: Possible Role in Human Obesity," *Science* 307, no. 4 (January 28, 2005): 584–86.

17. Centers for Disease Control and Prevention: U.S. Physical Activity Statistics, "1988–2005 No Leisure-Time Physical Activity Trend Chart," www.cdc.gov/nccdphp/ dnpa/physical/stats/leisure_time .htm (accessed August 12, 2007).

18. Walter Willett, *Eat, Drink, and Be Healthy: The Harvard Medical School Guide to Healthy Eating* (New York: Free Press, 2003), 35.

19. American Heart Association, "Abdominal Fat Distribution Predicts Heart Disease, Study Shows," *ScienceDaily* (December 11, 2007), www.sciencedaily.com.

20. Charles Mann, "Provocative Study Says Obesity May Reduce U.S. Life Expectancy," *Science* 307 (March 18, 2005): 1717.

21. S. J. Olshansky and others, "A Potential Decline in Life Expectancy in the United States in the 21st Century," *New England Journal of Medicine* 352, no. 11 (March 17, 2005): 1135–37.

22. Katherine Flegal and others, "Excess Deaths Associated with Underweight, Overweight, and Obesity," *Journal of the American Medical Association* 293, no. 15 (April 20, 2005) 1861–67.

23. Y. Takata and others, "Association Between Body Mass Index and Mortality in an 80-Year-Old Population," *Journal of the American Geriatric Society* 55, no. 6 (2007): 913–17.

24. Luigi Fontana and others, "Long-Term Calorie Restriction Is Highly Effective in Reducing the Risk for Atherosclerosis in Humans," *Proceedings of the National Academy of Sciences,* 101, no. 17 (April 27, 2004): 6659–63.

25. Carol O'Neil and Theresa Nicklas, "State of the Art Reviews: Relationship Between Diet/ Physical Activity and Health," *American Journal of Lifestyle Medicine,* Vol.1 (December 2007): 457–81.

26. Eugenia Calle and others, "Overweight, Obesity, and Mortality from Cancer in a Prospectively Studied Cohort of U.S. Adults," *New England Journal of Medicine* 348 (April 24, 2003): 1625–38.

27. Stuart P. Weisberg, "Obesity Is Associated with Macrophage Accumulation in Adipose Tissue," *Journal of Clinical Investigation* 112 (2003): 1796–1808.

28. USDA, "Popular Weight Loss Diets," U.S. Department of Agriculture White Paper (January 10, 2001).

29. Mayo Clinic, "Lose a Little: It Helps a Lot," Mayo Clinic, Consumer Health Tips and Products (January 6, 2005). www.mayoclinic.org.

30. M. A. Pelleymounter and others, "Effects of the Obese Gene Product on Body Weight Regulation in Ob/Ob Mice," *Science* 269, no. 5223 (July 28, 1995): 540–43.

31. P. A. Mole, "Exercise Reverses Depressed Metabolic Rate Produced by Severe Caloric Restriction," *Medical Science and Sports Exercise* 21, no. 1 (February 1989): 29–33. Also P. A. Mole, "Impact of Energy Intake and Exercise on Resting Metabolic Rate," *Sports Medicine* 10, no. 2 (August 1991): 72–87.

32. R. R. Wing and S. Phelan, "Long-Term Weight Loss Maintenance," *American Journal of Clinical Nutrition* 82, no. 1 (July 2005): 222S–25S.

33. K. Elfhag and S. Rossner, "Who Succeeds in Maintaining Weight Loss?" *Obesity Review* 6, no. 1 (February 2005): 67–85.

34. Ibid.

35. C. F. Smith and others, "Flexible versus Rigid Dieting Strategies: Relationship with Adverse Behavioral Outcomes," *Appetite* 32, no. 3 (June 1999): 295–305.

36. S. B. Moyers, "Medications as Adjunct Therapy for Weight Loss: Approved and Off-label Agents in Use," *Journal of the American Dietetic Association,* 105, no. 6 (June 2005): 948–59.

37. J. Kruger and others, "Weight Specific Practices Among U.S. Adults," *American Journal of Preventative Medicine* 26, no. 5 (June 2004): 402–6. Also J. Kruger and others, "Attempting to Lose Weight: Specific Practices Among U.S. Adults," *American Journal of Preventative Medicine* 26, no. 5 (January 2004): 402–6.

38. M. Schulz and others, "Weight Cycling and Hypertension," *Current Hypertension Reports* 7 (2005): 9–10.

39. A. Tsai and T. Wadden, "Systematic Review: An Evaluation of Major Commercial Weight Loss Programs in the U.S.," *Annals of Internal Medicine* 142, no. 1 (January 4, 2005): 56–66.

40. Sutter Health, "Eating Disorders," April 1, 2003.

41. R. Bachner-Melman and others, "Association Between a Vasopressin Receptor AVPR1A Promoter Region Microsatellite and Eating Behavior Measured by a Self-Report Questionnaire (Eating Attitudes Test) in a Family-Based Study of a Non-Clinical Population," *International Journal of Eating Disorders* 36, no. 4 (December 2004): 451–60.

Name:_____ Date: _____

Instructor: _____ Section: _____

Materials: Calculator, access to Internet (optional)

Purpose: To learn how to calculate energy balance and set realistic goals for calorie intake and energy expenditure.

Directions: Complete the following sections.

SECTION I: CALCULATING BMR AND ENERGY EXPENDITURE

Your **basal metabolic rate (BMR)** is the rate at which you burn calories to sustain life functions at rest at a normal room temperature. Your activities, fitness level, stress level, and many other things will affect your BMR.

1. **Calculate your BMR (the method shown here uses the Harris-Benedict formula):**

Men

(1) BMR = 66 + (6.3 × weight in pounds) + (12.9 × height in inches) − (6.8 × age in years)

(2) BMR = 66 + (   ) + (   ) − (   )

(3) BMR = _____ Calories (Cal)

Women

(1) BMR = 655 + (4.3 × weight in pounds) + (4.7 × height in inches) − (4.7 × age in years)

(2) BMR = 655 + (   ) + (   ) − (   )

(3) BMR = _____ Calories (Cal)

2. **Estimate your total energy expenditure (EE):**

Total energy expenditure takes into account your amount of activity within a 24-hour period. You can calculate your energy expenditure by keeping an activity log and adding up the calories expended during any nonsleep time. To do this, use the physical activity tracking tool on the MyPyramid website (www.mypyramidtracker.gov/). Another way to estimate total energy expenditure is to use the following calculations. Choose your level of activity on *average* and use that formula to calculate your energy expenditure (EE).

Multiply your BMR by the appropriate activity factor, completing ONE equation below:

- If you are **sedentary** (little or no exercise):

  EE = _____(BMR) × **1.2** = _____ Calories (Cal)

- If you are **lightly active** (light exercise/sports 1–3 days/week):

  EE = _____(BMR) × **1.375** = _____ Calories (Cal)

- If you are **moderately active** (moderate exercise/sports 3–5 days/week):

  EE = _____(BMR) × **1.55** = _____ Calories (Cal)

- If you are **very active** (hard exercise/sports 6–7 days/week):

  EE = _____(BMR) × **1.725** = _____ Calories (Cal)

- If you are **extra active** (very hard daily exercise/sports & physical job or 2×day training):

  EE = _____(BMR) × **1.9** = _____ Calories (Cal)

SECTION II: CALCULATING ENERGY BALANCE

1. Estimated **calorie INTAKE**

_____ Calories (Cal)

2. Estimated **calorie EXPENDITURE** (EE from Section I)

_____ Calories (Cal)

3. Subtract your EXPENDITURE (#2) from your INTAKE (#1) to get:

Out of balance calories = _____ Calories (Cal)

SECTION III: TOOLS FOR YOUR WEIGHT MANAGEMENT PLAN

1. What was your caloric intake from your dietary analysis? _____ What was your energy expenditure? _____ What was your overall energy balance?_____

- **Energy balance** (+/− 200 Cal): You are supplying your body with its energy needs and maintaining current weight.
- **Negative energy balance** (−201 Cal): You are expending more energy than you are eating and should be losing weight.
- **Positive energy balance** (+201 Cal): You are eating more energy than you are expending and should be gaining weight.

2. Do you want or need to lose body fat? **YES or NO**

3. What is your **goal** for your body fat percentage? _____

4. Complete the following calculations to figure out how many **pounds of fat** you need to lose in order to reach this goal:

- Find your **current fat weight:**

  _____ (current weight, lb) × _____ (current % body fat, expressed as a decimal) = _____ current fat weight (lb)

- Find your **lean body mass**

  (LBM): _____ (weight, lb) − _____ (fat weight, lb) = _____ LBM (lb)

- Find your **target body weight:**

  _____ (LBM) ÷ (1 − goal % body fat expressed as a decimal) = _____ target body weight (lb)

- Find the **lb of fat loss** needed to reach your body fat percentage goal:

  _____ (current weight, lb) − _____ (target weight, lb) = _____ fat loss needed (lb)

5. If you lose 1 pound of fat per week (500 Cal deficits per day), how many weeks will it take you to lose your desired fat weight? _____

6. Brainstorm ways that you can get to a −500 Calorie deficit per day through diet and exercise/activity changes.

DIET CHANGE (−250 Cal)   ACTIVITY CHANGE (−250 Cal)

_____   _____

_____   _____

_____   _____

_____   _____

_____   _____

Name:_____ Date: _____

Instructor: _____ Section: _____

Purpose: To encourage students to think critically about their dieting history, ways of controlling food consumption, and readiness for weight changes.

Directions: Complete the following sections to analyze your dieting patterns.

SECTION I: DIET HISTORY

1. **How many times have you been on a diet?**

0 times	1–3 times	4–10 times	11–20 times	more than 20

2. **How much weight did you lose?**

0 lb.	1–5 lb.	6–10 lb.	11–20 lb.	more than 20 lb.

3. **How long did you stay at the new lower weight?**

Under 1 mo.	2–3 mos.	4–6 mos.	6 to 12 mos.	Over 1 yr.

4. **Put a check mark by each dieting method you have tried:**

_____skipping breakfast _____skipping lunch or dinner
_____cutting out all snacks _____counting calories
_____cutting out most fats _____cutting out most carbohydrates
_____increasing regular exercise _____taking "weight loss" supplements
_____taking appetite suppressants _____using meal replacements such as Slim Fast
_____taking laxatives _____inducing vomiting
_____taking prescription appetite suppressants
_____other _____

SECTION II: READINESS TO START A WEIGHT-LOSS PROGRAM

If you are thinking about starting a weight-loss program, answer questions A–F:
   A. **How motivated are you to lose weight?**

1	2	3	4	5
Not at all motivated	Slightly motivated	Somewhat motivated	Quite motivated	Extremely motivated

   B. **How certain are you that you will stay committed to a weight-loss program long enough to reach your goal?**

1	2	3	4	5
Not at all certain	Slightly certain	Somewhat certain	Quite certain	Extremely certain

C. Taking into account other stresses in your life (school, work, and relationships), to what extent can you tolerate the effort required to stick to your diet plan?

1	2	3	4	5
Cannot tolerate	Can tolerate somewhat	Uncertain	Can tolerate well	Can tolerate easily

D. Assuming you should lose no more than 1 to 2 pounds per week, have you allotted a realistic amount of time for weight loss?

1	2	3	4	5
Very unrealistic	Somewhat unrealistic	Moderately realistic	Somewhat realistic	Realistic

E. While dieting, do you fantasize about eating your favorite foods?

1	2	3	4	5
Always	Frequently	Occasionally	Rarely	Never

F. While dieting, do you feel deprived, angry, upset?

1	2	3	4	5
Always	Frequently	Occasionally	Rarely	Never

Total your scores from questions A–F, circle your score category, and answer any questions below:
6 to 16: This may not be a good time for you to start a diet. Inadequate motivation and commitment and unrealistic goals could block your progress. Think about what contributes to your unreadiness. What are some of the factors? Consider changing these factors before undertaking a diet. How could you alter the most important ones?

17 to 23: You may be nearly ready to begin a program but should think about ways to boost your readiness. Regardless of readiness level, what are a few additional things you could do at this time to prepare?
24 to 30: The path is clear—you can decide how to lose weight in a safe, effective way.
Section II Comments:

SECTION III: HUNGER, APPETITE, AND EATING

Think about your hunger and the cues that stimulate your appetite or eating, and then answer parts A–C.

A. When food comes up in conversation or in something you read, do you want to eat, even if you are not hungry?

1	2	3	4	5
Never	Rarely	Occasionally	Frequently	Always

B. How often do you eat for a reason other than physical hunger?

1	2	3	4	5
Never	Rarely	Occasionally	Frequently	Always

C. When your favorite foods are around the house, do you succumb to eating them?

1	2	3	4	5
Never	Rarely	Occasionally	Frequently	Always

Total your scores from questions A–C, circle your score category, and answer any questions below:

3 to 6: You might occasionally eat more than you should, but it is due more to your own attitudes than to temptation and other environmental cues. Controlling your own attitudes toward hunger and eating may help you. What are some of these attitudes, and how could you control or change them?

7 to 9: You may have a moderate tendency to eat just because food is available. Losing weight may be easier for you if you try to resist external cues and eat only when you are physically hungry. What are some ways you could better resist external cues?

10 to 15: Some or much of your eating may be in response to thinking about food or exposing yourself to temptations to eat. Think of ways to minimize your exposure to temptations so you eat only in response to physical hunger.

Section III Comments:

SECTION IV: CONTROLLING EATING

How good are you at controlling overeating when you are on a diet? Answer parts A–C.

A. A friend talks you into going out to a restaurant for a midday meal instead of eating a brown-bag lunch. As a result, you:

1	2	3	4	5
Would eat much less	Would eat somewhat less	Would make no difference	Would eat somewhat more	Would eat much more

B. You "break" your diet by eating a fattening, "forbidden" food. As a result, for the day, you:

1	2	3	4	5
Would eat much less	Would eat somewhat less	Would make no difference	Would eat somewhat more	Would eat much more

C. You have been following your diet faithfully and decide to test yourself by taking a bite of something you consider a treat. As a result, for the day, you:

1	2	3	4	5
Would eat much less	Would eat somewhat less	Would make no difference	Would eat somewhat more	Would eat much more

Sum your scores from questions A–C, circle your score category, and answer any questions below:

3 to 7: You recover rapidly from mistakes. However, if you frequently alternate between out-of-control eating and very strict dieting, you may have a serious eating problem and should get professional help. Does that kind of alternation describe your pattern? If so, where on your college campus could you turn for professional guidance?

8 to 11: You do not seem to let unplanned eating disrupt your program. This is a flexible, balanced approach. Do "flexible" and "balanced" describe your dieting? How could you achieve even more flexibility and balance?

12 to 15: You may be prone to overeating after an event breaks your control or throws you off track. Your reaction to these problem-causing events could use improvement. What are some ways you could try to more effectively control an overeating reaction?

Section IV Comments:

SECTION V: REFLECTION

1. Were your previous dieting patterns successful? Why or why not? Was it hard to be consistent with these dieting methods?

2. Which dieting methods were challenging or did not work for you at all? Why were these methods more difficult? What would be the ideal dieting method for you?

Adapted from: "The Diet Readiness Test," in Kelly D. Brownell, "When and How to Diet," Psychology Today (June 1989) 41–46. Reprinted with permission from Psychology Today Magazine, copyright © 1989 (Sussex Publishers, Inc.).

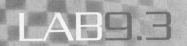

Name:_____   **Date:**_____

Instructor:_____   **Section:**_____

Materials: None

Purpose: To create an appropriate weight management goal, you must apply behavior change tools and make a plan to implement your goals.

Directions: Complete the following sections.

SECTION I: SHORT- AND LONG-TERM GOALS

1. Short-Term Goals

- My 3-month *or* 6-month (circle one) % body fat goal is _____.
- My 3-month *or* 6-month (circle one) weight goal is _____lb.
- My 3-month *or* 6-month (circle one) BMI goal is _____ kg/m².

2. Long-Term Goals

a. Based on my current weight, BMI, % body fat, and the tools gained in Lab 9.2:

- My 1-year % body fat goal is _____.
- My 1-year weight goal is _____lb.
- My 1-year BMI goal is _____ kg/m².

b. I plan to reach that goal by consuming about _____ Calories per day and adding _____ activity Calories per day.

SECTION II: DIET OBSTACLES AND STRATEGIES

1. Negative Food and Eating Triggers

Eating and food preferences can be triggered by emotions, social situations, and the sights and smells around you.

a. Fill out the following table exploring your negative food and eating triggers. For example, a situational trigger for you eating sugary foods may be "attending holiday parties."

Diet Behavior	Emotional Triggers	Social Triggers	Situational Triggers
Eating More Food			
Eating Late at Night			
Eating More Often			
Eating Sugary Foods			
Eating Fatty Foods			
Eating Fast Foods			
Eating Out			
Others:			

b. List three strategies to overcome or manage your food and eating triggers:

(1) _____

(2) _____

(3) _____

2. **Changing Food Patterns**

a. I need to eat LESS of the following foods and beverages:

_____

_____

b. For good nutrition and weight management goals, I will replace the above foods and beverages with the following that I need to get more of:

_____

_____

SECTION III: EXERCISE AND ACTIVITY OBSTACLES AND STRATEGIES

1. **Reducing Sedentary Behaviors**

a. Evaluate your sedentary activities in the space below. Not including time spent in class, list your top three sedentary activities, number of days per week you do them, and how many minutes per day.

	Sedentary Activity	Days/wk	Min/day
1			
2			
3			

b. Which sedentary activity could you replace with physical activity or even supplement with physical activity (such as exercising while you watch TV, or stretching while on your cell phone, etc.)? Write down three ideas for replacing sedentary activities with more active ones.

(1) _____

(2) _____

(3) _____

2. List a few of the obstacles to replacing sedentary activity with more energy-intensive physical activity, along with strategies for overcoming these obstacles:

Activity Obstacle	Strategy to Overcome
(1) _____	_____
(2) _____	_____
(3) _____	_____

SECTION IV: GETTING SUPPORT

1. **I feel supported in my weight goals by these people:**

_____

Here's what they do that assists me:

_____

2. I need additional support from these people:

_____

Here's what I need to ask for:

_____

3. **If I need group or medical support,** here are a few places to seek it: student health service, family physician, local hospital, local Weight Watchers chapter, online groups. If needed, I would be inclined to use

_____ for support.

SECTION V: REWARDS

1. When I make the **short-term** behavior change described above, my reward will be:

_____

Target date _____

2. When I make the **long-term** behavior change described above, my reward will be:

_____

Target date _____

CHAPTER 10

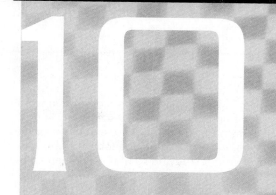

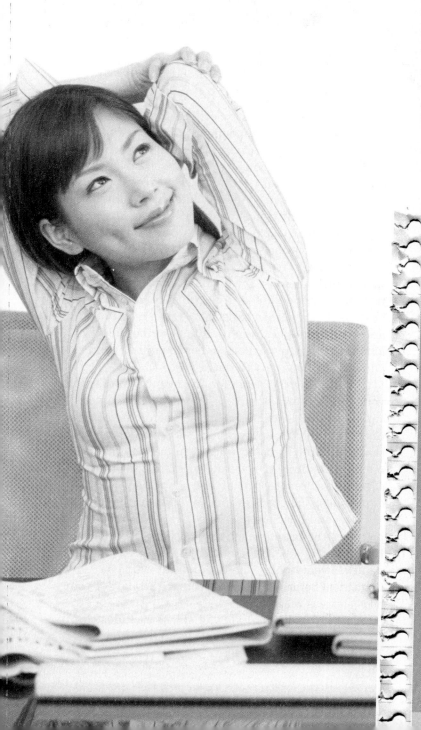

Managing Stress

OBJECTIVES

Understand how your body responds to stress.

Identify common sources of stress.

Describe effective tools for stress management.

Create your own stress management plan.

CASE STUDY

Cory

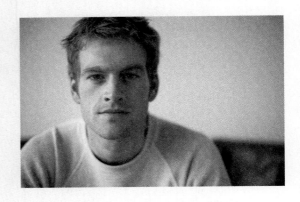

"Hi, I'm Cory. I'm a junior, majoring in biology. I'm from Denver, Colorado and just transferred schools in August to be closer to my dad, who lives alone and has diabetes. I take five classes, work part-time as a lab assistant, and I'm up late every night studying so that I can keep up my grades for applying to medical school. I've always felt like I was pretty good at working under pressure, but I have to admit, these past few months have been rough—I am constantly worn out, worried sick about my dad, and can hardly stay awake in class sometimes. I know that medical school will be even harder, so maybe I should just get used to living like this! But, man, I am so tired of being tired."

Everyone feels stress at least some of the time, be it from traffic, crowding, competition for schools and jobs, fast-changing technology, and/or a hectic pace that seems to accelerate yearly. Often we do not even realize how great our stress levels have become. Over time, however, stress can diminish not just our enjoyment of life, but our health and well-being, too. Thus, learning effective stress-management techniques is an important part of any complete wellness program.

This chapter explains the stress response, details the ways accumulated stress can affect your health, and proposes several helpful strategies you can use to counteract stress. Using the stress-management tools you'll discover in this chapter, you can better face the pressures of college life and beyond.

stress A term used to describe a physical, social, or psychological event or circumstance that disturbs the body's "normal" state and to which the body must try to adapt. Also used to describe the disturbed physical or emotional state experienced as a result of such events/circumstances.

stressor A physical, social, or psychological event or circumstance to which the body tries to adapt; stressors are often threatening, unfamiliar, disturbing, or exciting

stress response A set of physical and emotional reactions initiated by your body in response to a stressor

WHAT IS STRESS?

In a recent national survey, college students reported stress as the biggest impediment to their academic success, with a greater impact on achievement than colds, flu, sleep difficulty, relationship issues, and all other concerns.[1] But what, exactly *is* stress?

Stress is a term that is commonly used in many different ways. It is used to describe a *causative* physical, social, or psychological event (such as a threat, aggravation, or excitement) that disturbs an individual's "normal" physiological state and to which the body must try to adapt. Stress is also used to describe the disturbed physical and emotional state that a person experiences as a *result* of such an event.[2] Stress is even used to describe the *anticipation* of any event, real or imagined, that a person perceives as a threat.[3]

A more accurate term for any event that disrupts your body's "normal" state is **stressor.** A stressor can be physical, such as an angry roommate or an uncomfortably heavy backpack. It can also be emotional, like the fear and worry you feel before a major exam. A more accurate term for the physical *effect* of a stressor is the **stress response:** the set of physiological changes initiated by your body's nervous and hormonal signals. The stress response prepares the brain, heart, muscles, and other organs to respond to a perceived threat or demand. The dry mouth, sweaty palms, and pounding heart you might feel before giving a speech are all part of your body's stress response.

A more traditional view of stress includes the concepts of both positive stress and negative stress. Positive stress, or **eustress,** presents an opportunity for personal growth, satisfaction, and enhanced well-being. Eustress can invigorate us and motivate us to work harder and achieve more. Entering college, starting a new job, and developing a new relationship are all challenges that can produce eustress. Negative stress, or **distress,** can result from a buildup of negative stressors such as academic pressures, relationship discord, or money problems. It can even result from an overload of positive stressors such as getting married, moving to a new state, and starting a new job all in the same week. Distress can reduce wellness by promoting cardiovascular disease, impairing immunity, or causing mental and emotional dysfunction.

HOW DOES YOUR BODY RESPOND TO STRESS?

You file into the lecture hall to take your hardest midterm, sit down in an aisle seat, and teaching assistants start passing out the exam papers. As you take one and pass the pile to your right, you realize your heart is pounding, your breathing has quickened, your hands are sweating, you have "butterflies" in your stomach, and you feel a sense of dread. You are experiencing a stress response: a reaction involving nervous and hormonal activities that prepare both body and mind to deal with the disturbance to your normal state.

THE STRESS RESPONSE

Here's a simplified version of what happens during the seconds that the body initiates a stress response and in the minutes and hours as the response continues (Figure 10.1):

1. Your senses perceive and your brain interprets something as a threat; for example, the arrival of a test that will determine half your grade.

2. The threat triggers a region of your brain called the *hypothalamus* to release a hormone that in turn triggers your pituitary gland to secrete **adrenocorticotropic hormone** (ACTH) into your blood.

3. ACTH travels through the bloodstream and reaches the outer zone of each adrenal gland (located on top of each kidney). ACTH causes the adrenal glands to secrete **cortisol,** your body's main stress hormone.

At the same time, nerve signals from your brain and spinal cord reach and stimulate the central zone of each adrenal gland. Both adrenals respond by releasing **epinephrine** (also called *adrenalin*) and **norepinephrine,** two additional stress hormones that ready the body for quick action.

4. Traveling inside the bloodstream, cortisol reaches specific *target cells* within the body fat and within several organs, including the liver and intestines. Cortisol quickly triggers target cells to convert stored fat, protein, and carbohydrate molecules into glucose. Soon, more glucose is circulating in the blood, supplying the whole body—especially the brain and skeletal muscles—with the extra energy needed to respond to the stressor.

5. The epinephrine and norepinephrine released into the blood rapidly reach target cells in the heart, lungs, stomach, intestines, sense organs, and muscles. Along with signals from sympathetic nerves, these additional stress hormones ready the vital organs in ways that promote survival: fleeing from or confronting the threat. This physiological reaction is called the **fight-or-flight response.**

If you have ever jammed on the brakes to avoid an accident, you have probably felt a jolt of

---

eustress Stress based on positive circumstances or events; can present an opportunity for personal growth

distress Stress based on negative circumstances or events, or those perceived as negative; can diminish wellness

adrenocorticotropic hormone A hormone secreted by the pituitary gland that causes adrenal glands to secrete cortisol

cortisol Your body's main stress hormone, secreted by the cortex or outer layer of the adrenal glands located on top of the kidneys. Stimulates the sympathetic nervous system; can also damage or destroy neurons

epinephrine Also called *adrenaline;* one of two stress hormones released by adrenal glands that readies your body for quick action by stimulating sympathetic nerves

norepinephrine One of two stress hormones secreted by adrenal glands that readies your body for quick action by increasing arousal

fight-or-flight response A physiological reaction induced by nervous and hormonal signals that readies the heart, lungs, brain, muscles, and other vital organs and systems in ways that promote survival: fleeing from or confronting a threat

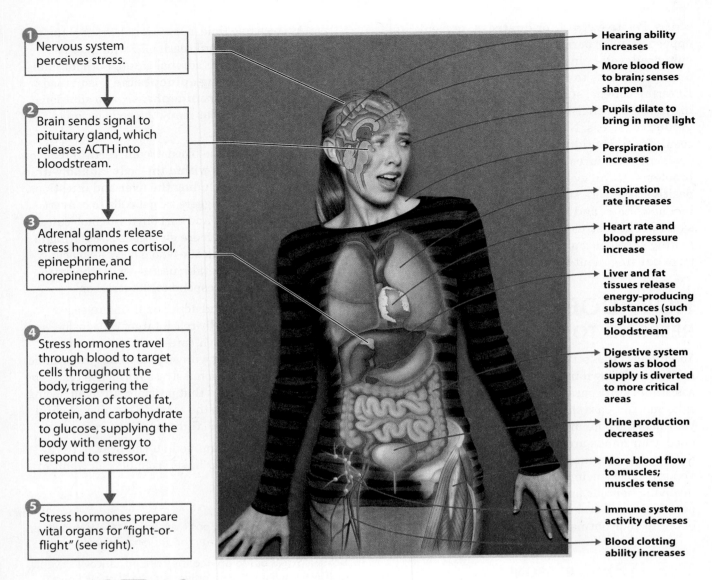

1. Nervous system perceives stress.

2. Brain sends signal to pituitary gland, which releases ACTH into bloodstream.

3. Adrenal glands release stress hormones cortisol, epinephrine, and norepinephrine.

4. Stress hormones travel through blood to target cells throughout the body, triggering the conversion of stored fat, protein, and carbohydrate to glucose, supplying the body with energy to respond to stressor.

5. Stress hormones prepare vital organs for "fight-or-flight" (see right).

Hearing ability increases

More blood flow to brain; senses sharpen

Pupils dilate to bring in more light

Perspiration increases

Respiration rate increases

Heart rate and blood pressure increase

Liver and fat tissues release energy-producing substances (such as glucose) into bloodstream

Digestive system slows as blood supply is diverted to more critical areas

Urine production decreases

More blood flow to muscles; muscles tense

Immune system activity decreses

Blood clotting ability increases

FIGURE 10.1
The stress response.

epinephrine. As part of the fight-or-flight response, your pupils dilate, enabling you to see more clearly. The air passages in your lungs also dilate, allowing more oxygen to enter. Your heart beats faster and pumps more blood to your muscles and brain. Your sweat glands release more sweat, and blood is directed away from your hands and feet toward your large muscles and body core; this can make your hands feel cold and clammy. Your digestive action slows or stops, and your bladder function slows, since neither process is crucial to short-term survival. Primed in all these ways, your body is ready to handle the stressor. Confronted by a car speeding toward you, your fight-or-flight response could save your life. Faced with financial hardship or excessive work pressures for years on end, your stress response can become chronic and start to harm your health.

After a perceived stressor subsides, your nervous system returns the body to its "normal" state with slower heartbeats, normal breathing rate, normal digestion, and so on. The stress-reduction techniques you will learn later deliberately encourage the body's return to this more relaxed state.

WHY DOES STRESS CAUSE HARM?

Why is chronic stress harmful? Two insightful models help explain how sustained stress can cause damage over time.

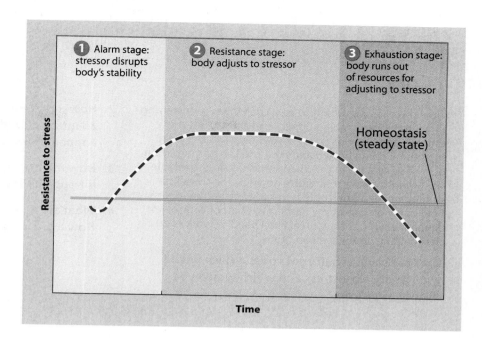

Homeostasis (steady state)

Resistance to stress

Time

FIGURE 10.2

Hans Seyle's general adaptation syndrome.

THE GENERAL ADAPTATION SYNDROME

In the 1930s, biologist Hans Selye studied the response of laboratory rats to painful physical or emotional stressors. He discovered that a wide variety of stressors—such as extreme heat, extreme cold, forced exercise, or surgery—all seemed to provoke the same general set of changes in the rats' bodies. Selye proposed a model he called the **general adaptation syndrome (GAS),** based on the reactions of the rats he observed.

Central to Seyle's GAS model is the idea that stress disrupts the body's stable internal environment, or *steady state*. Physiological mechanisms work to keep internal conditions (such as body temperature, blood-oxygen content, blood pH, and blood sugar levels) within certain "normal" ranges. Life scientists use the term **homeostasis** to describe the body's steady state. Seyle's general adaptation syndrome characterizes the stages of the body's response to stress as follows:

1. In the *alarm stage,* a stressor disrupts the steady state and triggers a *fight-or-flight response.* The body starts adapting to the stressor, but the effort can lower one's resistance to injury or disease (see Figure 10.2).[4]

2. In the *resistance stage,* a person's physiology and behavior adjusts, and resistance builds to the stressor. The body establishes a new level of homeostasis, despite the continued presence of the stressor.

3. In the hypothetical *exhaustion stage,* the body runs out of resources to successfully adapt to the stressor, resulting in physiological harm in the form of reduced immunity and increased susceptibility to physical or mental illness.

The general adaptation syndrome recognized that sustained stress can take a toll on wellness. However, scientists have since modified Seyle's concept of an "exhaustion stage" and the idea that illness results from running out of resources to adapt to a stressor. Rather, they now believe that over time, the stress response *itself* can damage the body and increase one's risk of developing illness, as we will examine in the next section.

ALLOSTATIC LOAD

Today's stress researchers use the term **allostasis** to describe the many simultaneous changes that

general adaptation syndrome (GAS) A historical model proposed by Hans Selye attempting to explain the body's stress response, consisting of alarm, resistance, and exhaustion stages

homeostasis A state of physiological equilibrium wherein various physiological mechanisms maintain internal conditions (such as pH, salt concentration, and temperature) within certain viable ranges

allostasis The many simultaneous changes that occur in the body to maintain homeostasis

CASE STUDY

Cory

"I knew this year was going to be a challenge—transferring to a new school and taking upper-level classes. But the first month actually went okay. I liked my classes, my dad seemed to be doing better, and I got used to getting by on 5 hours of sleep each night. Then sometime in the middle of fall, I caught a cold that didn't go away for 4 weeks! I was coughing all night, could barely pay attention in class, and did badly on one of my midterms. That, of course, just made me feel worse. Now I feel like I need to work even harder to make up for the bad grade."

1. List Cory's main sources of stress. Which would you classify as *eustress* and which would you classify as *distress*?

2. How might Hans Seyle have used general adaptation syndrome to explain what is happening with Cory?

3. How might the allostatic load model explain what is happening with Cory?

4. What are your own major sources of stress? How are you dealing with them?

---

occur in the body to maintain homeostasis, and they use the term **allostatic load** to refer to the long-term wear and tear on the body that is caused by prolonged allostasis.[5]

Allostatic load can result if your body's ability to shut off the stress response (after a stressor has disappeared) is impaired, allowing high levels of stress hormones to remain in the bloodstream. It can also develop when your body releases too *few* stress hormones and cannot mount an adequate stress response.[6] And it can build up if you experience a sustained string of stressful events over a long period of time. A classic example of a consequence of allostatic load is the development of stress-induced high blood pressure (hypertension.) As you will see shortly, chronically high blood pressure can damage arteries and increase one's risk of developing cardiovascular disease.[7]

A person's behavior and choices can also result in allostatic load. For example, some people respond to stress by exercising more, meditating, getting extra sleep, and avoiding drugs and alcohol. Others respond by exercising less, staying up late, drinking more, or starting smoking or taking drugs. Such counterproductive measures can result in allostatic load and increase one's susceptibility to developing illness.

allostatic load The long-term wear and tear on the body that is caused by prolonged allostasis

WHAT KINDS OF HARM CAN STRESS CAUSE?

Studies indicate that 40 percent of deaths and 70 percent of disease in the United States are related, in whole or in part, to stress.[8] The list of ailments related to chronic stress includes heart disease, diabetes, cancer, headaches, ulcers, low back pain, depression, and the common cold.

STRESS AND CARDIOVASCULAR DISEASE RISKS

Perhaps the most studied and documented health consequence of unresolved stress is cardiovascular disease (CVD). Research on this topic has demonstrated the impact of chronic stress on heart rate, blood pressure, heart attack, and stroke.[9] Historically, the increased risk of CVD from chronic stress has been linked to increased plaque buildup due to elevated cholesterol, hardening of the arteries, alterations in heart rhythm, and increased and fluctuating blood pressure. Recent research also points to metabolic abnormalities, insulin resistance, and inflammation in blood vessels as major contributors to heart disease.[10] In the past 15 to 20 years, researchers have identified direct links between the incidence and progression of CVD and stressors such as job strain, caregiving, bereavement, and natural disasters.[11] Whatever the mechanism, the evidence is clear that stress is a significant contributor to CVD morbidity and mortality.

STRESS AND DEPRESSION

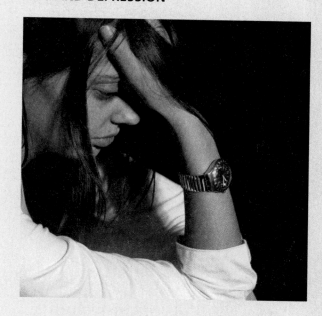

Stress and depression have complicated interconnections based on emotional, physiological, and biochemical processes. Prolonged stress can trigger depression in susceptible people, and prior periods of depression can leave individuals more susceptible to stress.[1]

The *physical* links between stress and depression are strong. During the stress response, the body is flooded with cortisol and with chemicals called *cytokines*. These factors promote inflammation as part of the body's immune response. Researchers think that exposure to both kinds of chemicals can damage or kill neurons in a part of the brain called the *hippocampus* and can alter nerve transmission within the brain. One result of hippocampal damage is impaired learning and memory.[2] Another is the onset of depression symptoms in genetically susceptible individuals.[3] Research confirms that loss of hippocampal neurons is present in many who suffer depression.[4]

Realizing the important interconnections between stress and depression can help you take appropriate steps to handling one or both. Because stress and depression symptoms overlap, applying the stress-management techniques outlined in this chapter may help alleviate depression. If depression symptoms become severe enough to interfere with studying or other aspects of daily life, you should seek help. Potential sources are the student health service, the campus counseling center, a doctor or mental health professional in your community, and your local depression or suicide hotline.

Sources:
1. M. A. Ilgen and K. E. Hutchison, "A History of Major Depressive Disorder and the Response to Stress," *Journal of Affective Disorders* 86, no. 2–3 (June 2005): 143–50.
2. F. A. Scorza and others, "Neurogenesis and Depression: Etiology or New Illusion?" *Review of Brazilian Psychiatry* 27, no. 3 (September 2005): 249–53.
3. See reference 1.
4. Prentiss Price, "Stress and Depression," *All About Depression* (September 9, 2004). www.allaboutdepression.com; David G. Myers, *Psychology.* 5th ed. (New York: Worth Publishers, 1998).

STRESS AND THE IMMUNE SYSTEM

A growing area of scientific investigation known as **psychoneuroimmunology (PNI)** explores the intricate relationship between the mind's response to stress and the immune system's ability to function effectively. Research suggests that too much stress over a long period can negatively regulate various aspects of the cellular immune response.[12] Whereas a short-term stress response is usually protective, prolonged fight-or-flight depresses the immune system. During prolonged stress, elevated levels of adrenal hormones (like cortisol) destroy or reduce the ability of certain white blood cells, known as killer T cells, to aid the immune response. When killer T cells aren't working correctly, the body becomes more susceptible to illness.

STRESS AND THE MIND

Stress may be one of the single greatest contributors to mental disability and emotional dysfunction in industrialized nations. Studies have shown that the rates of mental disorders, particularly depression and anxiety, are associated with various environmental stressors, including divorce, marital conflict, and economic hardship (see **Spotlight: Stress and Depression**).[13]

In severe cases, an individual's response to stress may develop into **post-traumatic stress disorder (PTSD).** PTSD generally develops within the first hours or days after a traumatic event, but in some cases symptoms do not begin until months or years later. Traumas that can trigger PTSD include wartime experiences, rape, near-death experiences in accidents, witnessing a

psychoneuroimmunology (PNI) Science of the interaction between the mind and the immune system

post-traumatic stress disorder (PTSD) An acute stress disorder caused by experiencing an extremely traumatic event

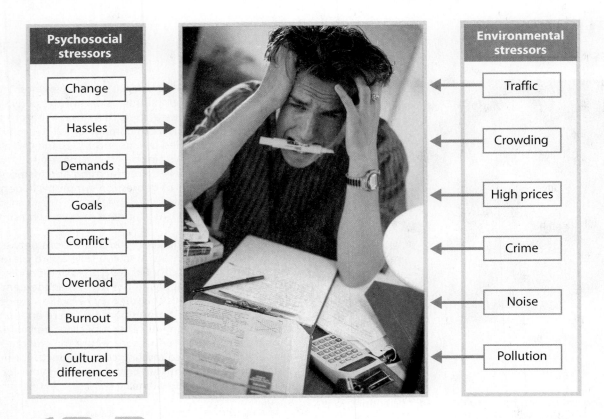

Psychosocial stressors		Environmental stressors
Change		Traffic
Hassles		Crowding
Demands		High prices
Goals		Crime
Conflict		Noise
Overload		Pollution
Burnout		
Cultural differences		

FIGURE 10.3

Stressors are often psychosocial or environmental in nature.

murder or death, being caught in a natural disaster, or a terrorist attack.

WHAT ARE THE MAJOR SOURCES OF STRESS?

College students tend to experience different stressors depending on age, sex, and year in school. First-year students, for example, primarily feel academic pressure.[14] Female freshmen also tend to report dieting and weight gain as stressful, while male students worry more about being underweight, relationship issues, and substance use (drugs, alcohol).[15] In addition, nontraditional students may experience other sources of stress, as described in the box **Understanding Diversity: Stress in Traditional and Nontraditional Students.**

What are your main sources of stress? Examining the many psychological, social, and environmental causes of stress may help you identify them (Figure 10.3).

PSYCHOSOCIAL SOURCES OF STRESS

Interactions with others, expectations we and others have of ourselves, and the social conditions we live in force us to readjust constantly. Some key psychosocial factors are:

Change Alterations from your normal routine can cause stress. The greater the change and your necessary adjustments to it, the more stress and the greater the potential impact on your immune system.[16] Certain kinds of life events predict increased risk for stress-related illness. Knowing them can help, as you'll discover in *Lab10.1.*

Hassles Petty annoyances and frustrations may seem unimportant if taken one by one: getting stuck in a long line at the bookstore, for example, or finding out that a school administrator has lost all your paperwork. However, minor hassles can build to major stress, if you perceive them negatively and let the feelings mount.[17] Regular release through stress management can counter this buildup.

UNDERSTANDING DIVERSITY

STRESS IN TRADITIONAL AND NONTRADITIONAL STUDENTS

As currently defined, *traditional students* are 18 to 24 years old, go right to college after high school, and are fully or partially supported by parents. *Nontraditional students* are 25 or older; have interrupted their educational sequence with working, traveling, or military service; are often married with children; and are self-supporting. Researchers have found notable differences in the way students in the two categories experience stressors at college.

Traditional students tend to experience stress mainly from course work, academic performance, and relationships.[1] Nontraditional students tend to be more stressed by juggling family responsibilities and schoolwork, commuting from off-campus, working at jobs, and feeling less involved with fellow students and detached from the institution they attend.[2] Research shows that wives or husbands who are supportive about the time demands on their college student spouses can help buffer some of the stress. According to those same studies, college and university counselors can and should play an increasingly important role in helping both traditional and nontraditional students overcome their unique stressors and thus complete their degrees.[3]

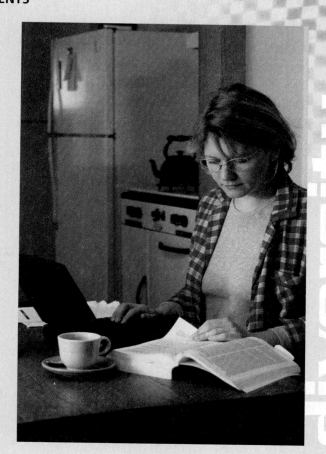

Sources:
1. H. Li and W. Kam, "Types and Characteristics of Stress on College Campus," *Psychological Science* 25, no. 4 (2002): 398–401.
2. Dawna-Cricket-Martita Meehan and Charles Negy, "Undergraduate Students' Adaptation to College: Does Being Married Make a Difference?" *Journal of College Development* (September–October 2003): 567–78.
3. Ibid.

Performance Demands We experience stress when we must speed up, intensify, or alter our behavior to meet higher standards or unfamiliar demands. We can lessen the impact of such demands by setting priorities and realistic deadlines.

Inconsistent Goals and Behaviors The negative effects of stress can be magnified when we don't match our goals with our actions. For instance, you may want good grades, and your family may expect them. But if you party and procrastinate throughout the term, your goals and behaviors are inconsistent. Behaviors that are consistent with your goals—for example, studying harder and partying less to achieve good grades—can help alleviate stress.

Conflict Conflict occurs when we have to choose between competing motives, behaviors, or impulses, or when we must face incompatible demands, opportunities, needs, or goals. For example, what if your best friend wanted you to help her cheat on an

exam, but you didn't feel right about it? College students often experience stress because their own developing set of beliefs conflicts with the values they learned from their parents.

Overload and Burnout Time pressure, responsibilities, course work, tuition, and high expectations for yourself and those around you—coupled with a lack of support—can lead to *overload:* a state of feeling overburdened, unable to keep up, and longing for escape. Overload pushes some students toward depression or substance abuse; others respond by using stress-management tools to alleviate tension before it piles up. Unrelieved overload can lead to *burnout,* a state of stress-induced physical and mental exhaustion. Teachers, nurses, and law enforcement officers, for example, experience high levels of burnout, and highly pressured professionals often apply stress-management techniques to avoid reaching this point.

Environmental Sources of Stress

Environmental stress results from events occurring in the physical environment. For example, people living in crowded urban environments tend to experience stress from traffic, housing density, a high cost of living, crime, noise, and pollution. Meanwhile, people living in rural areas may experience different stresses, including transportation difficulties, limited employment opportunities, reduced availability of services, and greater impact from weather and climatic events such as floods, fires, and tornadoes.

RACIAL, ETHNIC OR CULTURAL ISOLATION

Imagine what it would be like to come to campus and find yourself isolated, lacking friends, and ridiculed on the basis of who you are or how you look. Often, those who act, speak, or dress differently face additional pressures that do not affect more "typical" students. Students perceived as different—whether due to race, ethnicity, religious affiliation, age, physical handicap, or sexual orientation—may become victims of subtle and not-so-subtle forms of bigotry, insensitivity, harassment, or hostility.

appraisal The interpretation and evaluation of information provided to the brain by the senses

INTERNAL SOURCES OF STRESS

When you perceive that your coping resources are sufficient to meet life's demands, you experience little or no stress. By contrast, when you perceive that life's demands exceed your coping resources, you are likely to feel strain and distress.

Low Self-Esteem and Self-Efficacy

Several coping resources influence your **appraisal** of stress. Two of the most important are *self-esteem* and *self-efficacy*. Self-esteem is a sense of positive self-regard, or how you feel about yourself. Self-efficacy is a belief or confidence in personal skills and performance abilities. Researchers consider self-efficacy one of the most important personality traits that influence psychological and physiological stress responses.[18] Low self-esteem or low self-efficacy can lead you to feel helpless to cope with the stress in your life.

Type A Personality

So-called "Type A" personalities are characterized as hard-driving, competitive, time-driven perfectionists. "Type B" personalities, in contrast, are more relaxed, noncompetitive, and more tolerant of others. Historically, researchers believed that people with Type A characteristics were more prone to heart attacks than their Type B counterparts.[19] Researchers today believe that personality types are more complex than previously thought—most people are not one personality type all the time, and other variables must be explored.

According to psychologist Susanne Kobasa, *psychological hardiness* may negate self-imposed stress associated with Type A behavior. Psychologically hardy people are characterized by control, commitment, and an embrace of challenge.[20] People with a sense of control are able to accept responsibility for their behaviors and change those that they discover to be debilitating. People with a sense of commitment have good self-esteem and understand their purpose in life. People who embrace challenge see change as a stimulating opportunity for personal growth. The concept of hardiness has been studied extensively, and many researchers believe it is the foundation of an individual's ability to cope with stress and remain healthy.[21]

What stresses do you face, and how heavily are they affecting you? Lab 10.1 charts many common sources of stress for college students and others. Completing this lab will help you measure your current stress level and start learning some helpful stress-reduction strategies.

WHAT ARE EFFECTIVE TOOLS FOR STRESS MANAGEMENT?

Most college students do best with a low-key, multipronged approach to stress management.

EXERCISE AND PHYSICAL ACTIVITY

Improving your overall level of fitness may be the most helpful thing you can do to combat stress. Interestingly, research shows that exercise actually *stimulates* the stress response,[22] but that a well-exercised body adapts to the *eustress* of exercise, and as a result is able to tolerate greater levels of *distress* of all kinds. Compared to an unfit person, a fit individual develops a milder stress response to any given stressor.[23] Research also shows that exercise reduces both psychosocial stress and metabolic disturbances leading to belly fat, high blood pressure, high blood cholesterol, and vascular disease.[24]

Many physical activities relieve the feeling of stress and tension, while others—especially those that involve competition, high skill levels, or physical risk—may add to your stress load. Some activities are high in one value and low in the other, but many can build fitness and promote relaxation at the same time. The trick is to balance exercise, fun, and recreational activities in your free time so that you can stay fit and reduce chronic stress.

BASIC WELLNESS MEASURES

Many of the habits you cultivate to improve your wellness can also fight the negative effects of stress.

Eating Well

Eating Well Eating nutrient-dense foods rather than fast foods and junk foods gives you more mental and physical energy, improves your immune responses, and helps you stay at a healthy weight. Undereating, overeating, or eating nutrient-poor foods can contribute to your stress levels by diminishing your overall wellness. Most claims about vitamins and supplements that reduce stress are unsupported. Vitamin and mineral supplementation beyond your daily requirements may only add to your stress—financial stress, that is!

Getting Enough Sleep

Getting Enough Sleep Sleep is a central wellness component. As explained in the box **Spotlight: Sleep, Performance, and Stress,** sleep loss hinders learning, memory, academic work, and

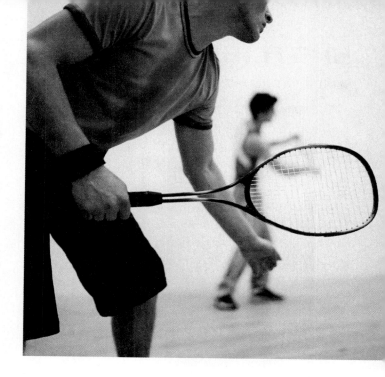

physical performance. It can also depress mood and prompt feelings of stress, anger, and sadness. *Sound* sleep is important, too. Some people find that inexpensive earplugs or eye masks from a drugstore block sleep-disturbing sound and light. Others require a quieter, darker room or more considerate roommates to solve their sleep problems.

Avoiding Tobacco and Alcohol

Avoiding Tobacco and Alcohol Both drinking and smoking can disrupt sleep patterns during the night. The nicotine in tobacco is highly addictive and acts as a mild stimulant. Tobacco use also impairs normal breathing and diminishes your ability to fight off colds and other infections.

CHANGING YOUR BEHAVIORAL RESPONSES

Realizing that stress is harming your fitness, wellness, relationships, or productivity is often the first step toward making positive changes. Start by assessing all aspects of a stressor, examining your typical response, determining ways to change it, and learning to cope. Often, you cannot change the stressors you face: the death of a loved one, the stringent requirements of your major, stacked-up course assignments, and so on. You can, however, change your reactions to them, and in so doing, help manage your stress.

Assess the Stressor

Assess the Stressor List and evaluate the stressors in your life. Can you change the stressor itself? If not, you can still change your behavior

SPOTLIGHT

SLEEP, PERFORMANCE, AND STRESS

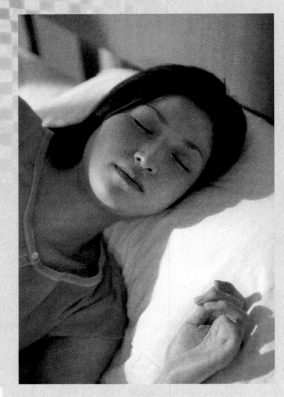

Sleep experts suggest that 18- to 20-year-olds need about 8.5 to 9.25 hours of sleep per night, while adults over 21 need about 7 to 9 hours of sleep (depending on individual physiology.)[1] In the 1980s, college students got an average of 7 to 7.5 hours of sleep per night. Today, however, that has slid to between 6 to 6.9 hours. In addition, the typical student sleeps less at the end of a semester than at the beginning due to the accumulation of assignments and exams.[2]

Losing an hour or two of sleep actually does matter, even to young, active, healthy college students. Research shows that sleep loss degrades learning and memory,

physical performance, and mood in both young and older adults. One piece of evidence for this is a German study that presented students with a math puzzle to work out. Most of those who "slept on it" realized a shortcut to solving the problem by morning and could solve the task much more quickly. Three-quarters of those who didn't "sleep on it" failed to intuit the way to a faster, simpler solution.[3] This was the first scientific proof that sleep can promote insight and problem solving.

Sleep deprivation can also increase feelings of stress, anger, and sadness. These emotional states can, in turn, make sleeping even harder. Feeling extremely stressed out and having a negative emotional response to that stress is, in fact, the best predictor that a student will have sleep problems.[4] Loneliness and limited social contacts are also correlated with higher stress levels and poorer sleep.[5]

Poor sleep is defined as getting fewer-than-recommended hours of sleep, having irregular bedtimes and rising times, and experiencing interrupted sleep. To improve your sleep and adopt better sleep habits,

- go to bed and wake up at as regular a time as possible;
- sleep in a room that is as quiet and dark as possible;
- get regular exercise but not too close to bedtime;
- avoid caffeine in the afternoon or evening;
- avoid taking naps;
- sleep where it is cool (not cold) and ventilated (but not drafty);
- avoid excess alcohol.

Sources:
1. National Sleep Foundation, "How Much Sleep Is Enough?" 2005. www.sleepfoundation.org.
2. J. Hawkins and P. Shaw, "Self-Reported Sleep Quality in College Students: A Repeated Measures Approach," *Sleep* 15, no. 6 (December 1992): 545–9.
3. Bruce Bower, "Sleeper Effects," *Science News* 165 (January 24, 2004): 53–54.
4. L. A. Verlander, J. O. Benedict, and D. P. Hanson, "Stress and Sleep Patterns of College Students," *Perceptual Motor Skills* 88, no. 3, pt. 1 (June 1999): 893–8.
5. S. D. Pressman and others, "Loneliness, Social Network Size, and Immune Response to Influenza Vaccination in College Freshman," *Health Psychology* 24, no. 3 (May 2005): 297–306.

and reactions to reduce the levels of stress you experience. For example, if you have a heavy academic workload, such as five term papers due for five different courses during the same quarter or semester, make a plan to start the papers early and space your work evenly so you can avoid panic over deadlines and all-night sessions to finish papers on time.

Change Your Response If something causes you distress—a habitually messy roommate, for example—you can (1) express your anger by yelling;

(2) pick up the mess yourself but then leave a nasty note; or (3) use humor to get your point across. Your first inclination may be counterproductive, so stop and ask yourself, "What will I gain from this approach?" Then think through the most effective choice. This technique requires practice and emotional control but reaps a large benefit.

Cognitive Coping Strategies Thinking things through before acting may help you avoid destructive or ineffective responses to potentially stressful events. Forethought and planning can also help you tolerate increasingly higher stress levels while limiting physical and mental wear and tear.

Prepare *Before* Stressful Events

Preparing yourself for an event that you know will be stressful can diminish its impact. For example, suppose you are nervous about giving a speech. Practicing in front of friends or taping yourself with a video camera may help you find and correct rough spots, and in turn, lower your levels of stress during the actual speech. The important thing is making the effort to plan and prepare.

Downshift

You may experience stress because you want to "have it all": a college diploma, a successful career, a family, a wide circle of friends, possessions, status in the community, and so on. But many people are starting to **downshift:** to step back to a simpler life by, for example, moving from a large urban area to a smaller town, from a hectic high-pressure career to a quieter one, or by scaling back to fewer, less-expensive possessions.

Consider some immediate and longer-term steps for simplifying your life:

- List and prioritize your goals. What must you do to reach your selected goals?

- Learn to say no. Decide who you want and need to spend time with, and which requests you can and cannot accommodate.

- Write out a financial plan for paying off credit cards and existing debt, and avoid unnecessary spending.

- Choose a career that you enjoy for itself, not primarily for the salary it commands. Some lower-paying jobs are less stressful and allow more free time for relaxation.

- Establish a savings plan, no matter how small; having a reserve for emergencies and future plans can ease tension.

- Clean drawers, closets, and desktops of clutter. Having fewer unnecessary, unused items means keeping track and taking care of that much less.

SEEKING SOCIAL SUPPORT

Making, keeping, and spending time with friends is a central stress-management tool that helps protect you against harmful stressors. Social interactions are such important buffers against the effects of stress that a person who is well-integrated socially is only half as likely to die from any cause at any age than is a person with few or no sources of social support.[25] This makes social connections a factor as large as being a nonsmoker versus a smoker! Married people are healthier and live longer than single or divorced people, and researchers attribute most of this effect to stress reduction.[26] Compared to students with a network of friends, lonely students experience more stress, poorer moods, and lower quality sleep.[27]

While friends can be important stress reducers, people sometimes need the help of a counselor or support group. Most colleges and universities offer counseling services at no cost for short-term crises. Clergy, instructors, and dorm supervisors also may be helpful resources. If university services are unavailable or if you are concerned about confidentiality, most communities offer low-cost counseling through mental health clinics. You may also be able to find and join a stress-reduction program or stress support group through one of these professional resources. Many individual counselors and stress-reduction classes teach tools like relaxation breathing, progressive muscle relaxation, mindfulness meditation, and cognitive stress reduction techniques to help you learn to change your thinking, behavior, or emotions. These help control your experience of stress and actually reduce stress hormone levels, and by so doing, slow the heart rate, relax the muscles, boost immunity, and help balance brain chemistry.

RELAXATION TECHNIQUES

Relaxation techniques tend to focus the mind and breathing while the body remains fairly stationary. Here are some of the most popular examples.

Relaxation Breathing

When we're tense, we often breathe shallowly in the upper chest or even hold our breath, but this kind of breathing can increase anxiety.[28] **Relaxation breathing**—inhaling deeply, rhythmically, and involving the abdominal muscles—can help relieve tension and increase oxygen levels in the blood. This, in turn, can boost energy and sharpen thinking. Relaxation breathing, also called

downshifting Forging new values that include stepping back to a simpler life

relaxation breathing Inhaling deeply and rhythmically, and expanding then relaxing the abdomen; this breathing technique can help relieve tension and increase oxygen intake

MINDFULNESS MEDITATION

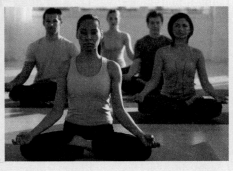

Meditation is a centuries-old practice that can promote relaxation, lessen damage from chronic stress, and help prevent stress-related illnesses. One of the easiest forms of meditation is called *mindfulness meditation,* which cultivates awareness, calms the body, and stops the mind from racing—at least for a while. You can start learning mindfulness meditation with 5-minute sessions, then build to frequent or daily sessions of 30 minutes or more. Many people find that meditating with a partner or in a small group helps reinforce their practice.

The following specific steps work for many beginning and experienced meditators.[1]

1. In a quiet place, sit cross-legged on the floor or upright in a chair, back straight but not stiff.

2. With eyes closed, breathe in slowly and fully and notice the sensation of air moving in and out of your nose, breathing passages, and lungs. Focus carefully on the abdomen rising. Then breathe out and note the abdomen falling. It helps some people to say silently, "Rising, rising . . . falling, falling . . ."

3. As you sit, you will inevitably experience sounds, smells, tastes, and other sensations. As they come up, notice them and label them (for example, "hearing, hearing . . ."). Then, gently return your concentration to your breathing and the rising and falling of your abdomen.

4. As you sit, your mind will inevitably become active with thoughts, images, plans, or worries. Notice them and label them (for example, "thinking, thinking . . .") and then return your focus to your breathing.

5. After meditating, open your eyes. Rise slowly and carefully, being aware of all the small changes in posture, movement, and effort.

Source: Sayadaw U Pandita Bhivamsa, "The Way to Practice Vipassana Meditation," www.Realization.org, May 20, 2000.

---

diaphragmatic breathing, is easy and can be done sitting in a chair or lying down, alone or in a small group, and for a few minutes or for a half hour or more. The object is to expand the chest fully by drawing downward with the diaphragm and outward with the abdomen, then releasing fully. Yoga, tai chi, meditation, and most other relaxation techniques rely on this or some similar form of deep, rhythmic breathing.

Progressive Muscle Relaxation

Progressive muscle relaxation (PMR) identifies tension stored in the muscles and releases it, muscle group by muscle group. To do PMR, lie down in a quiet, comfortable place and devote 10 or 20 minutes to gradually letting go of accumulated stiffness and tension in the affected muscles. *Lab10.2* teaches a simple method of tensing then relaxing isolated muscle groups. It will also teach you the specific order of muscle groups to follow. You can do this alone or in a group as a way to relax and refresh yourself fully. Some people also use it as a means of falling asleep.

Meditation

There are dozens of forms of meditation, but most involve sitting quietly for 15 to 30 minutes and focusing on deep breathing. Some involve assuming a particular posture like sitting cross-legged with back straight and hands resting gently on the thighs. Researchers have confirmed that meditation reduces the stress response and boosts the immune response.[29] Meditation also shifts brain activity from the right prefrontal lobe, associated with unhappiness, anger, and distress, and toward the left prefrontal lobe, associated with happiness and enthusiasm. The box **Tools for Change: Mindfulness Meditation** presents one of the easiest-to-learn meditation techniques.

Biofeedback

Biofeedback involves monitoring physical stress responses such as brain activity, blood pressure, muscle tension, or heart rate with a special machine and then learning to consciously alter these responses. Biofeedback is effective for several stress-related conditions, including high

progressive muscle relaxation (PMR) A stress-management technique that identifies tension stored in the muscles and releases it, one muscle group at a time

biofeedback A stress-management technique that teaches you to alter automatic physiological responses such as body temperature, heart rate, or sweating; uses a machine to monitor such responses and measure the success of conscious control attempts

blood pressure, headaches, irritable bowel syndrome, and asthma.[30]

Hypnosis
Hypnosis trains people to focus on one thought, object, or voice and to become unusually responsive to suggestion. A qualified hypnotherapist can implant a suggestion that directs a patient to resist habits such as smoking or overeating or to lessen phobias such as fear of snakes or air travel. The patient then learns to induce a state of self-hypnosis as a way to relax deeply and reinforce the behavioral changes.

People who get regular physical exercise and also practice one or more of these relaxation methods—relaxation breathing, progressive muscle relaxation, meditation, biofeedback, and hypnosis—can achieve very effective relief from stress symptoms.[31] Many will also see improvement in medical conditions that are worsened by stress.

MANAGING YOUR TIME, THOUGHTS, AND EMOTIONS

The world presents us with plenty of stressors. But we create some of our own as well through our ineffective time-management habits and our ways of thinking and reacting to events. Habits are learned behaviors, and you can *unlearn* or replace them with new habits that serve you better in managing stress. Here is what to aim for.

Manage Your Time
Time—or our perceived lack of it—is one of our biggest stressors. If you learn to handle demands in a more streamlined, efficient way, you can leave more time for other things, such as studying and having fun. The following tips can help:

- **Assess how you spend your time.** How do you spend the 168 hours in your week? Try keeping a time journal for 1 week. Tabulate the time you spend in productive pursuits, the time spent relaxing, and the time you may be wasting. Look for ways to tip the balance toward productivity.

- **Prioritize your tasks.** Make a daily "to do" list of things you must do today, must do soon, or could do later, if at all. Rank and assign deadlines to the more important tasks.

- **Single-task or multitask when appropriate.** It is usually unproductive to try to make phone calls, clean the bathroom, and write your term paper all at once. Term papers are singular tasks. Save multitasking for things that take less concentration such as doing the laundry and paying bills.

- **Break up big tasks.** Divide big tasks like finishing a term paper into smaller segments, then allocate a certain amount of time to each piece. If you find yourself floundering in a task, move on and come back to it when you are refreshed.

- **Clean your desk.** Periodically weed out unneeded papers and file the useful ones in separate folders. Try to handle papers just once: When bills come in, for example, take care of them immediately. Promptly read, respond to, file, or toss the other mail into the recycle bin.

- **Accommodate your natural rhythms.** Schedule activities to coincide with the time you are at your best. If you are a morning person, study and write papers in the morning, and take breaks when you start to slow down.

- **Avoid overcommitment.** Set your school and personal priorities and don't be afraid to say no to things you cannot or should not agree to do.

- **Avoid interruptions.** When you have a project that requires total concentration, schedule uninterrupted time. Go to a quiet room in the library or student union where no one will find you. Shut off your cell phone and let it take messages.

- **Reward yourself.** When you finish a task early, take a break and do something enjoyable that helps you recharge and refresh your energy levels.

Manage Your Thinking
Our "negative scripts" about ourselves contribute to our stress. When we see ourselves as unable to cope (that is, when we have low self-efficacy), we tend to handle life's problems and stresses more poorly. You can change negative scripts to more positive ones, however, and in the process reduce your stress responses. Successful stress management involves developing and practicing self-esteem skills, such as applying positive thinking and examining self-talk to reduce negative and irrational responses. Focus on your current capabilities rather than on past problems.

Here are specific actions you can take to develop better mental skills for stress management:

- **Worry constructively.** Don't waste time and energy worrying about things you can't change or events that may never happen.

---

hypnosis A medical and psychiatric tool that trains people to focus on one thought, object, or voice and to become unusually responsive to suggestion

- **Perceive life as changeable.** If you accept that change is a natural part of living and growing, the jolt of changes will become less stressful.

- **Consider alternatives.** Remember, there is seldom only one appropriate action. Anticipating options will help you plan for change and adjust more rapidly.

- **Moderate your expectations.** Aim high but be realistic about your circumstances and motivation.

- **Don't rush into action.** Think before you act. Tolerate mistakes by yourself and others. Rather than getting angry and stressed by mishaps, evaluate what happened, learn from them, and plan to avoid future occurrences.

- **Live simply.** Eliminate unnecessary possessions and obligations.

- **Take things less seriously.** Think about the times that you have spent getting all worked up about some perceived interpersonal slight, or concerns over what others may think or say. Lighten up—try to keep the real importance of these things in perspective. Ask yourself: How much will this matter in two weeks? Six months?

Manage Negative Emotions and Anger

Stress management involves learning to identify emotional reactions that are based on irrational beliefs and negative self-talk. Identifying those can allow you to deal with the belief or emotion in a healthy and appropriate way.

Learning how to manage anger is particularly important. Anger can be constructive if it mobilizes us to stand up for ourselves or to accomplish something others think we are incapable of. However, a habit of responding angrily when our wants or desires are thwarted can be destructive. Because anger triggers the fight-or-flight response, people who manage anger poorly operate with the stress response turned on longer than necessary.

Hotheaded, short-fused people are at risk for health problems. Numerous studies show that anger can significantly increase the risk of heart disease. Stress hormones released during anger may constrict blood vessels in the heart or actually promote clot formation, which can trigger a heart attack.[32] Strategies for controlling and redirecting anger include learning to forgive and forget; practicing problem-solving techniques in place of complaining; seeking objective opinions and constructive advice from friends; anticipating situations that trigger your anger and brainstorming solutions in advance; learning to express your feelings constructively; learning to de-escalate from anger by taking deep breaths or counting to 10; and keeping a journal to observe your own reactions and progress in controlling anger.

SPIRITUAL PRACTICE

Several medical studies have discovered correlations between spirituality and wellness. For example, prayer elicits the same relaxation response attained through other stress-management techniques: lowered blood pressure, heart rate, breathing and metabolism, and a more vigorous immune response.[33] Spirituality is also correlated with a reduced *perception* of stress in one's life.

Developing one's spirituality can be more than just an internal process. It can also be a social process that enhances your relationships with others. The ability to give and take, speak and listen, and forgive and move on is integral to any process of spiritual development.

The above techniques are summarized in Figure 10.4.

CASE STUDY

Cory

"Life was getting ridiculous. I was exhausted but would have trouble falling asleep, so that was a vicious cycle. I gained weight because I stopped working out—which I used to do twice a week but just didn't have the time for anymore. And I caught another cold at the end of October. My dad started joking that he was healthier than I was! Something had to give, so I dropped my one elective—Spanish, which I love. And I started going back to the gym, which actually seemed to give me some energy back. I honestly think just those two things alone helped me to get through the rest of the semester. Now, if I can just ace my MCATs . . ."

1. **What kinds of stress-related problems was Cory exhibiting?**

2. **Review the section on stress-management tools. Which strategies did Cory employ?**

3. **Which stress-management strategies do you use? What techniques seem to be the most effective for you?**

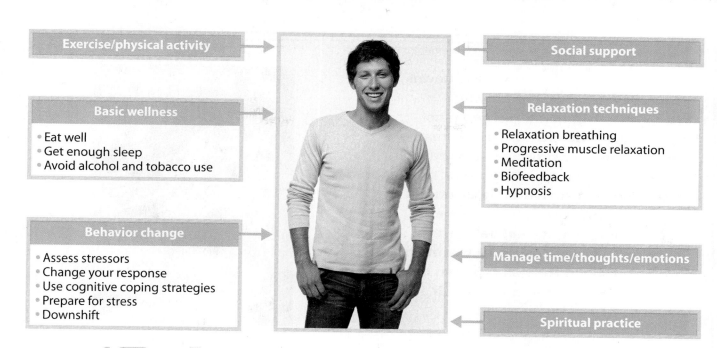

FIGURE 10.4

There are many effective techniques for helping you manage stress.

Exercise/physical activity

Basic wellness
- Eat well
- Get enough sleep
- Avoid alcohol and tobacco use

Behavior change
- Assess stressors
- Change your response
- Use cognitive coping strategies
- Prepare for stress
- Downshift

Social support

Relaxation techniques
- Relaxation breathing
- Progressive muscle relaxation
- Meditation
- Biofeedback
- Hypnosis

Manage time/thoughts/emotions

Spiritual practice

HOW CAN YOU CREATE YOUR OWN STRESS-MANAGEMENT PLAN?

You can use many of the fitness and wellness tools you read about in earlier chapters to help reduce your stress levels. These tools include self-assessment, drawing up a behavior change contract, and journaling.

STEP ONE: ASSESS YOURSELF

Lab 10.1 helps you assess situations that may leave you susceptible to stress. It also reveals signs of chronic stress. Using this information, target for change one or more behaviors that contribute to your increased stress.

Then, evaluate the behavior(s) you have chosen. Identify your stress-producing behavior patterns. What can you change now? What can you change in the near future?

STEP TWO: PLAN FOR CHANGE

Select one stress-producing behavior pattern that you want to change. Fill out the behavior change contract in Part V of *Lab 10.3*. As you learned earlier, your behavior change contract should include your long-term goal for change, your short-term goals, the rewards you will give yourself for reaching these goals, potential obstacles along the way, and strategies for overcoming these obstacles. Look for ways to apply wellness tools such as meditation, relaxation breathing, and progressive muscle relaxation (Lab 10.2).

STEP THREE: CHART YOUR PROGRESS

Chart your progress in your journal. At the end of a week, evaluate how successful you were in following your plan. What helped you be successful? What obstacles to change did you encounter? What will you do differently next week?

After you assess yourself, make a plan and revise it as needed. Are your short-term goals attainable? Are the rewards satisfying? Do you need to go beyond your own self-efforts and enlist the help of your peers or professionals? If you think you need professional support, start by consulting the student health service for advice and direction on finding suitable counselors, therapists, or stress-management support groups.

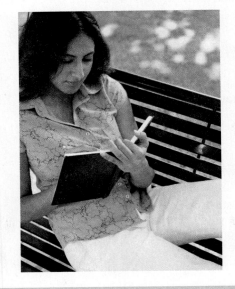

Try it NOW! Write it down! Journal writing is a great way to cleanse the mind, release emotions, and draft strategies for resolution. • The next time you are feeling stressed, write down the event or situation that activated your stress response, identify the emotions that accompany it, and list several options to bring closure to the event. • Writing these things down can be an effective means to cope with stressors.

CHAPTER IN REVIEW

REVIEW QUESTIONS

1. Graduating from college and moving to a new city can create stress as well as provide an opportunity for growth. This type of stress is called
   a. strain.
   b. distress.
   c. eustress.
   d. adaptive response.

2. The physiological instinct to flee from or confront a threat is called
   a. homeostasis.
   b. the fight-or-flight response.
   c. allostasis.
   d. allostatic load.

3. *Homeostasis* describes
   a. the body's "normal" or "steady state."
   b. long-term wear-and-tear on the body.
   c. sustained stress.
   d. the exhaustion stage of the general adaptation syndrome.

4. Hans Selye's general adaptation syndrome includes all of the following stages except
   a. the alarm stage.
   b. the resistance stage.
   c. the allostasis stage.
   d. the exhaustion stage.

5. Stress has been linked to all of the following except
   a. cardiovascular disease.
   b. immune system impairment.
   c. mental disorders.
   d. greater health.

6. Change, hassles, performance demands, and burnout are all examples of
   a. psychosocial sources of stress.
   b. environmental sources of stress.
   c. internal sources of stress.
   d. homeostasis.

7. *Allostatic load* refers to
   a. changes that occur in the body to maintain homeostasis.
   b. long-term wear-and-tear on the body caused by stress.
   c. the first stage of the general adaptation syndrome.
   d. eustress.

8. Effective tools for stress management include all of the following except
   a. getting by on little sleep.
   b. exercise and physical activity.
   c. eating well.
   d. avoiding alcohol and tobacco.

9. *Relaxation breathing* refers to
   a. inhaling deeply and rhythmically to relieve tension and increase oxygen levels in the blood.
   b. progressive muscle relaxation.
   c. monitoring physical stress responses and then consciously working to alter those responses.
   d. biofeedback.

10. What stress-fighting technique allows people to become unusually responsive to suggestion?
    a. Meditation
    b. Massage
    c. Biofeedback
    d. Hypnosis

CRITICAL THINKING QUESTIONS

1. Compare and contrast distress and eustress. In what ways are both types of stress potentially harmful?

2. Describe the body's physiological response to stress.

3. What are some of the health risks that result from chronic stress? Summarize the main points of the general adaptation syndrome and the allostatic load model.

4. What major factors seem to influence the nature and extent of a person's susceptibility to stress? Explain how social support, self-esteem, and personality may make a person more or less susceptible.

ONLINE RESOURCES

Please visit this book's website at **www.aw-bc.com/hopson** to access links related to topics in this chapter.

REFERENCES

1. American College Health Association, "National College Health Assessment. Reference Group Executive Summary Fall 2006," Baltimore: American College Health Association, 2007.

2. Mark A. Staal, "Stress, Cognition, and Human Performance: A Literature Review and Conceptual Framework," *National Aeronautics and Space Administration* (May 2004): NASA/TM-2004–212024.

3. Robert Sapolsky, *Why Zebras Don't Get Ulcers: An Updated Guide to Stress, Stress-Related Diseases, and Coping* (New York: Owl Books, 2004).

4. David G. Myers, *Psychology.* 5th ed. (New York: Worth Publishers, 1998): 518.

5. Bruce McEwen and Teresa Seeman, "Allostatic Load and Allostasis," John D. and Catherine T. MacArthur Research Network on Socioeconomic Status and Health (University of California at San Francisco 1999).

6. Ibid.

7. Robert Sapolsky, *Why Zebras Don't Get Ulcers: An Updated Guide to Stress, Stress-Related Diseases, and Coping* (New York: Owl Books, 2004).

8. A. Mokdal and others, "Actual Causes of Death in the United States 2000," *Journal of the American Medical Association* 291 (2004): 1238–45.

9. S. Das and J. H. O'Keefe, "Behavioral Cardiology: Recognizing and Addressing the Profound Impact of Psychosocial Stress on Cardiovascular Health," *Current Atherosclerosis Reports* 8, no. 2 (2006): 111–18; A. K. Ferketich and P. F. Binkley, "Psychological Distress and Cardiovascular Disease: Results from the 2002 National Health Interview Study," *European Heart Journal* 26, no. 18 (2005): 1923–29; S. Yusef and others, "Effect of Potentially Modifiable Risk Factors Associated with Myocardial Infarction in 52 Countries (The INTERHEART Study): Case-Control Study," *The Lancet* 364, no. 9438 (2004): 937–52.

10. J. R. Hapuarachchi and others, "Changes in Clinically Relevant Metabolites with Psychological Stress Parameters," *Behavioral Medicine* 29 (2003): 52–60; C. N. Merz and others, "Psychosocial Stress and Cardiovascular Disease: Pathophysiological Links," *Behavioral Medicine* 27 (2002): 141–48.

11. S. A. Everson-Rose and T. T. Lewis, "Psychosocial Risk Factors and Cardiovascular Disease," *Annual Review of Public Health* 26 (2005): 469–500.

12. S. C. Segerstrom and G. E. Miller, "Psychological Stress and the Human Immune System," *Psychological Bulletin* 130, no. 4 (2004): 601–30.

13. D. A. Katerndahl and M. Parchman, "The Ability of the Stress Process Model to Explain Mental Health Outcomes," *Comprehensive Psychiatry* 43 (2002): 351–60; R. C. Kessler and others, "The Epidemiology of Major Depressive Disorder," *Journal of the American Medical Association* 289 (2003): 3095–3105.

14. P. Jackson and M. Finney, "Negative Life Events and Psychological Distress Among Young Adults," *Social Psychology Quarterly* 65, no. 2 (June 2002): 186–201.

15. Ibid.

16. T. Holmes and R. Rahe, "The Social Readjustment Rating Scale," *Journal of Psychosomatic Research* 11 (1967): 213–18.

17. R. Lazarus, "The Trivialization of Distress," in *Preventing Health*

Risk Behaviors and Promoting Coping with Illness, eds. J. Rosen and L. Solomon (Hanover, NH: University Press of New England, 1985): 279–98.

18. A. D. Von and others, "Predictors of Health Behaviors in College Students," *Journal of Advanced Nursing* 48, no. 5 (2004): 463–74.

19. M. Friedman and R. H. Rosenman, *Type A Behavior and Your Heart* (New York: Knopf, 1974).

20. S. Kobasa, "Stressful Life Events, Personality, and Health: An Inquiry Into Hardiness," *Journal of Personality and Social Psychology* 37 (1979): 1–11.

21. B. J. Crowley and others, "Psychological Hardiness and Adjustment to Life Events in Adulthood," *Journal of Adult Development* 10 (2003): 237–48; S. R. Maddi, "The Story of Hardiness: Twenty Years of Theorizing, Research, and Practice," *Consulting Psychology Journal: Practice and Research* 54 (2002): 173–86.

22. A. Leal-Cerro and others, "Mechanisms Underlying the Neuroendocrine Response to Physical Exercise," *Journal of Endocrinological Investigation* 26, no. 9 (September 2003): 879–85.

23. U. Rimmele and others, "Trained Men Show Lower Cortisol, Heart Rate, and Psychological Responses to Psychosocial Stress Compared with Untrained Men," *Psycho-neuroendocrinology* 32, no. 6 (July 2007): 627–35.

24. A. Tsatsoulis and S. Fountoulakis, "The Protective Role of Exercise on Stress System Dysregulation and Comorbidities," *Annals of the New York Academy of Sciences* 1083 (November 2006): 196–213.

25. S. Levine, D. M. Lyons, and A. F. Schatzberg, "Psychobiological Consequences of Social Relationships," *Annals of the New York Academy of Sciences* 89, no. 7 (1999): 210–18.

26. J. Holmes, "Healthy Relationships: Their Influence on Physical Health," BC Council for Families, 2004. www.bccf.bc.ca/learn/health_relations.htm.

27. S. D. Pressman and others, "Loneliness, Social Network Size, and Immune Response to Influenza Vaccination in College Freshmen," *Health Psychology* 24, no. 4 (July 2005): 348.

28. A. Conrad and others, "Psycho-physiological Effects of Breathing Instructions for Stress Management," *Applied Psychophysiology and Biofeedback* 32, no. 2 (June 2007): 89–98.

29. S. Jain and others, "A Randomized Controlled Trial of Mindfulness Meditation Versus Relaxation Training: Effects on Distress, Positive States of Mind, Rumination, and Distraction," *Annals of Behavioral Medicine* 33, no. 1 (February 2007): 11021, R. J. Davidson and others, "Alterations in Brain and Immune Function Produced by Mindfulness Meditation," *Psychosomatic Medicine* 65, no. 4 (July–August 2003): 564–70.

30. Mayo Clinic, "Biofeedback: Using Your Mind to Improve Your Health," January 26, 2006. www.mayoclinic.com/health/biofeedback/SA00083.

31. Mayo Clinic, "Relaxation Techniques: Learn Ways to Calm Your Stress," March 7, 2007. www.mayoclinic.com/health/relaxation-technique/SR00007. Also, "Exercise: Rev Up Your Routine to Reduce Stress," MayoClinic.com, July 20, 2006. www.mayoclinic.com/print/exercise-and-stress/SR00036/METHOP=print.

32. L. D. Kubzansky and others, "Shared and Unique Contributions of Anger, Anxiety, and Depression to Coronary Heart Disease: A Prospective Study in the Normative Aging Study," *Annals of Behavioral Medicine* 31, no. 1 (February 2006): 21–9; I. Kawachi and others, "A Prospective Study of Anger and Coronary Heart Disease. The Normative Aging Study," *Circulation* 94, no. 9 (November 1, 1996): 2090–5.

33. D. K. Reibel and others, "Mindfulness-Based Stress Reduction and Health-Related Quality of Life in a Heterogeneous Patient Population," *General Hospital Psychiatry* 23, no. 4 (July–August 2001): 183–92, R. Sethness and others, "Cardiac Health: Relationships Among Hostility, Spirituality, and Health Risk," *Journal of Nursing Care Quality* 20, no. 1 (January–March 2005): 81–9. And L. E. Carlson and others, "Mindfulness-Based Stress Reduction in Relation to Quality of Life, Mood, Symptoms of Stress and Levels of Cortisol, Dehyroepiandrosterone Sulfate (DHEAS) and Melatonin in Breast and Prostate Cancer Outpatient," *Psychoneuro-endocrinology* 29, no. 4 (May 2004): 448–74.

Name: _____ **Date:** _____

Instructor: _____ **Section:** _____

Purpose: To uncover your major stressors and your stress levels during the last year

Directions: The following Life Experiences Survey lists events that can cause a buildup of chronic stress. If you did not experience a listed event, circle the zero in front of a statement. If you experienced the event but feel that it had a positive impact on your life, also mark a zero. If you experienced an event and feel it had a *negative* impact, use the scale below and circle a 1, 2, or 3.

Life Experience Survey

3 = Extremely negative impact

2 = Moderately negative impact

1 = Somewhat negative impact

0 = No impact or a positive impact

College

☐ 0 1 2 3   Beginning a new school experience at a higher academic level.

☐ 0 1 2 3   Changing to a new school at same academic level

☐ 0 1 2 3   Academic probation

☐ 0 1 2 3   Failing an important exam

☐ 0 1 2 3   Changing a major

☐ 0 1 2 3   Failing a course

☐ 0 1 2 3   Dropping a course

☐ 0 1 2 3   Joining a fraternity/sorority

☐ 0 1 2 3   Ending formal college education

☐ 0 1 2 3   Financial problems concerning college

Family

☐ 0 1 2 3   Marriage

☐ 0 1 2 3   Death of spouse

Death of a close family member

  ☐ 0 1 2 3   Mother

  ☐ 0 1 2 3   Father

  ☐ 0 1 2 3   Brother

  ☐ 0 1 2 3   Sister

  ☐ 0 1 2 3   Child

  ☐ 0 1 2 3   Grandmother

  ☐ 0 1 2 3   Grandfather

  ☐ 0 1 2 3   Other _____

  _____

☐ 0 1 2 3   Male: Wife/girlfriend's pregnancy

☐ 0 1 2 3   Female: Pregnancy

Serious illness or injury of close family member:

  ☐ 0 1 2 3   Father

  ☐ 0 1 2 3   Mother

  ☐ 0 1 2 3   Sister

  ☐ 0 1 2 3   Brother

  ☐ 0 1 2 3   Grandmother

  ☐ 0 1 2 3   Grandfather

  ☐ 0 1 2 3   Spouse

  ☐ 0 1 2 3   Child

  ☐ 0 1 2 3   Other _____

  _____

☐ 0 1 2 3   Trouble with in-laws

☐ 0 1 2 3   Major change in closeness of family members (decreased or increased)

☐ 0 1 2 3   Gaining a new family member (birth, adoption, member moving away)

☐ 0 1 2 3   Separation from spouse due to work, travel, school, etc.

☐ 0 1 2 3   Marital separation from mate (due to conflict)

☐ 0 1 2 3   Marital reconciliation with mate

☐ 0 1 2 3   Major change in number of arguments with spouse (a lot more, a lot fewer)

☐ 0 1 2 3   Married male: Change in wife's work outside the home (beginning work, loss of job, changing job, retirement, etc.)

☐ 0 1 2 3   Married female: Change in husband's work (beginning work, loss of job, changing job, retirement, etc.)

☐ 0 1 2 3   Male: Wife/girlfriend having abortion

☐ 0 1 2 3   Female: Having an abortion

☐ 0 1 2 3	Major change in living condition of family (new home, remodeling, damage to home, loss of home)	
☐ 0 1 2 3	Divorce	
☐ 0 1 2 3	Son or daughter leaving home	
☐ 0 1 2 3	Leaving home for first time	

Fitness/Wellness Issues

☐ 0 1 2 3	Major changes in sleeping habits (much more or much less sleep)
☐ 0 1 2 3	Major change in eating habits (much more or much less food intake)
☐ 0 1 2 3	Major personal illness or injury
☐ 0 1 2 3	Sexual difficulties

Social Issues

☐ 0 1 2 3	Detention in jail or comparable institution
☐ 0 1 2 3	Minor law violation (traffic ticket, disturbing the peace, etc.)
☐ 0 1 2 3	Death of a close friend
☐ 0 1 2 3	Change of residence (moving)
☐ 0 1 2 3	Major change in church activities (increased or decreased attendance)
☐ 0 1 2 3	Major change in usual type or amount of recreation
☐ 0 1 2 3	Major change in social activities, such as parties, movies, visiting (increased or decreased participation)

☐ 0 1 2 3	Serious injury or illness of close friend
☐ 0 1 2 3	Breaking up with boyfriend/girlfriend
☐ 0 1 2 3	Engagement
☐ 0 1 2 3	Reconciliation with boyfriend/girlfriend

Money Matters

☐ 0 1 2 3	Foreclosure on mortgage or loan
☐ 0 1 2 3	Major change in financial status (a lot better off, a lot worse off)
☐ 0 1 2 3	Borrowing more than $10,000 (buying a home, business, etc.)
☐ 0 1 2 3	Borrowing less than $10,000 (buying a car, TV, getting a school loan)

Work

☐ 0 1 2 3	New job
☐ 0 1 2 3	Changed work situation (different working conditions, working hours, etc.)
☐ 0 1 2 3	Trouble with employer (in danger of losing job, being suspended, demoted, etc.)
☐ 0 1 2 3	Being fired from job
☐ 0 1 2 3	Retirement from work

Additional Factors

Other experiences that have had a negative impact on your life in the past year.

RESULTS

Sum of negative scores: _____

Use the table below to find the rating of your score and write it here: _____

Life Experience Survey Scores

Sum of Negative Score	Interpretation	Action
< 6	Below-normal stress	None needed
6–9	Average stress	Consider improving your fitness and wellness
9–13	Above-average stress	Consider improving fitness and applying stress-reduction techniques
14 +	Much-above-average stress	Consider improving fitness, reducing stress, and seeking counseling or group support

Source: Adapted from I.G. Sarason and others, "Assessing the Impact of Life Changes: Development of the Life Experiences Survey." Journal of Consulting and Clinical Psychology 46:932–946, 1978. Copyright 1978 by the American Psychological Association.

Name: _____ Date: _____

Instructor: _____ Section: _____

Purpose: To learn to tense and then relax a sequence of muscle groups. This technique helps you identify tense muscles, release the tightness, and reduce overall feelings of stress and tension.

Directions: Individually or in a small group, practice tensing and then relaxing specific muscle groups in the sequence outlined here. Take 15 to 20 minutes to complete the whole series. Once learned, you can use PMR daily or whenever you need it to reduce stress and tension.

Position yourself: Lie down in a quiet place without distractions such as the telephone, doorbell, or people entering the room. Rest your arms comfortably along your sides.

SECTION I: GETTING READY

You may want to record the steps of PMR on a tape recorder. Some prefer to memorize the sequence of muscle groups and repeat the instructions mentally. Alternatively, ask another person to speak these instructions to you and to monitor your responses and reactions.

SECTION II: LEARN THE BASIC TECHNIQUE

For each muscle group, you will carry out the same set of actions as you lie with eyes closed:

1. As an example, focus on the toe muscles of your right foot.

2. You will isolate and tense just those muscles as you inhale to the count of 5.

3. Pause for 3 seconds, holding the tension.

4. Now release the tension in your right toe muscles as you exhale to the count of 8.

5. Finally, take a moment to feel the relaxation like a wave of warming and softening that spreads slowly. Notice the blood pulsing in the area. Notice the absence of tension.

Hint: When you isolate and tense a muscle group, be sure not to contract too tightly. This can cause cramping, especially in your toes, feet, calves, and neck.

SECTION III: REPEAT THE BASIC TECHNIQUE WITH OTHER MUSCLE GROUPS

Remember, for each group; inhale and tense for 5 seconds; hold for 3 seconds; exhale and release for 8 seconds; stop and feel the relaxation.

The suggested order of muscle groups to isolate, tense, and relax is right toes, left toes, right foot, left foot, right calf, left calf, right thigh, left thigh, whole right leg, whole left leg, abdominal muscles, chest muscles, right hand, left hand, right forearm, left forearm, right upper arm, left upper arm, whole right arm, whole left arm, both shoulders, neck, and face.

SECTION IV: REFLECTION AND EVALUATION

1. Describe any changes in sensation (seeing, hearing, etc.) or in your thinking once you finish practicing progressive muscle relaxation.

_____

_____

2. Did you find this technique difficult or easy to do? Why?

_____

_____

3. Did you feel a significant relaxation after performing some or all of this sequence? Describe the sensations.

_____

_____

LAB10.3

Name: _____ Date: _____

Instructor: _____ Section: _____

Purpose: To develop a stress-management plan that targets the key sources of stress in your life.

SECTION I: EXAMINE YOUR BEHAVIOR AND ATTITUDES

1. Enter your results from Lab 10.1 here:

Score: _____ Interpretation: _____

Action:

_____

2. Do you feel that stress is a problem in your life right now? ☐ Yes ☐ No

If you scored above average in Lab 10.1, indicating relatively high exposure to stressors and fairly high stress levels, and yet you don't see stress as an issue to address, consider your readiness for change.

SECTION II: IDENTIFY MAJOR SOURCES OF STRESS

After reviewing your entries in the Life Experiences Survey in Lab 10.1, describe your main sources of stress, grouping them into the following categories:

College _____

_____

Family _____

_____

Fitness/Wellness Issues _____

_____

Social Issues _____

_____

Money Matters _____

_____

Time-Management Issues _____

_____

SECTION III: SET REALISTIC GOALS

Use this chart to rank your top five stressors from Section II, in order of urgency. Note ways to modify or eliminate each stressor. Note stress-reduction techniques that you can apply when the stressor arises.

	Stressors	Can I Modify or Eliminate the Stressor? Y/N	Can I Reduce Stress Symptoms? Y/N
Most urgent	1.		
⇓	2.		
⇓	3.		
⇓	4.		
Least urgent	5.		

SECTION IV: DEVISE A STRATEGY AND AN ACTION PLAN

Use this section to target the most urgent source of stress in your life first, then address additional stressors as you feel ready to work on them.

1. Stressor: _____

2. Is it possible that I will need help from others? ☐ Y   ☐ N

If yes, ask yourself the following:

What professional resources are available where I live, work, or go to school? _____

_____

_____

How can I get my friends or family involved? _____

_____

3. List general strategies for modifying or eliminating environmental stressors that apply to more than one of your most urgent examples: _____

_____

4. What stress-management techniques can I use to relieve my own ongoing or recurrent symptoms of stress? (Consider relaxation breathing, progressive muscle relaxation, visual imagery, meditation, yoga, improved fitness, improved diet, better time-management skills, and enhanced spiritual connectedness.) _____

_____

5. How can I plan ahead to avoid this stressor in the future? _____

_____

6. How will I reward myself for sticking to my plan? _____

_____

SECTION V: CREATE A BEHAVIOR CHANGE CONTRACT

Use the information from Part IV to develop a behavior change contract that targets the stressor(s) you selected. The format of a basic behavior change contract appears on page 27, as well as at the front of this book.

CHAPTER 11

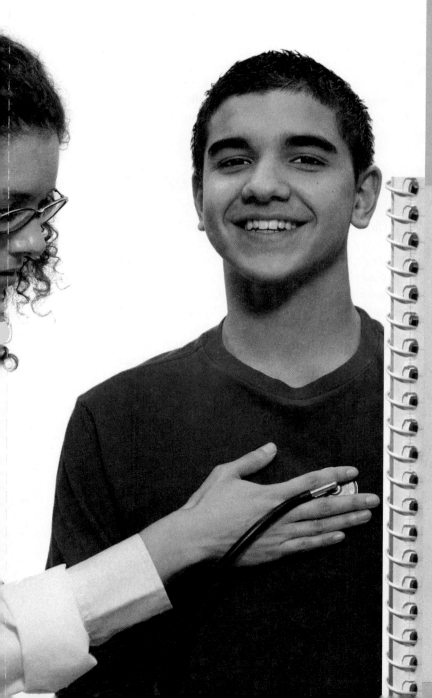

Reducing Your Risk of Cardiovascular Disease

OBJECTIVES

Identify the major forms of cardiovascular disease and describe how they affect the heart and blood vessels.

Identify cardiovascular disease risk factors that you can control.

Create a plan and apply behavior-change skills to reduce your own risk for cardiovascular disease.

CASE STUDY

Daryl

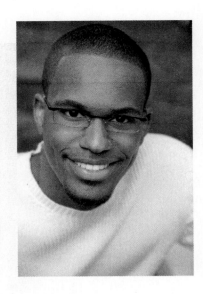

"Hi, I'm Daryl. I'm a junior, majoring in education. I'm also a jazz pianist and play at clubs around town about three times a week. I love jazz, and the gigs help me pay for tuition.

"I think I'm pretty healthy—I've never been hospitalized for anything in my life—but I do have a family history of heart disease. Both of my grandfathers died from heart attacks during their 30s. My dad died of a stroke when I was 10, and my mom is currently getting treatment for high blood pressure and high cholesterol. I know I'm still young, but given the family history, I'm worried. Are there things I can be doing to protect myself? And is there anything I can do to help my mom?"

C ardiovascular disease (CVD) is the broad term used to describe diseases of the heart and the blood vessels. CVD can bring on potentially devastating consequences, such as a heart attack or stroke, which are two of the leading causes of death in America.[1] About 9 to 15 percent of women and men under age 40 have some form of CVD (see Figure 11.1).[2] The prevalence rises to about 40 percent in middle-aged adults of both sexes and then climbs sharply after age 60, involving a large majority of older Americans.[3] Among Americans of all age groups, approximately one out of every three has some form of cardiovascular disease.[4]

WHY WORRY ABOUT CARDIOVASCULAR DISEASE?

As a college student, your most pressing concerns are probably things like getting good grades, paying tuition, and landing that first job. Cardiovascular disease is likely the furthest thing from your mind. However, it is not too early to start learning about CVD. For many people, the earliest manifestations of heart and blood vessel diseases take root during childhood and early adulthood.[5] While genetic predisposition plays an important role, lifestyle choices that you make now—such as whether or not to smoke, how often to exercise, your stress level, and what you eat—can also greatly influence your risk for developing cardiovascular disease later.

CARDIOVASCULAR DISEASE
IS AMERICA'S BIGGEST KILLER

Cardiovascular disease killed 36.3 percent of all those who died in the United States in 2004—more than any other single cause of death in America.[6] In fact, cardiovascular disease has been the leading cause of death in the U.S. every year since 1900, except in 1918, when pandemic flu killed more Americans. If we were to completely eliminate CVD in the United States, experts estimate that our life expectancy would rise by almost 7 years.[7] CVD is the leading cause of death in America for both men *and* women (see the box **Understanding Diversity: Men, Women, and Cardiovascular Disease** on page 324).

Figure 11.2 shows a breakdown of deaths resulting from heart attack, stroke, and other forms of CVD, while Figure 11.3 shows the prevalence of CVD throughout the country.

Cardiovascular disease costs Americans an estimated $438.5 billion each year, a figure that includes the costs of actual care (physicians, hospitals, nursing homes, and medications) as well as lost productivity.[8]

cardiovascular disease (CVD) A disease of the heart and/or blood vessels

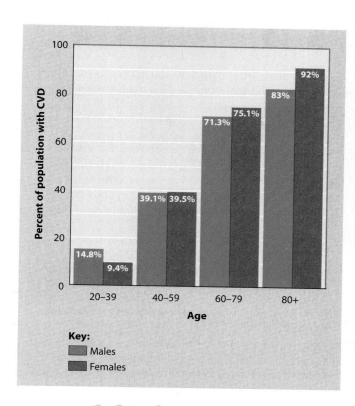

FIGURE 11.1

Prevalence of cardiovascular disease in adults aged 20 and older, by age and sex.

Source: American Heart Association, Heart Disease and Stroke Statistics 2008 Update-at-a-Glance.

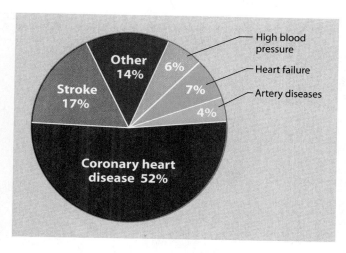

FIGURE 11.2

More people die from coronary heart disease (CHD) than from any other form of cardiovascular disease.

Source: American Heart Association, Heart Disease and Stroke Statistics 2008 Update-at-a-Glance.

FIGURE 11.3

Cardiovascular disease age-adjusted death rates by state.

Source: American Heart Association, Heart Disease and Stroke Statistics 2008 Update-at-a-Glance.

Among developed nations, eastern European countries such as Russia, Bulgaria, and Romania have the highest incidence of deaths attributed to CVD, with over 500 deaths per 100,000 population per year.[9] France, Japan, Switzerland, Spain, and Italy are at the bottom of the list, with about 200 deaths or fewer per 100,000 population. The United States is in the middle—along with countries such as England, Denmark, New Zealand, and Germany—with 300 to 400 deaths per 100,000 population per year, depending on demographic groups within the populations.[10]

CARDIOVASCULAR DISEASE CAN GREATLY DECREASE QUALITY OF LIFE

The potential of cardiovascular disease to cause death is obviously its most serious consequence, but even when it is not fatal, it can seriously impact daily life. Heart attack and stroke survivors may lose their ability to walk, talk, read, exercise, or carry out other daily activities normally. Cardiovascular disease can cause chest pain, shortness of breath, and damage to internal organs. It can also necessitate the taking of expensive drugs, which have their own negative side effects.

UNDERSTANDING DIVERSITY

MEN, WOMEN, AND CARDIOVASCULAR DISEASE

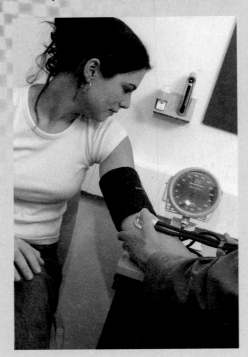

Many people are aware that cardiovascular disease is the leading cause of death in men, claiming 410,600 male victims in 2005.[1] Few people realize, however, that cardiovascular disease is the leading cause of death in women as well—and in fact kills more women than men each year. CVD claimed 459,100 female victims in 2005. This figure is higher than the number of female lives lost in 2005 due to cancer, Alzheimer's, diabetes, and accidents *combined*.[2]

Even physicians can harbor some of the same misconceptions about women and cardiovascular disease. In one study, fewer than one doctor in five knew that CVD kills more women than men each year.[3] Another study has shown that doctors are more likely to screen male patients for heart disease and make recommendations

for intervention than they are to screen or treat female patients for the same.[4]

Researchers have also found significant differences in the ways that men and women tend to express patterns and symptoms of cardiovascular disease. For example:

• Men tend to develop heart disease 10 to 15 years earlier than women. Women rarely have heart attacks before menopause (early 50s); then they show rates of CVD two or three times higher after menopause than before.

• While having a heart attack, men tend to experience the classic "squeezing" sensation in the chest, pain in the chest or arm, and/or shortness of breath. Women, however, are less likely to feel these symptoms. Instead, they are more likely to experience dizziness, nausea, and a feeling of pressure between the shoulder blades.

• Men with CVD are more likely to have heart attacks, while women with CVD are more likely to have strokes. This is perhaps based on the smaller size of blood vessels throughout the body, including the brain.[5]

• Doctors have long prescribed daily aspirin to both sexes as a way to prevent heart attacks. Recent studies, however, have shown that aspirin seems to prevent some heart attack deaths in men and some stroke deaths in women but does not seem to prevent stroke deaths in men or heart attack deaths in women.[6]

Sources:
1–2. American Heart Association, Heart Disease and Stroke Statistics, 2008 Update-at-a-Glance.
3. L. Mosca and others, "National Study of Physician Awareness and Adherence to Cardiovascular Disease Prevention Guidelines," *Circulation* 111, no. 4 (February 1, 2005): 449–510.
4. J. H. Mieres, "Review of the American Heart Association's Guidelines for Cardiovascular Disease Prevention in Women," *Heart* 92, Suppl 3 (May 2006): iii10–3.
5. T. Kurth and others, "Migraine and Risk of Cardiovascular Disease in Women," *Journal of the American Medical Association* 296, no. 3 (July 19, 2006); 283–91, Kurth and others, "Healthy Lifestyle and the Risk of Stroke in Women," *Archives of Internal Medicine* 166, no. 13 (July 10, 2006): 1403–9.
6. J. S. Berger and others, "Aspirin for the Primary Prevention of Cardiovascular Events in Women and Men: A Sex-Specific Meta-analysis of Randomized Controlled Trials," *Journal of the American Medical Association* 295, no. 3 (January 18, 2006): 306–13.

One form of CVD, **hypertension** (high blood pressure), may cause cognitive declines—especially in processing speed—and may even predispose a person to dementia later in life.[11] High blood pressure can begin in one's 20s or 30s (even earlier in some cases) and is common by the time people reach their 40s and 50s.[12]

hypertension Sustained high blood pressure

CARDIOVASCULAR DISEASE
CAN BEGIN EARLY IN LIFE

Cardiovascular disease can begin in adolescence or earlier.[13] Studying blood vessel tissue from 3,000 young people between the ages of 15 and 34 who had died of accidents, homicides, or suicides, researchers found glistening streaks of fat and fatty, waxy buildup in some of the vessel specimens—deposits that marked the unmistakable beginnings of cardiovascular disease. The researchers found

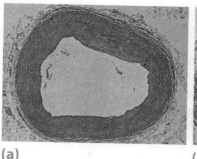
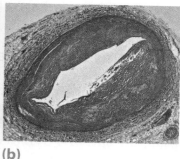

FIGURE 11.4

(a) Cross section of a normal coronary artery.
(b) A coronary artery narrowed by plaque.

(a)   (b)

early signs of CVD in 2 percent of males aged 15 to 19. They also observed advanced markers of CVD in 20 percent of 30- to 34-year-old males, and 8 percent of females in the same age group. In examining the subjects' health records, the researchers found evidence of the same kinds of habits that contribute to cardiovascular disease in middle-aged and older adults—including smoking, poor diet, lack of exercise, and high body mass index.[14]

HOW DOES
CARDIOVASCULAR DISEASE AFFECT THE BODY?

Learning about how cardiovascular disease affects the body is useful for understanding why it causes the symptoms that it does, as well as what you can do to keep your cardiovascular system healthy.

CARDIOVASCULAR DISEASE
AFFECTS THE HEART AND BLOOD VESSELS

Your body contains trillions of living cells, all needing a continuous supply of oxygen and energy compounds. The circulatory system—the heart and blood vessels—does the critical work of delivering that oxygen and energy to your cells. It also removes carbon dioxide and other wastes *from* your cells. To review the anatomy of the circulatory system, see Chapter 4.

In a healthy 10-year-old, the heart is almost adult size. The blood vessel walls are smooth inside and out. The walls of the arteries are strong and elastic, while the walls of the veins are thinner and more fixed in diameter. The long narrow opening down the middle of each vessel is clear and free-flowing. The ventricles fill smoothly and forcibly push blood out. Tight-closing *valves* help prevent blood from flowing backward. The circulating blood reaches all the distant capillary beds in the brain, limbs, kidneys, skin, and other organs, then returns quickly through the venous system.

Starting at age 10 or even earlier, however, changes can accumulate in the blood vessels that diminish the distribution of oxygenated blood and the removal of carbon dioxide and other wastes from body cells. This condition is known as **atherosclerosis** (from the Greek words "athero," meaning gruel, and "sclerosis," meaning hardness.) Both lifestyle and genetic factors can allow a sludgelike layer of fatty, waxy debris to accumulate inside arteries and smaller arterioles, narrowing their inner channels. This narrowing is called **arterial stenosis.** Minute injuries to the inner walls of arteries can also allow pinpoint areas of accumulation called **plaques** to build at the injury sites, grow larger, and bulge inward. Plaques can eventually grow large enough to block or occlude blood passage through the vessel (see Figure 11.4) or even cause the vessel to rupture. The buildup process can take decades, but early signs of atherosclerosis can start in childhood, especially in the overweight and obese.[15]

Arteries with a narrowed channel or bulging side-wall plaques transport less blood and are stiffer and less flexible. Just as the pressure builds up in a hose if you prevent normal water flow with your thumb, channel narrowing and plaque buildup can increase pressure within the blood vessels. High blood pressure (or hypertension, as mentioned earlier) is technically a form of cardiovascular disease, in and of itself. It is also a contributor to other forms of

atherosclerosis Hardening or stiffening of the arteries as plaque accumulates at injury sites in the inner linings of arteries

arterial stenosis A narrowing of the inner channel of arteries and smaller arterioles due to the buildup of a sludgelike layer of fatty, waxy debris

plaque A pinpoint area of fatty, waxy debris that accumulates at a site (usually of an injury) along the inner wall of an artery or arteriole. As immune system cells and inflammation enlarge the mass, plaque can pile up, bulge inward, and partially or fully block blood flow through the channel.

CVD, as it can cause blood vessel damage and promote the development of plaques.

Symptoms of Cardiovascular Disease

It is possible to have cardiovascular disease and experience no symptoms. When symptoms *are* present, they usually reflect the response of organs or tissues to oxygen deprivation and a dearth of energy compounds. People with CVD can feel fatigue, chest pain, chest tightness, or shortness of breath. Occluded or damaged vessels in the arms and legs can result in numbness or pain in those extremities; in the kidneys or eyes, they can cause organ failure or vision loss, respectively. Blocked arteries in or to the brain can lead to dizziness, headaches, and double vision. If a blockage or rupture triggers a stroke, the result can be damaged brain tissue and loss of function.

CARDIOVASCULAR DISEASE TAKES MANY FORMS

Table 11.1 identifies the most common forms of cardiovascular disease and their prevalence in American adults. Let's look at each of these forms of CVD in detail.

Hypertension

Hypertension, or sustained high blood pressure, is the most common form of cardiovascular disease. It is also considered a risk factor for other forms of CVD. About one-third of all Americans have hypertension.[16] Many are unaware of having the condition, causing experts to refer to it as a "silent killer."

Hypertension can result from consuming too much sodium in the diet, leading to water retention and increased blood volume. As mentioned earlier, arterial stenosis and plaque deposits can increase resistance to blood flow throughout the circulatory system and can cause blood pressure to rise. Other causes of hypertension include kidney or heart abnormalities, aging, inherited tendencies, obesity, sleep apnea, stress, or certain kinds of tumors.

A blood pressure device can help diagnose hypertension. Such devices measure your blood pressure in two parts, expressed as a fraction—for example, 120/80. Both values are measured in millimeters

systolic pressure The pressure being applied to the walls of the arteries when the heart contracts

diastolic pressure The pressure applied to the walls of the arteries during the heart's relaxation phase

TABLE 11.1

Major Types of Cardiovascular Disease and Prevalence of Each

Type of Cardiovascular Disease	Prevalence in the United States
Hypertension	73 million
Coronary heart disease (including heart attack)	16 million
Angina pectoris	9 million
Arrhythmia	Over 2.2 million
Congestive heart failure	5 million
Congenital heart disease	One out of every 1,000 live births
Stroke	780,000 new or recurrent cases of stroke each year

Data from the American Heart Association, Heart Disease and Stroke Statistics, 2008 Update-at-a-Glance.

of mercury (mm Hg). The first number refers to **systolic pressure,** or the pressure being applied to the walls of the arteries when the heart contracts, pumping blood to the rest of the body. The second value is **diastolic pressure,** or the pressure applied to the walls of the arteries during the heart's relaxation phase. During this phase, blood is reentering the heart's chambers, preparing for the next heartbeat.

Normal blood pressure varies, depending on weight, age, physical condition, gender, and ethnic background. Systolic blood pressure tends to increase with age, while diastolic blood pressure tends to increase until age 55, and then decline. Generally, men have a greater risk for high blood pressure than women until age 55; at that point, the risks become about equal. After age 75, women are more likely to have high blood pressure than men.[17]

For the "average" person, normal systolic blood pressure is less than 120, and normal diastolic blood pressure is less than 80.[18] A physician may diagnose *prehypertension* or the potential beginnings of hypertension when systolic pressure is between 120 and 139 and diastolic pressure is between 80 and 89. *High blood pressure* (HBP) is usually diagnosed when systolic pressure is 140 or above and diastolic pressure is 90 or above (although the latter reading may not necessarily be elevated). When only systolic pressure is high, the condition is known as *isolated*

TABLE 11.2

Blood Pressure Readings

Classification	Systolic Reading (mm Hg)	Diastolic Reading (mm Hg)
Normal	< 120	< 80
Prehypertension	120–139	80–89
Hypertension		
Stage 1	140–159	90–99
Stage 2	≥ 160	≥ 100

Note: If systolic and diastolic readings fall into different categories, treatment is determined by the highest category. Readings are based on the average of two or more properly measured, seated readings on each of two or more health care provider visits.

Source: National Heart, Lung, and Blood Institute, *Seventh Report of the Joint National Committee on Prevention, Detection, Evaluation, and Treatment of High Blood Pressure* (NIH Publication No. 03-5233) (Bethesda, MD: National Institutes of Health, May 2003).

systolic hypertension (ISH), the most common form of high blood pressure in older Americans. If your blood pressure exceeds 140/90, you need to work with your physician to lower it through diet, exercise, stress reduction, and prescription drugs. Table 11.2 presents a summary of blood pressure values.

Atherosclerosis As discussed earlier, *atherosclerosis* describes a thickening and hardening of the arteries. Plaque contains fatty and waxy compounds, cholesterol, cellular waste products, calcium, and natural blood-clotting agents. Things that can "nick" the inner linings of arteries (causing the damage that can lead to plaque buildup) include hypertension and chemicals in alcohol or tobacco. High levels of cholesterol intake and the presence of other fats in the blood also contribute to plaque buildup.

In recent years, medical researchers have studied the role of *inflammation* in atherosclerosis. Inflammation is an immune response that causes redness and swelling in response to injury. Researchers think that LDL (low-density lipoprotein) cholesterol, cigarette smoking, hypertension, diabetes mellitus, and disease-causing bacteria may all promote inflammation. The most likely infectious agents are *Chlamydia pneumoniae* (a sexually transmitted infection), *Helicobacter pylori* (which causes ulcers), herpes simplex virus (which the majority of Americans are exposed to by the age of 5), and cytomegalovirus (another herpes virus transmitted through body fluids and infecting most Americans before the age of 40).

During an inflammatory reaction, researchers can often detect high levels of two or more substances. One is a set of proteins called *C-reactive proteins* (CRPs), the other is an amino acid called *homocysteine*. These substances may inflame the inner linings of arteries and promote plaque deposits and blood-clot formation. At the very least, their presence is an indicator of inflammation. In the near future, physicians may be able to order sensitive tests that detect CRPs and homocysteine as markers of atherosclerosis.[19] Lifestyle changes such as regular exercise, weight management, non-smoking, moderation of alcohol intake, and eating less saturated fat and cholesterol appear to reduce inflammation and its markers in the blood.

Coronary Heart Disease When atherosclerosis occurs in the heart's main blood vessels, it is called **coronary artery disease (CAD)** or **coronary heart disease (CHD).** When it occurs in the feet, ankles, calves, hands, or forearms, it is called *peripheral artery disease.* Of all the types of cardiovascular disease, CHD is the greatest killer. An estimated 1.2 million Americans will suffer a coronary attack this year, and over 450,000 will die.[20]

A heart attack, also called a **myocardial infarction (MI),** involves an area of the heart that suffers permanent damage after its normal blood supply has been blocked. The blockage can be caused by a blood clot in a coronary artery or by atherosclerotic narrowing. When blood flow slows dramatically or stops, the surrounding tissue is deprived of oxygen. If the blockage is extremely minor, an otherwise healthy heart will adapt over time as small blood vessels reroute needed blood through other areas.

When heart blockage is more severe, a person can experience the symptoms of a heart attack and will require life-saving support. The box **Spotlight: In the Event of a Heart Attack, Stroke, or Cardiac Arrest** describes how you should respond if you recognize such symptoms in someone else or yourself.

coronary artery disease (CAD) Atherosclerosis (the buildup of plaque deposits) in the main arteries that supply oxygen and other materials to the heart muscle. Also called **coronary heart disease (CHD)**

myocardial infarction (MI) Medical term for a heart attack; involves permanent damage to an area of the heart muscle brought on by a cessation of normal blood supply

SPOTLIGHT

IN THE EVENT OF A HEART ATTACK, STROKE, OR CARDIAC ARREST

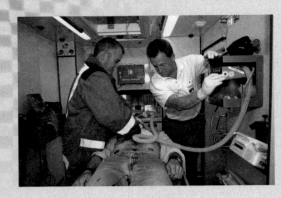

Knowing how to act in a cardiovascular emergency could save a friend's life—or your own.

WARNING SIGNS OF A HEART ATTACK

- Uncomfortable pressure, fullness, squeezing, or pain in the center of the chest, lasting 2 minutes or longer
- Jaw pain and/or shortness of breath
- Pain spreading to the shoulders, neck, or arms
- Dizziness, fatigue, fainting, sweating, and/or nausea

Not all of these warning signs occur in every heart attack. For instance, a woman's heart attack may show up as shortness of breath, fatigue, and jaw pain, stretched out over hours rather than minutes. If any of these symptoms appear, don't wait. Get help immediately!

WARNING SIGNS OF A STROKE

- Sudden numbness or weakness, especially on one side of the body. Can affect face, arm, and/or leg
- Sudden mental confusion, especially trouble speaking or understanding words
- Sudden vision problems in one or both eyes
- Sudden dizziness, loss of balance, lack of coordination, or trouble walking
- Sudden severe headache without apparent cause

WARNING SIGNS OF A CARDIAC ARREST

- Sudden loss of responsiveness (won't respond if tapped on either shoulder)
- Stops normal breathing (tilt head up; check for breathing for 5 seconds)

KNOW WHAT TO DO BEFORE AN EMERGENCY STRIKES

- Find out which hospitals in your area have 24-hour emergency cardiac care.
- Determine (in advance) the hospital or medical facility that is nearest your home and office, and tell your family and friends to call this facility in an emergency.
- Keep a list of emergency rescue service numbers next to your telephone and in your pocket, wallet, or purse. Remember 911 if you don't have time to call emergency rescue numbers.
- If you have chest or jaw discomfort that lasts more than 2 minutes, call the emergency rescue service or 911. Do not drive yourself to the hospital unless there is no other alternative.

BE A LIFESAVER DURING A CRISIS

- If you are with someone who is showing signs of a heart attack, stroke, or cardiac arrest and the warning signs last for 2 minutes or longer, act immediately.
- Expect a denial. It is normal for a person with chest discomfort to deny the possibility of anything as serious as a heart attack. Don't take no for an answer. Insist on taking prompt action.
- Call 911 or an emergency rescue service, or get to the nearest hospital emergency room that offers 24-hour emergency cardiac care.
- Give CPR (mouth-to-mouth breathing and chest compression) if necessary and if you are properly trained.
- An automated external defibrillator may save a person during cardiac arrest.

Source: American Heart Association, "Heart Attack, Stroke, and Cardiac Arrest Warning Signs," www.americanheart.org/, August 22, 2006.

---

ischemia A damaging reduction in the blood (and therefore the oxygen supply) to a region of the heart, brain, or other organ

angina pectoris Chest pain due to ischemia, or reduction in blood flow to the heart muscle and surrounding tissues

Angina Pectoris Atherosclerosis and other circulatory impairments often reduce the heart's blood and oxygen supply and cause a condition called **ischemia.** People with ischemia often suffer from varying degrees of chest pain, also called **angina pectoris.** The American Heart Association estimates that over 9 million Americans suffer from angina.[21] Many people experience short episodes of angina whenever they exert themselves physically. Symptoms may range from slight indigestion to a feeling that the heart is being crushed. Generally, the more serious the oxygen deprivation, the more severe the pain.

Doctors currently use several methods of treating angina. In mild cases, they prescribe rest. To treat more serious chest pain, they may recommend nitroglycerin tablets to relax veins and lessen the heart's workload. Calcium channel blockers can also relieve angina caused by spasms of the coronary arteries. Drugs called *beta blockers* can control potential overactivity of the heart muscle.

Arrhythmias

An **arrhythmia,** or irregular heartbeat, is relatively common: Over 2.2 million Americans experience it each year.[22] The disturbance of heartbeat rhythm can take several forms: a racing heart in the absence of exercise or anxiety (called *tachycardia*); an abnormally slow heartbeat (called *bradycardia*); or a sporadic, quivering pattern called **fibrillation.** Fibrillation renders the heart extremely inefficient at pumping blood through the vessels. If a fibrillation incident or series of incidents go untreated, the condition may be fatal. Even without cardiovascular disease, you may feel heart arrhythmias from drinking too much caffeine or from the nicotine in tobacco. Mild cases like this are seldom life-threatening. If you develop a severe case due to disease, you may require drug therapy or a pacemaker.

Congestive Heart Failure

Over 5 million Americans suffer from **congestive heart failure (CHF).**[23] In CHF, the heart muscle is damaged or overworked, the pumping chambers are often taxed to the limit, and the heart lacks the strength to keep blood circulating normally through the body. Damage to the heart muscle can result from pneumonia, heart attack, other cardiovascular problems, or even treatments for cancer. The weakened heart pumps less blood out through the arteries. As a result, the "return" blood can't flow back through the veins to the heart in normal amounts. As the blood begins to back up, it causes congestion in body tissues. Blood pooling enlarges the heart, making it even less efficient, and fluid accumulates in the legs, ankles, or lungs, where it can cause swelling or difficulty in breathing.

Congestive heart failure can be fatal if untreated, but most cases respond well to drug treatment. Diuretics (water pills) increase urination and reduce fluid accumulation, drugs such as digitalis increase

the heart's pumping action, and vasodilators expand blood vessels so blood can flow through more easily and reduce the heart's workload.

Congenital Heart Disease

Congenital heart disease, meaning heart disease present at birth, affects 9 out of every 1,000 live births.[24] A baby may be born with a slight *heart murmur,* an audible sound based on an irregular heart valve that allows turbulent blood flow through the heart. Some children outgrow such heart murmurs and have no further problems. Others, however, can have more serious congenital irregularities with heart anatomy or function that require surgical repair. Causes may include hereditary factors, a mother's case of rubella or certain other infections during pregnancy, or the mother's use of alcohol or drugs during fetal development. Advances in treatment have been continually improving the prospects for children with congenital heart defects.

Stroke

We saw that a heart attack can occur when a blocked vessel prevents a region of the heart from getting enough oxygenated blood. In a similar way, a **stroke** is a sudden loss of function in a region of the brain caused by blockage in or rupture of a blood vessel, leading to oxygen deprivation and cell damage or death. *Ischemic* strokes are the result of a plaque-blocked vessel or a floating blood clot that lodges in a vessel and cuts off blood supply to a brain region. *Hemorrhagic* strokes occur when a blood vessel bursts, spilling oxygenated blood rather than transporting it to a distal brain region, allowing that unsupplied area to become damaged through oxygen deprivation. Atherosclerosis, heart

---

arrhythmia Irregular heartbeat; can involve abnormally fast or slow heartbeat or the disorganized, sporadic beat of fibrillation

fibrillation A sporadic, quivering heartbeat pattern that results in very inefficient pumping of blood

congestive heart failure (CHF) A cardiovascular disease in which the heart muscle is damaged or overworked, the pumping chambers are often taxed to the limit, and the heart lacks the strength to keep blood circulating normally through the body

congenital heart disease Heart disease present at birth

stroke A sudden loss of function in a region of the brain caused by blockage in or rupture of a blood vessel, leading to oxygen deprivation, cell damage, or death

disease, congestive heart failure, hypertension, smoking, diabetes, and other factors can all contribute to triggering strokes.[25]

Some strokes are mild and cause only temporary dizziness or slight weakness or numbness. If an affected area is large or is in a crucial part of the brain, stroke may cause speech impairments, memory problems, loss of motor control, or death. Stroke killed 150,147 Americans in 2004 and is the third leading cause of death after heart disease and cancer.[26] Each year, about 780,000 people experience a new or recurrent stroke—that's about one person every 40 seconds.[27]

About 1 in 10 major strokes is preceded days, weeks, or months earlier by *transient ischemic attacks (TIAs)*, brief interruptions of the blood supply to the brain that cause only temporary dizziness, weakness, paralysis, numbness, or other symptoms. Deaths due to strokes have decreased in recent years, thanks to better diagnosis, better surgical options, new clot-busting drugs that can be injected immediately after a stroke has occurred, and better aftercare for stroke patients. Campaigns to teach awareness and avoidance of risk factors could prevent up to half of annual strokes if people followed them carefully.

WHAT ARE THE MAIN RISK FACTORS FOR CARDIOVASCULAR DISEASE?

The prevalence of cardiovascular disease is an unfortunate reality. However, many risk factors are controllable. By identifying which controllable risks you may have (see *Lab11.1*), you can learn to modify risk-promoting behaviors and lower your chances of developing a CVD.

RISKS YOU CAN CONTROL

Experts have identified at least 10 significant risk factors for CVD: tobacco use, hypertension, high blood fats, obesity/overweight, physical inactivity, type 2 diabetes, metabolic syndrome, heavy alcohol consumption, poor diet, and uncontrolled stress. Since lifestyle choices underlie many of these risk factors, changes to daily habits can often reduce the chances of developing cardiovascular disease. Many people have multiple risk factors for CVD; the more risk factors they have, the greater their chances of experiencing a heart attack, stroke, angina, atherosclerosis, and other specific forms of CVD.[28] Let's look at each of these risk factors more closely.

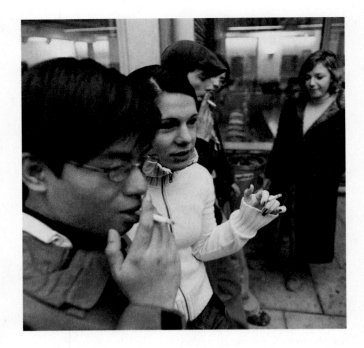

Tobacco Use In 1964, the Surgeon General of the United States asserted that smoking was the greatest risk factor for heart disease. Today, more than one in five deaths from CVD are directly related to smoking. The risk for cardiovascular disease is 70 percent greater for smokers than for nonsmokers. Smokers who have a heart attack are more likely to die suddenly (within 1 hour) than are nonsmokers. Evidence also indicates that an estimated 35,052 *non*smokers die from cardiovascular disease each year as a result of chronic exposure to environmental tobacco smoke.[29]

How does tobacco use damage the cardiovascular system? Researchers have several plausible explanations. One is that the nicotine in all forms of tobacco (cigarettes, cigars, chewing tobacco, etc.) increases heart rate, heart output, blood pressure, and oxygen use by the heart muscle. Another is that cigarette smoke is filled with carbon monoxide, which displaces oxygen in heart tissue, requiring a smoker's heart to work harder to obtain enough oxygen. Chemicals in smoke can cause injuries to arteries that lead to both plaque formation and inflammation. Finally, smokers have a higher level of a natural blood-clotting factor, and these increased levels may contribute to the blood clots that trigger heart attacks and strokes.[30]

Hypertension We have seen that hypertension can damage artery walls and lead to atherosclerosis. It can also weaken artery walls and lead to an *aneurysm*, an abnormal, blood-filled bulge in a blood vessel that has the potential to rupture.

Hypertension can damage coronary arteries, enlarge the heart, or weaken the heart muscle. By affecting blood vessels in the brain, hypertension can cause strokes and TIAs, promote dementia, and impair cognitive functioning. By damaging delicate blood vessels in the kidneys or eyes, hypertension can lead to kidney damage or failure, or to impaired vision or vision loss. In addition, hypertension can reduce sexual function, disrupt sleep, and magnify the bone loss of osteoporosis.[31] Reducing dietary sodium, blood fats, and excess weight can help lower blood pressure, as can managing stress and taking certain prescription drugs. For unknown reasons, increasing numbers of young adults (particularly males) seem to be experiencing hypertension.[32]

High Levels of Blood Fats
Hyperlipidemia—or high levels of cholesterol, triglycerides, and other fats in the blood—is correlated with increased risk of several cardiovascular diseases. According to a report by the National Heart, Lung, and Blood Institute, nearly 36 million people in the United States—one-fifth of all adults—have such high blood cholesterol levels that they require medications to avoid cardiovascular problems.[33] Unfortunately, many of these medications carry significant risks of their own. Additionally, many people use these medications as "crutches" and continue to eat high fat foods, assuming that the medications will keep any risks from CVD at bay.

Diets high in saturated or *trans* fats can raise blood cholesterol levels and contribute to atherosclerosis. They can also switch on the body's blood-clotting system, making the blood thicker and stickier. All of these blood changes increase the risk of heart attack or stroke.

Increases in blood cholesterol can also contribute to hardening of the arteries or atherosclerosis with its long-term effects on CVD. Table 11.3 shows recommended levels for blood cholesterol. People with several risk factors for CVD should follow the most stringent range of the guidelines.[34]

Total cholesterol levels are just one measure of cardiovascular disease risks. Another is the ratio of "bad" to "good" cholesterol. Low-density lipoprotein (LDL), often referred to as "bad" cholesterol, is believed to contribute to plaque buildup on artery walls. However, high-density lipoprotein (HDL), or "good" cholesterol, appears to remove plaque from artery walls, thus serving as a protector. In theory, if LDL levels get too high relative to HDL levels, plaque will tend to accumulate inside arteries and lead to cardiovascular problems. The LDL/HDL ratio can increase because of too much saturated fat

TABLE 11.3

LDL, Total, and HDL Cholesterol (mg/dL) Levels for Adults

LDL Cholesterol

< 100	Optimal
100–129	Near optimal/above optimal
130–159	Borderline high
160–189	High
= 190	Very high

Total Cholesterol

< 200	Desirable
200–239	Borderline high
= 240	High

HDL Cholesterol

< 40	Low
≥ 60	Desirable

Triglycerides

< 150	Normal
150–199	Borderline high
200–499	High
= 500	Very high

Source: National Heart, Lung, and Blood Institute, "Detection, Evaluation, and Treatment of High Blood Cholesterol in Adults" (NIH Publication No. 02-5215), 2002.

in the diet, lack of exercise, high stress levels, or genetic predisposition.

It can be useful to obtain an accurate assessment of your total cholesterol and LDL and HDL levels. This analysis requires a fasting blood test (no eating or drinking for 12 hours prior to the test) administered by a reputable health provider. You can compare your numbers to Table 11.3 and discuss their significance with your physician. In general, the best method of evaluating risk from blood cholesterol is to examine the ratio of HDL to total cholesterol, or the percentage of HDL in total cholesterol. If the HDL level is lower than 35, the risk increases dramatically.

A second type of blood fat called *triglycerides* also appears to promote atherosclerosis. As people get older, heavier, or both, their triglyceride and cholesterol levels tend to rise. No one has yet proved that high triglyceride levels cause atherosclerosis and thus underlie CVD. However, these blood fats may contribute to faster plaque development.

Overweight and Obesity

Being overweight or obese can strain the heart, forcing it to push blood through "extra" miles of capillaries that supply each pound of fat. A heart that must continuously move blood through an overabundance of vessels has to work harder and may become weakened or damaged. The same high-fat, high-sugar, and high-calorie diets that lead to overweight and obesity can also contribute to plaque formation.

Overweight people are more likely to develop heart disease and stroke even if they have no other CVD risk factors.[35] Losing even 5 to 10 pounds can make a significant difference to CVD risk. This is especially true for people who tend to store fat around the upper body and waist (an "apple" shape) as opposed to those who tend to store fat around the hips and thighs (a "pear" shape.) Men tend to have "apple" shapes and women "pear" shapes, but there are many exceptions.

Physical Inactivity

A sedentary lifestyle is one of the largest risk factors for CVD. Elevating the heart rate and blood flow through moderate to vigorous activity benefits the heart muscle and helps prevent plaque deposits on artery walls. Conversely, inactivity decreases the efficiency of the heart muscle and allows plaque buildup to occur more easily. Even modest levels of low-intensity physical activity—walking, gardening, housework, dancing—are beneficial if done regularly and over the long term. Despite the clear benefits of regular exercise, only 30.9 percent of Americans over age 18 engage in any regular physical activity.[36]

Diabetes Mellitus

The interrelated nature of chronic diseases is especially clear when it comes to diabetes and cardiovascular disease. Diabetes significantly increases one's risk for CVD even if blood sugar levels are well controlled. When uncontrolled, the risks are even higher. At least 65 percent of people with diabetes mellitus die from some form of CVD.[37] In fact, the risk is so great, many physicians consider someone with pre-diabetes or early diabetes to have the same risks as someone who has already had their first heart attack. Because overweight people have a higher risk for diabetes, it can be difficult to separate the effects of the two conditions. Diabetics also tend to have elevated blood fat levels, increased atherosclerosis, and a tendency toward deterioration of small blood vessels, particularly in the eyes and extremities.

Metabolic Syndrome

Metabolic syndrome refers to a cluster of obesity-related risk factors associated with CVD and type 2 diabetes.[38] A common characteristic of patients with metabolic syndrome is abdominal obesity or a large waistline (more than 40 inches in men or 35 inches in women). People with metabolic syndrome also have elevated blood fats, low levels of "good cholesterol" (HDLs), hypertension, and high blood sugar. An estimated 47 million American adults have metabolic syndrome.[39] By definition, they have multiple risk factors for CVD, and thus their overall risk of developing cardiovascular illness is high.

Other Controllable Factors

Stress can act as a risk factor for CVD. Your body's stress response can cause blood pressure to rise and can trigger blood-clotting and heart rhythm abnormalities. Stress can also foster habits that promote CVD, such as overeating or smoking. One person in five appears to have an exaggerated cardiovascular reaction to stressful stimulation.[40]

Poor nutrition also increases CVD risk. Too much saturated fat, salt, and refined carbohydrates, and too little fiber and too few fruits and vegetables all heighten risk, while improved nutrition lowers risk.

Although some studies have suggested that *moderate* amounts of alcohol may help lower the risk of cardiovascular disease, excessive alcohol consumption can raise blood triglycerides, trigger arrhythmias, raise blood pressure, promote obesity,

CASE STUDY

Daryl

"I took my mom in for a checkup the other day. The good news is that her blood pressure and cholesterol have both come down since her last visit. While I was sitting in the waiting room, though, I read a brochure about risk factors for heart disease. I knew genetics was a factor, but I was surprised at how many other risk factors I had: not being very active (unless you count playing the piano!), breathing in other people's smoke at jazz clubs, too much fast food, and stress."

1. What else could Daryl do to assess his risk for cardiovascular disease?

2. What risk factors for cardiovascular disease do you have? Which ones are controllable? How could you change your lifestyle to reduce them?

and contribute to heart failure and strokes. Stimulant drugs, such as amphetamines or cocaine, can also trigger strokes—even in young people.[41]

RISKS YOU CANNOT CONTROL

Unfortunately, not all risk factors for cardiovascular disease are controllable. Such factors include the following:

Heredity A family history of cardiovascular disease—that is, CVD in several generations of an extended family—appears to increase risk significantly. Researchers are unsure whether the increase is due to genetics, to the environment in which you were raised (including diet, exercise, and stress levels), or both.

Age Seventy-five percent of all heart attacks occur in people over age 65. The risk for CVD increases with age for both sexes.

Gender Men are at greater risk for CVD until about age 60. Women under 35 have a fairly low risk unless they have high blood pressure, kidney problems, or diabetes. Being a smoker while using oral contraceptives also increase a woman's risk. Hormonal factors appear to protect women before menopause; after menopause or after estrogen levels decline due to hysterectomy or ovary disease, a woman's LDL levels tend to rise and with them, the chances of developing cardiovascular disease.

Race Members of certain racial/ethnic groups may be susceptible to increased cardiovascular disease risk. Among Caucasian Americans, 37.2 percent of men and 35 percent of women have CVD.[42] Among African Americans, 44.6 percent of men and 49 percent of women have CVD. Among Mexican Americans, 31.6 percent of men and 34.4 percent of women have CVD. Rates for Asian Americans are below 25 percent (see Figure 11.5).[43]

HOW CAN YOU AVOID CARDIOVASCULAR DISEASE?

People often wait until they get a scary medical diagnosis before changing their habits. If you have risk factors for cardiovascular disease, the earlier you confront them, the better your chances of avoiding CVD later.

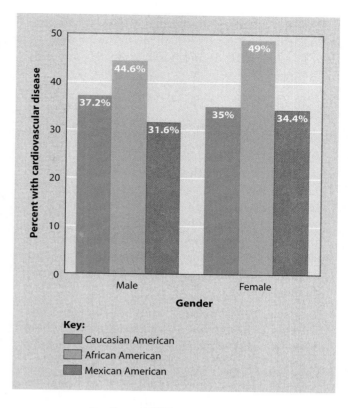

FIGURE 11.5

Cardiovascular disease affects a disproportionate percentage of African Americans.

Data from Heart Disease and Stroke Statistics 2008 Update-at-a-Glance. Comparable data on Hispanic American and Asian American populations were not available in this report.

LOWER YOUR CONTROLLABLE RISKS

Here are specific behavioral tips for avoiding cardiovascular disease by reducing the risk factors you can control.

Don't Use Tobacco According to the American Heart Association, smoking is the greatest preventable cause of disease and death. Even light smoking—just two cigarettes per day—increases your CVD risk. When people stop smoking, regardless of how long or how much they have smoked, their risk of heart disease declines rapidly. Three years after quitting, the risk of death from heart disease and stroke for people who smoked a pack a day or less is almost the same as for people who never smoked. Women appear to recover lung function more fully than men.[44] Since secondhand smoke is a potent risk factor, avoid smoky places when possible. Avoid all forms of tobacco, since nicotine increases blood pressure, heart rate, blood clotting, and plaque buildup.

Eat Well There are numerous ways you can promote cardiovascular health through better nutrition. The American Heart Association recommends the following:[48]

- Aim to use up at least as many calories as you consume.

- Eat a wide variety of foods from all the basic food groups.

- Aim to have a diet that consists of mainly nutrient-rich foods such as vegetables, fruits, and whole-grain products. Fruits and vegetables are high in vitamins, minerals, and fiber, and are low in calories. Meanwhile, the fiber in unrefined whole-grain foods can help lower cholesterol and help you feel full (which can help with weight management).

- Eat fish at least twice a week. The omega-3 fatty acids in fish such as salmon and trout may help lower the risk of death from coronary artery disease.

- Consume lean meats without skin, and cook them without added saturated and *trans* fat.

- Consume fat-free, 1 percent fat, and low-fat dairy products.

- Reduce your consumption of foods containing partially hydrogenated vegetable oils to lower the amount of *trans* fat in your diet.

- Cut back on foods high in dietary cholesterol. Aim to eat less than 300 milligrams of cholesterol each day.

- Cut back on beverages and foods with added sugars.

- Reduce your intake of sodium to 2,300 milligrams or less per day. People with elevated blood pressure should cut back to 1,500 milligrams or less per day.

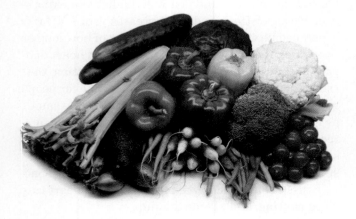

- Drink alcohol in moderation.

- Be aware of portion sizes, especially while dining out.

If you have (or are at risk of developing) hypertension, your physician may suggest that you adopt the DASH (Dietary Approaches to Stop Hypertension) diet. Following this diet can help lessen your risk of hypertension and other forms of cardiovascular disease. The box **Tools for Change: The DASH Diet** discusses the diet's specific recommendations.

Exercise Regularly Regular cardiovascular exercise strengthens the heart muscles and helps keep the blood vessels resilient. Performing 30 to 60 minutes or more of moderate activity most days of the week will help prevent cardiovascular disease, especially if you reach your *target heart rate* (see page 85). Strength training and flexibility are also important components of your exercise plan for cardiovascular wellness, helping you to maintain muscle mass, speed metabolism, control weight, and prevent injury.

Manage Your Stress The physiological stress response raises blood pressure, speeds the heart rate, and floods the bloodstream with glucose. All of these, in turn, can promote cardiovascular disease by damaging the blood vessels and directly contributing to atherosclerosis, and by weakening the heart through electrical and hormonal overstimulation. Learning specific techniques for stress reduction, relaxation, and anger management can give you important tools for lowering your risk of cardiovascular disease.

Control Diabetes Because elevated sugar levels in the blood greatly increase the risk for heart disease, stroke, and artery disease, people with diabetes are at tremendous risk. The very factors that contribute to the development of diabetes (obesity, hypertension, elevated blood cholesterol and triglycerides, inactivity) are additional risks for CVD and help explain why three-quarters of all diabetics die of heart disease, stroke, or vessel deterioration, particularly in the eyes and extremities. Recent National Institutes of Health guidelines underscore the unique CVD risks for people with diabetes, especially those who have taken insulin for several years. Careful diet, increased exercise, and medication help most diabetics lower their CVD risk.

Avoid Alcohol and Drug Abuse If you drink, keep your consumption below one drink per day for women and two per day for men. Greater

THE DASH DIET

The DASH (Dietary Approaches to Stop Hypertension) diet is a set of nutritional guidelines designed to reduce blood pressure.[1] Recommended by the National Heart, Lung, and Blood Institute and the American Heart Association, it is characterized by the following:

- Reduced consumption of saturated fat, total fat, red meats, sodium, sweets, added sugars, and sugar-containing beverages

- Increased consumption of fruits, vegetables, fat-free or low-fat dairy products, whole-grain foods, fish, poultry, and nuts

- Special care to consume recommended levels of potassium, magnesium, calcium, protein, and fiber

A person on the DASH diet who eats about 2,100 calories per day would follow the nutrient goals summarized below:[2]

Total Fat	27% of Calories
Saturated fat	6% of calories
Protein	18% of calories
Carbohydrate	55% of calories
Cholesterol	150 mg
Sodium	2,300 mg (1,500 for older individuals or those with hypertension)
Potassium	4,700 mg
Calcium	1,250 mg
Magnesium	500 mg
Fiber	30 gm

The diet also provides daily serving recommendations for various food groups.[3] People eating 1,600 or 2,600 calories per day would aim for these amounts:

Food Groups	Servings per Day at 1,600-Calorie Level	Servings per Day at 2,600-Calorie Level
Whole grains	6	10–11
Vegetables	3–4	5–6
Fruits	4	5–6
Fat-free or low-fat dairy products	2–3	3
Lean meats, poultry, and fish	3–6	6
Nuts, seeds, and legumes	3/week	1
Fats and oils	2	3
Sweets and added sugars	0	2 or less

In addition to these guidelines, the DASH diet provides tips for reducing sodium—often hidden in processed foods—that can benefit virtually everyone:

- Buy the low- or reduced-sodium versions of soups, condiments, crackers, and other packaged foods. Read labels carefully and watch for sodium in such items as breakfast cereals and salad dressings.

- Choose fresh or frozen vegetables. If buying canned, look for no- or low-sodium versions.

- Watch out for canned, smoked, cured, or processed meats, and brined foods such as pickles and olives, which are usually very high in sodium. Rinse when practical to wash away some of the salt.

- Some processed foods have so much sodium you may simply have to avoid them; examples include packaged cake and sauce mixes, pizzas, and frozen dinners.[4]

Sources:
1–4. U.S. Department of Health and Human Services, National Institutes of Health, National Heart, Lung, and Blood Institute, *DASH Eating Plan: Lower Your Blood Pressure* (NIH Publication #06-4082, Revised April, 2006).

consumption raises blood sugar and triglyceride levels. Avoid recreational drugs, especially stimulants.

WHAT IS YOUR PLAN FOR AVOIDING CARDIOVASCULAR DISEASE?

Identifying the controllable risk factors for cardiovascular disease in your life, and making simple changes to reduce them, will give you a head start toward protecting your cardiovascular health throughout adulthood. Lab 11.1 will help you assess the risk factors in your life.

REVIEW QUESTIONS

1. All of the following are examples of cardiovascular disease (CVD) except
   a. hypertension.
   b. atherosclerosis.
   c. coronary heart disease.
   d. systolic pressure.

2. Which of the following accurately describes *hypertension*?
   a. Sustained high blood pressure
   b. A thickening or hardening of the arteries
   c. Heart blockage
   d. Irregular heartbeat

3. Symptoms of cardiovascular disease include
   a. chest pain.
   b. numbness or pain in the extremities.
   c. having no symptoms at all.
   d. All of the above

4. When atherosclerosis occurs in the heart's main blood vessels, it is called
   a. peripheral artery disease.
   b. coronary artery disease or coronary heart disease.
   c. inflammation.
   d. homocysteine.

5. Significant risk factors for CVD include
   a. tobacco use.
   b. uncontrolled stress.
   c. obesity.
   d. All of the above

6. All of the following are characteristic of *metabolic syndrome* except
   a. abdominal obesity or a large waistline.
   b. elevated blood fats.

   c. high levels of "good" cholesterol (HDLs).
   d. high blood sugar.

7. Which of the following statements is true?
   a. The earliest manifestations of cardiovascular disease often take root during childhood.
   b. Young adults don't need to worry about cardiovascular disease.
   c. Heavy alcohol consumption will not affect your risks for developing cardiovascular disease.
   d. Thin people who do not exercise are not at risk for cardiovascular disease.

8. Low-density lipoprotein (LDL) is often referred to as
   a. "good" cholesterol.
   b. "bad" cholesterol.
   c. diabetes mellitus.
   d. metabolic syndrome.

9. At least _____ percent of people with diabetes mellitus die from some form of CVD.
   a. 30
   b. 45
   c. 50
   d. 65

10. *Systolic pressure* refers to
    a. the pressure applied to the walls of the arteries when the heart contracts.
    b. the pressure applied to the walls of the arteries when the heart relaxes.
    c. high blood pressure.
    d. inflammation.

CRITICAL THINKING QUESTIONS

1. List six different forms of CVD. Compare and contrast their risk factors, symptoms, and prevention.

2. Discuss the evidence that people in your age group are at risk for developing CVD.

3. Discuss specific ways that exercise and dietary changes can help prevent CVD.

ONLINE RESOURCES

Please visit this book's website at **www.aw-bc.com/hopson** for a list of websites that have additional resources about cardiovascular wellness, disease, and prevention.

REFERENCES

1. National Center for Health Statistics (NCHS) Fastats, www.cdc.gov/nchs/fastats/lcod.htm (accessed September 9, 2007).

2. National Center for Health Statistics (NCHS), National Health and Nutrition Examination Survey Data, 1999–2004.

3. Ibid.

4. American Heart Association, Heart Disease and Stroke Statistics, 2008 Update-at-a-Glance.

5. M. L. Daviglus and others, "Favorable Cardiovascular Risk Profile in Young Women and Long-Term Risk of Cardiovascular and All-Cause Mortality," *Journal of the American Medical Association* 292, no. 13 (October 6, 2004): 1588–92.

6–8. See note 4.

9. World Health Organization, "Cardiovascular Disease: Prevention and Control," World Health Organization Global Strategy on Diet, Physical Activity, and Health, www.who.int/dietphysicalactivity/publications/facts/cvd/en/ (accessed August 2007).

10. Ibid.

11. H. E. King and R. E. Miller, "Hypertension: Cognitive and Behavioral Considerations," *Neuropsychological Review* 1, no. 1 (March 1990): 31–73; J. Birns and L. Kalra, "Blood Pressure and Vascular Cognitive Impairment: The Debate Continues," *Journal of Human Hypertension* 20 (2006): 1–3; Lena Kilander and others, "Hypertension Is Related to Cognitive Impairment," *Hypertension* 31 (1998): 780–86.

12. P. K. Elias and others, "Blood Pressure-Related Cognitive Decline: Does Age Make a Difference?" *Hypertension* 44 (November 2004): 631–36.

13. Henry C. McGill and others, "Association of Coronary Heart Disease Risk Factors with Microscopic Qualities of Coronary Atherosclerosis in Youth," *Circulation* 102 (2000): 374.

14. Henry C. McGill and others, "Origin of Atherosclerosis in Childhood and Adolescence," *American Journal of Clinical Nutrition* 72, no. 5 (November 2000): 1307S–1315S.

15. D. H. Whincup and J. E. Deanfield, "Childhood Obesity and Cardiovascular Disease: The Challenge Ahead," *Nature: Clinical Practice in Cardiovascular Medicine* 2, no. 9 (September 2005): 432–33.

16. See note 4.

17. American Heart Association, "What Is High Blood Pressure?" July 20, 2007.

18. Ibid.

19. L. Best and others, "C-Reactive Proteins as a Predictor of Cardiovascular Risk in a Population with High Prevalence of Diabetes," *Circulation* 112, no. 9 (2005): 1289–95; C. Boos and G. Lip, "Elevated High Sensitive C-Reactive Protein, Large Arterial Stiffness and Atherosclerosis: A Relationship between Inflammation and Hypertension," *Journal of Human Hypertension* 19, no. 7 (2005): 511–13.

20. See note 4.

21. American Heart Association, "Heart Attack and Angina Statistics," www.americanheart.org/presenter.jhtml?identifier=4591 (accessed April 1, 2008).

22. American Heart Association, "Arrhythmia," www.americanheart.org/presenter.jhtml?identifier=10845 (accessed April 1, 2008).

23. American Heart Association, "What is Congestive Heart Failure?" www.americanheart.org (accessed April 1, 2008).

24. See note 4.

25. Christopher Skidmore and Irene Katzan, "Stroke," Cleveland Clinic Medical Index (May 30, 2002).

26–27. See note 4.

28. Australian Institute of Health and Welfare, "Living Dangerously: Australians with Multiple Risk Factors for Cardiovascular Disease," *Bulletin* 24 (February 24, 2005).

29. Morbidity and Mortality Weekly Report 54 (2005): 625–28.

30. Victor Tapson, "The Role of Smoking in Coagulation and Thromboembolism in Chronic Obstructive Pulmonary Disease," *Proceedings of the American Thoracic Society* 2 (2005): 71–77.

31. Mayo Clinic, "High Blood Pressure Dangers: Hypertension's Effects on Your Body," Mayo Clinic, www.mayoclinic.com January 24, 2007.

32. Medco Health Solutions, Inc., "Younger Adults Increasingly Treated for Heart-Disease Related Conditions," Medco News Releases, October 30, 2007.

33. National Heart, Lung, and Blood Institute, "Third Report of the National Cholesterol Education Program (NCEP) Expert Panel on Detection, Evaluation and Treatment of High Blood Cholesterol in Adults (Adult Treatment Panel III)," www.nhlbi.nih.gov/guidelines/cholesterol/index/htm, May 2001.

34. Ibid.

35–39. See note 4.

40. R. Eliot, "Changing Behavior: A New Comprehensive and Quantitative Approach" (keynote address, Annual Meeting of the American College of Cardiology on Stress and the Heart, Jackson Hole, WY, July 3, 1987).

41. Arthur N. Westover, Susan McBride, and Robert W. Haley, "Stroke in Young Adults Who Abuse Amphetamines or Cocaine," *Archives of General Psychiatry* 64 (2007): 495–502.

42–43. See note 4.

44. N. R. Anthonisen and others, "The Effects of a Smoking Cessation Intervention on 14.5 Year Mortality: A Randomized Controlled Trial," *Annals of Internal Medicine* 142 (2005): 223–39.

45. American Heart Association, "Our 2006 Diet and Lifestyle Recommendations," www.americanheart.org/presenter.jhtml?identifier=851 (accessed April 1, 2008).

Name: _____   Date: _____

Instructor: _____   Section: _____

Purpose: To engage students in critical thinking about their own risk factors for CVD.

Directions: Complete each of the following questions about CVD risk and total your points in each section—the higher the score, the greater your risk. If you answered "don't know" for any question, talk to your parents or other family members as soon as possible to find out if you have any unknown risks.

SECTION I: ASSESS YOUR FAMILY RISK FOR CVD

1. Do any of your primary relatives (mother, father, grandparents, siblings) have a history of heart disease or stroke?

| YES _____ (1 point) | NO _____ (0 points) | Don't Know _____ |

2. Do any of your primary relatives (mother, father, grandparents, siblings) have diabetes?

| YES _____ (1 point) | NO _____ (0 points) | Don't Know _____ |

3. Do any of your primary relatives (mother, father, grandparents, siblings) have high blood pressure?

| YES _____ (1 point) | NO _____ (0 points) | Don't Know _____ |

4. Do any of your primary relatives (mother, father, grandparents, siblings) have a history of high cholesterol?

| YES _____ (1 point) | NO _____ (0 points) | Don't Know _____ |

5. During the time you lived at home, did your family consume red meat and high-fat dairy products several times per week?

| YES _____ (1 point) | NO _____ (0 points) | Don't Know _____ |

Total Points [_____]

SECTION II: ASSESS YOUR LIFESTYLE RISK FOR CVD

1. Do you have high blood pressure?

YES _____ (1 point)	NO _____ (0 points)	Don't Know _____

2. Is your total cholesterol level higher than recommended? (See Table 11.3)

YES _____ (1 point)	NO _____ (0 points)	Don't Know _____

3. Have you been diagnosed as prediabetic or diabetic?

YES _____ (1 point)	NO _____ (0 points)	Don't Know _____

4. Do you smoke three or more cigarettes per day?

YES _____ (1 point)	NO _____ (0 points)	Don't Know _____

5. Would you describe your life as being highly stressful?

YES _____ (1 point)	NO _____ (0 points)	Don't Know _____

Total Points [_____]

SECTION III: ASSESS YOUR ADDITIONAL RISKS FOR CVD

1. How would you best describe your current BMI?
   a. Below 18.5 (1 point)
   b. Between 18.5 and 24.9 (0 points)
   c. Above 25 (1 point)
   d. Above 30 (2 points)

2. How would you describe your level of exercise?
   a. Moderate activity for 30 to 60 minutes on fewer than 3 days per week, plus fewer than three cardio workouts per week and fewer than two strength-training workouts per week (1 point)
   b. Moderate activity for 30 to 60 minutes most days of the week, plus three cardio workouts and two strength-training workouts per week (0 points)
   c. Moderate activity for 60 minutes or more most days of the week, plus more than three cardio workouts and two strength-training workouts per week (0 points)

3. How would you describe your dietary behaviors?
   a. I eat about the recommended number of calories/day for my age, BMI, and activity level. (0 points)
   b. I eat fewer than the recommended number of calories each day. (0 points)
   c. I eat more than the recommended number of calories each day. (1 point)

4. Which of the following best describes your typical dietary behavior?

   a. I eat from the major food groups, trying hard to get the recommended fruits and vegetables. (0 points)

   b. I eat several servings of red meat per week and consume saturated fat from other meats and high-fat dairy products most days. (1 point)

   c. Whenever possible, I try to substitute olive oil or canola oil for other forms of dietary fat. (0 points)

5. Which of the following best describes you?

   a. I watch my sodium intake. (0 points)

   b. I try to reduce stress in my life. (0 points)

   c. I try to eat 5 to 10 milligrams of soluble fiber each day. (0 points)

   d. I substitute a soy product for an animal product in my diet at least once each week. (0 points)

Total Points [   ]

SECTION IV: REFLECTION

1. What are your risk factors for CVD? Identify any behaviors that put you at risk for CVD. What can you change right now? What can you change in the future to reduce your risk?

2. Which risk factors for CVD are outside of your control? What can you do to reduce your risk of CVD, even though you have some uncontrollable risk factors?

From Access to Health, 10th ed. by Rebecca J. Donatelle. Copyright © 2008. Reprinted by permission of Pearson Education, Inc.

APPENDIX A

ANSWERS TO END-OF-CHAPTER QUESTIONS

CHAPTER 1
1.b; 2.b; 3.c; 4.a; 5.d; 6.d; 7.b; 8.c; 9.a; 10.d

CHAPTER 2
1.b; 2.c; 3.d; 4.c; 5.a; 6.b; 7.c; 8.b; 9.d; 10.d

CHAPTER 3
1.c; 2.d; 3.b; 4.c; 5.a; 6.b; 7.d; 8.c; 9.b; 10.d

CHAPTER 4
1.c; 2.b; 3.a; 4.d; 5.c; 6.a; 7.d; 8.c; 9.a; 10.c

CHAPTER 5
1.d; 2.c; 3.a; 4.d; 5.a; 6.b; 7.c; 8.b; 9.d; 10.c

CHAPTER 6
1.a; 2.c; 3.b; 4.b; 5.d; 6.b; 7.c; 8.b; 9.c; 10.a

CHAPTER 7
1.c; 2.d; 3.b; 4.b; 5.b; 6.c; 7.b; 8.c; 9.b; 10.a

CHAPTER 8
1.d; 2.d; 3.c; 4.d; 5.d; 6.b; 7.a; 8.d; 9.b; 10.d

CHAPTER 9
1.a; 2.b; 3.c; 4.a; 5.c; 6.d; 7.a; 8.d.; 9.a; 10.b

CHAPTER 10
1.c; 2.b; 3.a; 4.c; 5.d; 6.a; 7.b; 8.a; 9.a; 10.d

CHAPTER 11
1.d; 2.a; 3.d; 4.b; 5.d; 6.c; 7.a; 8.b; 9.d; 10.a

SAMPLE BEGINNER CARDIORESPIRATORY FITNESS PROGRAMS

The following sample programs—organized around walking, jogging/running, cycling, and swimming—provide you with a starting point for developing your own cardiorespiratory fitness routine. These programs are designed for beginners and assume that you have been medically cleared for exercise. Please also be sure that you have read and understood the basic fitness principles and procedures for starting a fitness program outlined in Chapters 2 and 3.

While these programs are focused on cardiorespiratory fitness, remember that a well-rounded fitness program should also include muscle strength, muscle endurance, flexibility, and back health exercises.

FITNESS WALKING
4-WEEK STARTER WALKING PROGRAM**

Phase One: Start walking a couple of days a week and work up to a 10–15 minute continuous walk.

Phase Two: Follow the chart below.

Phase Three: After you have completed Phase Two, increase your walks by 2–5 minutes each week until you reach your goal. Aim to walk for at least 30 minutes on most days of the week.

	MON		TUE		WED		THURS		FRI		SAT		SUN	
	TIME*	INTENSITY*	TIME	INTENSITY	TIME	INTENSITY	TIME	INTENSITY	TIME	INTENSITY	TIME	INTENSITY	TIME	INTENSITY
Week 1	15	12			15	12			15	14				
Week 2	15	13			20	12			15	13	15	14		
Week 3	15	14	20	13	15	14			20	13	15	15		
Week 4	20	14	15	16	20	15			20	14	25	13		

*Time is in minutes and intensity is in Rating of Perceived Exertion (RPE) (see Ch. 2). Time does not include warm-up or cool-down time.
**Adjust time, intensity, and days of the walks to suit your personal fitness level and schedule.

JOGGING AND RUNNING
4-WEEK STARTER JOGGING/RUNNING PROGRAM**

Phase One: Start a walking program and work up to a 30-minute fast-paced walk, 4–5 times per week.

Phase Two: Walk for 5 minutes, jog for 1 minute and repeat 3–4 times. Do this 3–4 times per week. Decrease your walking and increase your running by 1–2 minutes each time until you are jogging for 9 minutes continuously at least 3 times per week.

Phase Three: Follow the chart below. You can start at this phase if you can already jog for 9 minutes without stopping. After you have completed the following program, increase your runs by 2–5 minutes each week until you reach your goal. A typical maintenance running program consists of four 30 minute runs per week.

	MON		TUE		WED		THURS		FRI		SAT		SUN	
	TIME*	INTENSITY*	TIME	INTENSITY	TIME	INTENSITY	TIME	INTENSITY	TIME	INTENSITY	TIME	INTENSITY	TIME	INTENSITY
Week 1	10	14			10	14			10	14				
Week 2	15	14			15	14			15	14	15	14		
Week 3	15	14			20	14			15	15	20	14		
Week 4	20	14			15	16			20	14	25	13		

*Time is in minutes and intensity is in Rating of Perceived Exertion (RPE) (see Ch. 2). Time does not include warm-up or cool-down time.
**Adjust time, intensity, and days of the runs to suit your personal fitness level and schedule.

CYCLING
4-WEEK STARTER CYCLING PROGRAM**

Phase One: Start bicycling and work up to a continuous 15 minute bike ride 3 times per week.

Phase Two: Follow the chart below. You can start at this phase if you can already bike for 15–20 minutes continuously. After you have completed the following program, increase your rides by 5–10 minutes each week until you reach your goal. Aim for a fitness cycling program that consists of four 45-minute rides per week at a minimum.

	MON		TUE		WED		THURS		FRI		SAT		SUN	
	TIME*	INTENSITY*	TIME	INTENSITY	TIME	INTENSITY	TIME	INTENSITY	TIME	INTENSITY	TIME	INTENSITY	TIME	INTENSITY
Week 1	20	12			20	13			20	13				
Week 2	25	12			20	13			25	13	20	14		
Week 3	25	13			30	14			25	15	30	13		
Week 4	35	13			30	15			30	14	35	13		

*Time is in minutes and intensity is in Rating of Perceived Exertion (RPE) (see Ch. 2). Time does not include warm-up or cool-down time.
**Adjust time, intensity, and days of the rides to suit your personal fitness level and schedule.

SWIMMING
4-WEEK STARTER SWIMMING PROGRAM**

Phase One: Become comfortable with the water and learn to swim.

Phase Two: Walk through the pool 2–4 times (25 yard or meter length pool), jog through the pool 2–4 times, swim a comfortable stroke across the pool 1–2 times. Repeat this process 3–5 times for an overall workout time of 15–30 minutes. Do this workout 2 times per week. Decrease your pool walking/running lengths and increase your swimming lengths until you are swimming an easy stroke continuously 8–10 times across the pool (200–250 yards or meters).

Phase Three: Follow the chart below. You can start at this phase if you can already swim 200 yards or meters continuously. After you have completed the following program, increase your swimming by 100 yards or meters each week until you reach your goal. Aim to swim for 30 minutes 2–3 times per week (distances will vary greatly depending upon swim skill/speed).

	MON		TUE		WED		THURS		FRI		SAT		SUN	
	TIME*	INTENSITY*	TIME	INTENSITY	TIME	INTENSITY	TIME	INTENSITY	TIME	INTENSITY	TIME	INTENSITY	TIME	INTENSITY
Week 1			15	13			15	14						
Week 2			20	14			20	13			15	15		
Week 3			20	14			25	14			20	15		
Week 4			25	14			30	13			25	15		

*Time is in minutes and intensity is in Rating of Perceived Exertion (RPE) (see Ch. 2). Time does not include warm-up or cool-down time.
**Adjust time, intensity, and days of the swims to suit your personal fitness level and schedule.

For more sample programs, as well as web resources and tools for tracking your progress online, visit www.aw-bc.com/hopson.

NUTRITIVE VALUE OF SELECTED FOODS AND FAST FOODS

This section presents nutritional information about a wide array of foods, including many fast foods. Values are given for calories, protein, carbohydrates, fiber, fat, saturated fat, and cholesterol for common foods and serving sizes. Use this information to assess your diet and make improvements.

MDA CODE	FOOD NAME	AMT	WT (G)	ENER (KCAL)	PROT (G)	CARB (G)	FIBER (G)	FAT (G)	SAT (G)	CHOL (G)
BEVERAGES										
ALCOHOLIC BEVERAGES										
22831	Beer	12 fl. oz	360	157	1	13		0	0	
34053	Beer, light	12 fl. oz	353	105	1	5	0	0	0	
22606	Beer, nonalcoholic	12 fl. oz	353	73	1	14	0	0	0	
22884	Wine, red	1 fl. oz	29	24	0	1		0	0	
22861	Wine, white	1 fl. oz	29.3	24	0	1		0	0	
22514	Gin, 80 proof	1 fl. oz	27.8	64	0	0	0	0	0	
22593	Rum, 80 proof	1 fl. oz	27.8	64	0	0	0	0	0	
22515	Tequila, 80 proof	1 fl. oz	27.8	64	0	0	0	0	0	
22594	Vodka, 80 proof	1 fl. oz	27.8	64	0	0	0	0	0	
22670	Whiskey, 80 proof	1 fl. oz	27.8	64	0	0	0	0	0	
COFFEE, TEA, AND DAIRY DRINK MIXES										
20012	Coffee, brewed	1 cup	237	2	0	0	0	0	0	0
20686	Coffee, decaffeinated, brewed	1 cup	237	0	0	0	0	0	0	0
20439	Coffee, espresso	1 cup	237	5	0	0	0	0	0.2	0
20402	Coffee, from mix, French vanilla, sugar & fat free	1 ea	7	25	0	5	0	0	0.1	0
85	Chocolate milk, prepared w/syrup	1 cup	282	254	9	36	1	8	4.7	25
46	Hot cocoa, w/aspartame, sodium, vitamin A, prepared w/water	1 cup	256	74	3	14	1	1	0	0
48	Hot cocoa, prep from dry mix with water	1 cup	275	151	2	32	1	2	0.9	3
166	Hot cocoa, w/marshmallows, from dry packet	1 ea	28	112	1	24	1	1	0.4	2
39	Chocolate flavor, dry mix, prepared w/milk	1 cup	266	226	9	32	1	9	4.9	24
41	Strawberry flavor, dry mix, prepared w/milk	1 cup	266	234	8	33	0	8	5.1	32

MDA CODE	FOOD NAME	AMT	WT (G)	ENER (KCAL)	PROT (G)	CARB (G)	FIBER (G)	FAT (G)	SAT (G)	CHOL (G)
20014	Tea, brewed	1 cup	237	2	0	1	0	0	0	0
20036	Tea, herbal (not chamomile) brewed	1 cup	237	2	0	0	0	0	0	0

FRUIT AND VEGETABLE BEVERAGES AND JUICES

MDA CODE	FOOD NAME	AMT	WT (G)	ENER (KCAL)	PROT (G)	CARB (G)	FIBER (G)	FAT (G)	SAT (G)	CHOL (G)
71080	Apple juice, canned or bottled, unsweetened	1 ea	262	123	0	31	0	0	0	0
20277	Capri Sun All Natural Juice, Drink Fruit Punch	1 ea	210	99	0	26	0	0	0	0
5226	Carrot juice, canned	1 cup	236	94	2	22	2	0	0.1	0
3042	Cranberry juice cocktail	1 cup	253	137	0	34	0	0	0	0
20024	Fruit punch, canned	1 cup	248	117	0	30	0	0	0	0
20035	Fruit punch, from frozen concentrate	1 cup	247	114	0	29	0	0	0	0
20101	Grape drink, canned	1 cup	250	153	0	39	0	0	0	0
3053	Grapefruit juice, from frozen concentrate, unsweetened	1 cup	247	101	1	24	0	0	0	0
20045	Lemonade flavor drink, from dry mix	1 cup	266	112	0	29	0	0	0	0
20047	Lemonade w/aspartame, low kcal, from dry mix	1 cup	237	5	0	1	0	0	0	0
20070	Orange drink, canned	1 cup	248	122	0	31	0	0	0	0
20004	Orange flavor drink, from dry mix	1 cup	248	122	0	31	0	0	0	0
71108	Orange juice, canned, unsweetened	1 ea	263	110	2	26	1	0	0	0
3090	Orange juice, fresh	1 cup	248	112	2	26	0	0	0.1	0
3091	Orange juice, from frozen concentrate, unsweetened	1 cup	249	112	2	27	0	0	0	0
5397	Tomato juice, canned w/o salt	1 cup	243	41	2	10	1	0	0	0
20849	Vegetable and fruit, mixed juice drink	4 oz	113	33	0	8	0	0	0	0
20080	Vegetable juice cocktail, canned	1 cup	242	46	2	11	2	0	0	0

SOFT DRINKS

MDA CODE	FOOD NAME	AMT	WT (G)	ENER (KCAL)	PROT (G)	CARB (G)	FIBER (G)	FAT (G)	SAT (G)	CHOL (G)
20006	Club soda	1 cup	237	0	0	0	0	0	0	0
20685	Low-calorie cola, with aspartame, caffeine free	12 fl. oz	355	4	0	1	0	0	0	0
20843	Cola, with higher caffeine	12 fl. oz	370	152	0	39	0	0	0	0
20008	Ginger ale	1 cup	244	83	0	21	0	0	0	0
20032	Lemon-lime soft drink	1 cup	246	98	0	25	0	0	0	0
20027	Pepper-type soft drink	1 cup	246	101	0	26	0	0	0.2	0
20009	Root beer	1 cup	246	101	0	26	0	0	0	0

OTHER

MDA CODE	FOOD NAME	AMT	WT (G)	ENER (KCAL)	PROT (G)	CARB (G)	FIBER (G)	FAT (G)	SAT (G)	CHOL (G)
20033	Soy milk	1 cup	245	127	11	12	3	5	0.6	0
20041	Water, tap	1 cup	237	0	0	0	0	0	0	0

BREAKFAST CEREALS

MDA CODE	FOOD NAME	AMT	WT (G)	ENER (KCAL)	PROT (G)	CARB (G)	FIBER (G)	FAT (G)	SAT (G)	CHOL (G)
40095	All-Bran/Kellogg	0.5 cup	30	78	4	22	9	1	0.2	0
40032	Cap'n Crunch/Quaker	0.75 cup	27	108	1	23	1	2	0.4	0

MDA CODE	FOOD NAME	AMT	WT (G)	ENER (KCAL)	PROT (G)	CARB (G)	FIBER (G)	FAT (G)	SAT (G)	CHOL (G)
40297	Cheerios/Gen Mills	1 cup	30	111	4	22	4	2	0.4	0
40126	Cinnamon Toast Crunch/ Gen Mills	0.75 cup	30	127	2	24	1	3	0.5	0
40195	Corn Flakes/Kellogg	1 cup	28	101	2	24	1	0	0.1	0
40089	Corn Grits, instant, plain, prepared/Quaker	1 pkg	137	93	2	21	1	0	0	0
40206	Corn Pops/Kellogg	1 cup	31	117	1	28	0	0	0.1	0
40179	Cream of Rice, prepared w/salt	1 cup	244	127	2	28	0	0	0	0
40182	Cream of Wheat, instant, prepared w/salt	1 cup	241	149	4	32	1	1	0.1	0
40104	Crispix/Kellogg	1 cup	29	109	2	25	0	0	0.1	0
40218	Froot Loops/Kellogg	1 cup	30	118	2	26	1	1	0.5	0
40217	Frosted Flakes/Kellogg	0.75 cup	31	114	1	28	1	0	0	0
11916	Frosted Mini-Wheats, bite size/Kellogg	1 cup	55	189	6	45	6	1	0.2	0
40209	Raisin Bran/Kellogg	1 cup	61	195	5	47	7	2	0.3	0
40210	Rice Krispies/Kellogg	1.25 cup	33	128	2	28	0	0	0.1	0
60887	Shredded wheat, large biscuit	2 ea	37.8	127	4	30	5	1	0.2	0
40211	Special K/Kellogg	1 cup	31	117	7	22	1	0	0.1	0

DAIRY AND CHEESE

MDA CODE	FOOD NAME	AMT	WT (G)	ENER (KCAL)	PROT (G)	CARB (G)	FIBER (G)	FAT (G)	SAT (G)	CHOL (G)
500	Cream, half & half	2 Tbs	30	39	1	1	0	3	2.1	11
11	Milk, condensed, sweetened, canned	2 Tbs	38.2	123	3	21	0	3	2.1	13
19	Milk, lowfat, 1% fat, chocolate	1 cup	250	158	8	26	1	2	1.5	8
218	Milk, 2%, w/added vitamins A & D	1 cup	245	130	8	13	0	5	3	
6	Milk, nonfat/skim, w/added vitamin A	1 cup	245	83	8	12	0	0	0.1	5
1	Milk, whole, 3.25%	1 cup	244	146	8	11	0	8	4.6	24
20	Milk, whole, chocolate	1 cup	250	208	8	26	2	8	5.3	30
72088	Yogurt, fruit variety, nonfat	1 cup	245	230	11	47	0	0	0.3	5
1287	American cheese, nonfat slices	1 pce	21.3	32	5	2	0	0	0.1	3
13349	Cheez Whiz cheese sauce/Kraft	2 Tbs	33	91	4	3	0	7	4.3	25
1014	Cottage cheese, 2% fat	0.5 cup	113	102	16	4	0	2	1.4	9
1015	Cream cheese	2 Tbs	29	101	2	1	0	10	6.4	32
1452	Cream cheese, fat free	2 Tbs	29	28	4	2	0	0	0.3	2
1016	Feta, crumbled	0.25 cup	37.5	99	5	2	0	8	5.6	33
47887	Mozzarella, whole milk, slice	1 ea	34	102	8	1	0	8	4.5	27
1075	Parmesan, grated	1 Tbs	5	22	2	0	0	1	0.9	4
1024	Ricotta, part skim	0.25 cup	62	86	7	3	0	5	3.1	19
1064	Ricotta, whole milk	0.25 cup	62	108	7	2	0	8	5.1	32

EGGS AND EGG SUBSTITUTES

MDA CODE	FOOD NAME	AMT	WT (G)	ENER (KCAL)	PROT (G)	CARB (G)	FIBER (G)	FAT (G)	SAT (G)	CHOL (G)
19525	Egg substitute, liquid	0.25 cup	62.8	53	8	0	0	2	0.4	1
19506	Egg, white, raw	1 ea	33.4	17	4	0	0	0	0	0
19509	Egg, whole, fried	1 ea	46	92	6	0	0	7	2	210
19515	Egg, whole, hard boiled	1 ea	37	57	5	0	0	4	1.2	157

MDA CODE	FOOD NAME	AMT	WT (G)	ENER (KCAL)	PROT (G)	CARB (G)	FIBER (G)	FAT (G)	SAT (G)	CHOL (G)
19521	Egg, whole, poached	1 ea	37	54	5	0	0	4	1.1	156
19516	Egg, whole, scrambled	1 ea	61	101	7	1	0	7	2.2	215
19508	Egg, yolk, raw, fresh	1 ea	16.6	53	3	1	0	4	1.6	205

FRUIT

MDA CODE	FOOD NAME	AMT	WT (G)	ENER (KCAL)	PROT (G)	CARB (G)	FIBER (G)	FAT (G)	SAT (G)	CHOL (G)
72101	Apricots, canned, heavy syrup, drained	1 cup	182	151	1	39	5	0	0	0
3164	Fruit cocktail canned in juice	1 cup	237	109	1	28	2	0	0	0
71079	Apple w/skin, raw	1 cup	125	65	0	17	3	0	0	0
3331	Applesauce w/added vitamin C	0.5 cup	128	97	0	25	2	0	0	0
3657	Apricot, raw	1 cup	165	79	2	18	3	1	0	0
3210	Avocado, California, peeled, raw	1 ea	173	289	3	15	12	27	3.7	0
71082	Banana, peeled, raw	1 ea	81	72	1	19	2	0	0.1	0
71976	Grapefruit, fresh	0.5 ea	154	60	1	16	6	0	0	
3055	Grapes, Thompson seedless, fresh	0.5 cup	80	55	1	14	1	0	0	4
3642	Melon, fresh, wedge	1 pce	69	23	1	6	1	0	0	5
3168	Mixed fruit (prune, apricot, & pear) dried	1 oz	28.4	69	1	18	2	0	0	0
3216	Nectarine, raw	1 cup	138	61	1	15	2	0	0	0
3726	Peach, peeled, raw	1 ea	79	31	1	8	1	0	0	0
3106	Pear, raw	1 ea	209	121	1	32	6	0	0	0
3766	Raisins, seedless	50 ea	26	78	1	21	1	0	0	0
72113	Pineapple, fresh, slice	1 pce	84	38	0	10		0		5
3085	Orange, fresh	1 ea	184	86	2	22	4	0	0	
3135	Strawberries, halves/slices, raw	1 cup	166	53	1	13	3	0	0	0

GRAIN PRODUCTS

BREADS, ROLLS, AND BREAD CRUMBS

MDA CODE	FOOD NAME	AMT	WT (G)	ENER (KCAL)	PROT (G)	CARB (G)	FIBER (G)	FAT (G)	SAT (G)	CHOL (G)
71170	Bagel, cinnamon-raisin	1 ea	26	71	3	14	1	0	0.1	0
71167	Bagel, egg	1 ea	26	72	3	14	1	1	0.1	6
71152	Bagel, plain/onion/poppy/ sesame, enriched	1 ea	26	67	3	13	1	0	0.1	0
42433	Biscuit, w/butter	1 ea	82	280	5	27	0	17	4	0
71192	Biscuit, Plain or Buttermilk, refrig dough, baked, reduced fat	1 ea	21	63	2	12	0	1	0.3	0
42004	Bread crumbs, dry, plain, grated	1 Tbs	6.8	27	1	5	0	0	0.1	0
49144	Bread, crusty Italian w/garlic	1 pce	50	186	4	21	10	2.4	6	
70964	Bread, garlic, frozen/Campione	1 pce	28	101	2	12	1	5	0.8	
42069	Bread, oat bran	1 pce	30	71	3	12	1	1	0.2	0
42095	Bread, wheat, reduced kcal	1 pce	23	46	2	10	3	1	0.1	0
71247	Bread, white, commercially prepared, crumbs/cubes/slices	1 pce	9	24	1	5	0	0	0.1	0
42084	Bread, white, reduced kcal	1 pce	23	48	2	10	2	1	0.1	0
26561	Buns, hamburger, Wonder	1 ea	43	117	3	22	1	2	0.4	
42021	Hamburger/hot dog bun, plain	1 ea	43	120	4	21	1	2	0.5	0

MDA CODE	FOOD NAME	AMT	WT (G)	ENER (KCAL)	PROT (G)	CARB (G)	FIBER (G)	FAT (G)	SAT (G)	CHOL (G)
42115	Cornbread, prepared from dry mix	1 pce	60	188	4	29	1	6	1.6	37
71227	Pita bread, white, enriched	1 ea	28	77	3	16	1	0	0	0
71228	Pita bread, whole wheat	1 ea	28	74	3	15	2	1	0.1	0
71368	Roll, dinner, plain, homemade w/reduced fat (2%) milk	1 ea	43	136	4	23	1	3	0.8	15
42161	Roll, French	1 ea	38	105	3	19	1	2	0.4	0
71056	Roll, hard/kaiser	1 ea	57	167	6	30	1	2	0.3	0
42297	Tortilla, corn, w/o salt, ready to cook	1 ea	26	58	1	12	1	1	0.1	0
90645	Taco shell, baked	1 ea	5	23	0	3	0	1	0.2	0

CRACKERS

MDA CODE	FOOD NAME	AMT	WT (G)	ENER (KCAL)	PROT (G)	CARB (G)	FIBER (G)	FAT (G)	SAT (G)	CHOL (G)
71451	Cheez-its/Goldfish crackers, low sodium	55 pce	33	166	3	19	1	8	3.2	4
43507	Oyster/soda/soup crackers	1 cup	45	193	4	32	1	5	0.7	0
70963	Ritz crackers/Nabisco	5 ea	16	79	1	10	0	4	0.6	0
43587	Saltine crackers, original premium/Nabisco	5 ea	14	59	2	10	0	1	0.3	0
43545	Sandwich crackers, cheese filled	4 ea	28	134	3	17	1	6	1.7	1
43546	Sandwich crackers, peanut butter filled	4 ea	28	138	3	16	1	7	1.4	0
44677	Snackwell Wheat Cracker/Nabisco	1 ea	15	62	1	12	1	2		
43581	Wheat Thins, baked/Nabisco	16 ea	29	136	2	20	1	6	0.9	0
43508	Whole wheat cracker	4 ea	32	142	3	22	3	6	1.1	0

MUFFINS AND BAKED GOODS

MDA CODE	FOOD NAME	AMT	WT (G)	ENER (KCAL)	PROT (G)	CARB (G)	FIBER (G)	FAT (G)	SAT (G)	CHOL (G)
42723	English muffin, plain	1 ea	57	132	5	26		1	0.2	
62916	Muffin, blueberry, commercially prepared	1 ea	11	30	1	5	0	1	0.2	3
44521	Muffin, corn, commercially prepared	1 ea	57	174	3	29	2	5	0.8	15
44514	Muffin, oatbran	1 ea	57	154	4	28	3	4	0.6	0
44518	Toaster muffin, blueberry	1 ea	33	103	2	18	1	3	0.5	2

NOODLES AND PASTA

MDA CODE	FOOD NAME	AMT	WT (G)	ENER (KCAL)	PROT (G)	CARB (G)	FIBER (G)	FAT (G)	SAT (G)	CHOL (G)
38048	Chow mein noodles, dry	1 cup	45	237	4	26	2	14	2	0
38047	Egg noodles, enriched, cooked	0.5 cup	80	110	4	20	1	2	0.3	23
38060	Spaghetti, whole wheat, cooked	1 cup	140	174	7	37	6	1	0.1	0
38251	Egg noodles, enriched, cooked w/salt	0.5 cup	80	110	4	20	1	2	0.3	
38102	Macaroni noodles, enriched, cooked	1 cup	140	221	8	43	3	1	0.2	
38118	Spaghetti noodles, enriched, cooked	0.5 cup	70	111	4	22	1	1	0.1	4

GRAINS

MDA CODE	FOOD NAME	AMT	WT (G)	ENER (KCAL)	PROT (G)	CARB (G)	FIBER (G)	FAT (G)	SAT (G)	CHOL (G)
38076	Couscous, cooked	0.5 cup	78.5	88	3	18	1	0	0	0
38080	Oats	0.25 cup	39	152	7	26	4	3	0.5	0

MDA CODE	FOOD NAME	AMT	WT (G)	ENER (KCAL)	PROT (G)	CARB (G)	FIBER (G)	FAT (G)	SAT (G)	CHOL (G)
38010	Rice, brown, long grain, cooked	1 cup	195	216	5	45	4	2	0.4	0
38256	Rice, white, long grain, enriched, cooked w/salt	1 cup	158	205	4	45	1	0	0.1	0
38019	Rice, white, long grain, instant, enriched, cooked	1 cup	165	193	4	41	1	1	0	0
PANCAKES, FRENCH TOAST, AND WAFFLES										
42156	French toast, homemade, w/reduced fat (2%) milk	1 pce	65	149	5	16	1	7	1.8	75
45192	Pancake/waffle, buttermilk/ Eggo/Kellogg	1 ea	42.5	99	3	16	0	3	0.6	5
45117	Pancakes, plain, homemade	1 ea	77	175	5	22	1	7	1.6	45
45193	Waffle, lowfat, homestyle, frozen	1 ea	35	83	2	15	0	1	0.3	9
MEAT AND MEAT SUBSTITUTES										
BEEF										
10093	Beef, average of all cuts, lean & fat (1/4" trim), cooked	3 oz	85.1	260	22	0	0	18	7.3	75
10705	Beef, average of all cuts, lean (1/4" trim), cooked	3 oz	85.1	184	25	0	0	8	3.2	73
10133	Beef, whole rib, roasted, 1/4" trim	3 oz	85.1	305	19	0	0	25	10	71
58129	Ground beef (hamburger), 25% fat, cooked, pan-browned	3 oz	85.1	236	22	0	0	15	6	76
58119	Ground beef (hamburger), 15% fat, cooked, pan-browned	3 oz	85.1	218	24	0	0	13	5	77
58109	Ground beef (hamburger), 5% fat, cooked, pan-browned	3 oz	85.1	164	25	0	0	6	2.9	76
10791	Porterhouse steak, lean & fat (1/4" trim), broiled	3 oz	85.1	280	19	0	0	22	8.7	61
58257	Rib eye steak, small end (ribs 10–12), 0" trim, broiled	3 oz	85.1	210	23	0	0	13	4.9	94
58094	Skirt steak, trimmed to 0" fat, broiled	3 oz	85.1	187	22	0	0	10	4	51
58328	Strip steak, top loin, 1/8" trim, broiled	3 oz	85.1	171	25	0	0	7	2.7	67
10805	T-Bone steak, lean & fat (1/4" trim), broiled	3 oz	85.1	260	20	0	0	19	7.6	55
11531	Veal, average of all cuts, cooked	3 oz	85.1	197	26	0	0	10	3.6	97
CHICKEN										
15057	Chicken breast, w/o skin, fried	3 oz	85.1	159	28	0	0	4	1.1	77
15080	Chicken, dark meat, w/skin, roasted	3 oz	85.1	215	22	0	0	13	3.7	77
15026	Chicken, dark meat, w/o skin, fried	3 oz	85.1	203	25	2	0	10	2.7	82
15042	Chicken drumstick, w/o skin, fried	3 oz	85.1	166	24	0	0	7	1.8	80
15048	Chicken, wing, w/o skin, fried	3 oz	85.1	180	26	0	0	8	2.1	71

MDA CODE	FOOD NAME	AMT	WT (G)	ENER (KCAL)	PROT (G)	CARB (G)	FIBER (G)	FAT (G)	SAT (G)	CHOL (G)
15059	Chicken, wing, w/o skin, roasted	3 oz	85.1	173	26	0	0	7	1.9	72
TURKEY										
51151	Turkey bacon, cooked	1 oz	28.4	108	8	1	0	8	2.4	28
51098	Turkey patty, breaded, fried	1 ea	42	119	6	7	0	8	2	26
16110	Turkey breast w/skin, roasted	3 oz	85.1	130	25	0	0	3	0.7	77
16038	Turkey breast, no skin, roasted	3 oz	85.1	115	26	0	0	1	0.2	71
16101	Turkey, dark meat w/skin, roasted	3 oz	85.1	155	24	0	0	6	1.8	100
16003	Turkey, ground, cooked	1 ea	82	193	22	0	0	11	2.8	84
LAMB										
13604	Lamb, average of all cuts (1/4" trim), cooked	3 oz	85.1	250	21	0	0	18	7.5	83
13616	Lamb, average of all cuts, lean (1/4" trim), cooked	3 oz	85.1	175	24	0	0	8	2.9	78
PORK										
12000	Bacon, broiled, pan-fried, or roasted	3 pcs	19	103	7	0	0	8	2.6	21
28143	Canadian bacon	1 pce	56	68	9	1		3	1	27
12211	Ham, cured, boneless, regular fat (11% fat), roasted	1 cup	140	249	32	0	0	13	4.4	83
12309	Pork, average of retail cuts, cooked	3 oz	85.1	232	23	0	0	15	5.3	77
12097	Pork, ribs, backribs, roasted	3 oz	85.1	315	21	0	0	25	9.4	100
12099	Pork, ground, cooked	3 oz	85.1	253	22	0	0	18	6.6	80
LUNCHMEATS										
13000	Beef, thin slices	1 oz	28.4	42	5	0	0	2	0.8	20
58275	Bologna, beef and pork, low fat	1 ea	14	32	2	0	0	3	1	5
13157	Chicken breast, oven roasted deluxe	1 oz	28.4	29	5	1	0	1	0.2	14
13306	Corned beef, cooked, chopped, pressed	1 ea	71	101	14	1	0	5	2	46
13264	Ham, slices, regular (11% fat)	1 cup	135	220	22	5	2	12	4	77
13101	Pastrami, beef, cured	1 oz	28.4	41	6	0	0	2	0.8	19
13215	Salami, beef, cotto	1 oz	28.4	59	4	1	0	4	1.9	24
16160	Turkey breast slice	1 pce	21	22	4	1	0	0	0.1	9
58279	Turkey ham, sliced, extra lean, prepackaged or deli-sliced	1 cup	138	163	27	2	0	5	1.8	92
SAUSAGE										
13070	Chorizo, pork & beef	1 ea	60	273	14	1	0	23	8.6	53
57877	Frankfurter, beef	1 ea	45	148	5	2	0	13	5.3	24
13012	Frankfurter, turkey	1 ea	45	102	6	1	0	8	2.7	48
57890	Italian sausage, pork, cooked	1 ea	83	286	16	4	0	23	7.9	47
13021	Pepperoni sausage	1 pce	5.5	26	1	0	0	2	0.9	6
13185	Pork sausage links, cooked	2 ea	48	165	8	0	0	15	5.1	37
58227	Sausage, pork, precooked	3 oz	85	321	12	0	0	30	9.9	63
58007	Turkey sausage, breakfast links, mild	2 ea	56	132	9	1	0	10	4.4	34

MDA CODE	FOOD NAME	AMT	WT (G)	ENER (KCAL)	PROT (G)	CARB (G)	FIBER (G)	FAT (G)	SAT (G)	CHOL (G)
MEAT SUBSTITUTES										
7509	Bacon substitute, vegetarian, strips	3 ea	15	46	2	1	0	4	0.7	0
7722	Garden patties, frozen/ Worthington, Morningstar	1 ea	67	119	11	10	4	4	0.5	1
7674	Harvest burger, original flavor, vegetable protein patty	1 ea	90	138	18	7	6	4	1	0
90626	Sausage, vegetarian, meatless	1 ea	28	72	5	3	1	5	0.8	0
7726	Spicy Black Bean Burger/ Worthington, Morningstar	1 ea	78	115	12	15	5	1	0.2	1
NUTS										
4519	Cashews, dry roasted w/salt	0.25 cup	34.2	196	5	11	1	16	3.1	0
4728	Macadamia nuts, dry roasted, unsalted	1 cup	134	962	10	18	11	102	16	0
4592	Mixed nuts, w/peanuts, dry roasted, salted	0.25 cup	34.2	203	6	9	3	18	2.4	0
4626	Peanut butter, chunky w/salt	2 Tbs	32	188	8	7	3	16	2.6	0
4756	Peanuts, dry roasted w/o salt	30 ea	30	176	7	6	2	15	2.1	0
4696	Peanuts, raw	0.25 cup	36.5	207	9	6	3	18	2.5	0
4540	Pistachio nuts, dry roasted, salted	0.25 cup	32	182	7	9	3	15	1.8	0
SEAFOOD										
17029	Bass, freshwater, cooked w/dry heat	3 oz	85.1	124	21	0	0	4	0.9	74
17037	Cod, Atlantic, baked/broiled (dry heat)	3 oz	85.1	89	19	0	0	1	0.1	47
19036	Crab, Alaskan King, boiled/ steamed	3 oz	85.1	83	16	0	0	1	0.1	45
17090	Haddock, baked or broiled (dry heat)	3 oz	85.1	95	21	0	0	1	0.1	63
17291	Halibut, Atlantic & Pacific, baked or broiled (dry heat)	3 oz	85.1	119	23	0	0	3	0.4	35
17181	Salmon, Atlantic, farmed, cooked w/dry heat	3 oz	85.1	175	19	0	0	11	2.1	54
17099	Salmon, Sockeye, baked or broiled (dry heat)	3 oz	85.1	184	23	0	0	9	1.6	74
71707	Squid, fried	3 oz	85.1	149	15	7	0	6	1.6	221
17066	Swordfish, baked or broiled (dry heat)	3 oz	85.1	132	22	0	0	4	1.2	43
56007	Tuna salad, lunchmeat spread	2 Tbs	25.6	48	4	2	0	2	0.4	3
17151	White tuna, canned in H_2O, drained	3 oz	85.1	109	20	0	0	3	0.7	36
17083	White tuna, canned in oil, drained	3 oz	85.1	158	23	0	0	7	1.1	26
VEGETABLES AND LEGUMES										
BEANS										
7038	Baked beans, plain or vegetarian, canned	1 cup	254	239	12	54	10	1	0.2	0
5197	Bean sprouts, mung, canned, drained	1 cup	125	15	2	3	1	0	0	0

MDA CODE	FOOD NAME	AMT	WT (G)	ENER (KCAL)	PROT (G)	CARB (G)	FIBER (G)	FAT (G)	SAT (G)	CHOL (G)
7012	Black beans, boiled w/o salt	1 cup	172	227	15	41	15	1	0.2	0
5862	Beets, boiled w/salt, drained	0.5 cup	85	37	1	8	2	0	0	0
90018	Cowpeas, cooked w/salt	1 cup	171	198	13	35	11	1	0.2	0
7081	Hummus, garbanzo or chickpea spread, homemade	1 Tbs	15.4	27	1	3	1	1	0.2	0
7087	Kidney beans, canned	1 cup	256	210	13	37	11	2	0.2	0
7006	Lentils, boiled w/o salt	1 cup	198	230	18	40	16	1	0.1	0
7051	Pinto beans, canned	1 cup	240	206	12	37	11	2	0.4	0
6748	Snap green beans, raw	10 ea	55	17	1	4	2	0	0	0
5320	Snap yellow beans, raw	0.5 cup	55	17	1	4	2	0	0	0
90026	Split peas, boiled w/salt	0.5 cup	98	116	8	21	8	0	0.1	0
7054	White beans, canned	1 cup	262	307	19	57	13	1	0.2	0
FRESH VEGETABLES										
9577	Artichokes (globe or French) boiled w/salt, drained	1 ea	20	10	1	2	1	0	0	0
6033	Arugula/roquette, raw	1 cup	20	5	1	1	0	0	0	0
90406	Asparagus, raw	10 ea	35	7	1	1	1	0	0	0
5558	Broccoli stalks, raw	1 ea	114	32	3	6	4	0	0.1	0
5036	Cabbage, raw	1 cup	70	17	1	4	2	0	0	0
90605	Carrots, baby, raw	1 ea	15	5	0	1	0	0	0	0
5049	Cauliflower, raw	0.5 cup	50	12	1	3	1	0	0	0
90436	Celery, raw	1 ea	17	2	0	1	0	0	0	0
7202	Corn, white, sweet, ears, raw	1 ea	73	63	2	14	2	1	0.1	0
5900	Corn, yellow, sweet, boiled w/salt, drained	0.5 cup	82	89	3	21	2	1	0.2	0
5908	Eggplant (brinjal) boiled w/salt, drained	1 cup	99	35	1	9	2	0	0	0
5087	Lettuce, looseleaf, raw	2 pcs	20	3	0	1	0	0	0	0
51069	Mushrooms, brown, Italian, or crimini, raw	2 ea	28	6	1	1	0	0	0	0
90472	Onions, chopped, raw	1 ea	70	29	1	7	1	0	0	0
5116	Peas, green, raw	1 cup	145	117	8	21	7	1	0.1	0
7932	Peppers, jalapeno, raw	1 cup	90	27	1	5	2	1	0.1	0
90493	Peppers, sweet green, chopped/sliced, raw	10 pcs	27	5	0	1	0	0	0	0
6990	Pepper, sweet red, raw	1 ea	10	3	0	1	0	0	0	0
9251	Potatoes, red, flesh and skin, baked	1 ea	138	123	3	27	2	0	0	0
9245	Potatoes, russet, flesh and skin, baked	1 ea	138	134	4	30	3	0	0	0
5146	Spinach, raw	1 cup	30	7	1	1	1	0	0	0
90525	Squash, zucchini w/skin, slices, raw	1 ea	118	19	1	4	1	0	0	0
6924	Sweet potato, baked in skin w/salt	0.5 cup	100	90	2	21	3	0	0.1	0
5180	Tomato sauce, canned	0.5 cup	123	39	2	9	2	0	0	0

MDA CODE	FOOD NAME	AMT	WT (G)	ENER (KCAL)	PROT (G)	CARB (G)	FIBER (G)	FAT (G)	SAT (G)	CHOL (G)
90532	Tomato, red, ripe, whole, raw	1 pce	15	3	0	1	0	0	0	0
5306	Yam, peeled, raw	0.5 cup	75	88	1	21	3	0	0	0
SOY AND SOY PRODUCTS										
7564	Tempeh	0.5 cup	83	160	15	8	9	1.8	0	
7015	Soybeans, cooked	1 cup	172	298	29	17	10	15	2.2	0
7542	Tofu, firm, silken, 1" slice	3 oz	85.1	53	6	2	0	2	0.3	0
MEALS AND DISHES										
92216	Tortellini with cheese filling	1 cup	108	332	15	51	2	8	3.9	45
57658	Chili con carne w/beans, canned entree	1 cup	222	269	16	25	9	12	3.9	29
57703	Chili, vegetarian chili w/beans, canned entree/Hormel	1 cup	247	205	12	38	10	1	0.1	0
57068	Macaroni and cheese, unprepared/Kraft	1 ea	70	259	11	48	1	3	1.3	10
70958	Stir fry, rice & vegetables, w/soy sauce/Hanover	1 cup	137	130	5	27	2	0		
70943	Beef & bean burrito/Las Campanas	1 ea	114	296	9	38	1	12	4.2	13
16195	Chicken & vegetables/Lean Cuisine	1 ea	297	252	19	32	5	6	1	24
70917	Hot Pockets, beef & cheddar, frozen	1 ea	142	403	16	39		20	8.8	53
70918	Hot Pockets, croissant pocket w/chicken, broccoli, & cheddar, frozen	1 ea	128	301	11	39	1	11	3.4	37
56757	Lasagna w/meat sauce/Stouffer's	1 ea	215	277	19	26	3	11	4.7	41
11029	Macaroni & beef in tomato sauce/Lean Cuisine	1 ea	283	249	14	37	3	5	1.6	23
5587	Mashed potatoes, from granules w/milk, prep w/water & margarine	0.5 cup	105	122	2	17	1	5	1.3	2
70898	Pizza, pepperoni, frozen	1 ea	146	432	16	42	3	22	7.1	22
56703	Spaghetti w/meat sauce/Lean Cuisine	1 ea	326	313	14	51	6	6	1.4	13
SNACK FOODS										
10051	Beef jerky	1 pce	19.8	81	7	2	0	5	2.1	10
63331	Breakfast bars, oats, sugar, raisins, coconut	1 ea	43	200	4	29	1	8	5.5	0
61251	Cheese puffs and twists, corn based, low fat	1 oz	28.4	123	2	21	3	3	0.6	0
44032	Chex snack mix	1 cup	42.5	181	5	28	2	7	2.4	0
23059	Granola bar, hard, plain	1 ea	24.5	115	2	16	1	5	0.6	0
23104	Granola bar, soft, plain	1 ea	28.4	126	2	19	1	5	2.1	0
44012	Popcorn, air-popped	1 cup	8	31	1	6	1	0	0.1	0
44076	Potato chips, plain, no salt	1 oz	28.4	152	2	15	1	10	3.1	0
5437	Potato chips, sour cream & onion	1 oz	28.4	151	2	15	1	10	2.5	2

MDA CODE	FOOD NAME	AMT	WT (G)	ENER (KCAL)	PROT (G)	CARB (G)	FIBER (G)	FAT (G)	SAT (G)	CHOL (G)
44015	Pretzels, hard	5 pcs	30	114	3	24	1	1	0.1	0
44021	Rice cake, brown rice, plain, salted	1 ea	9	35	1	7	0	0	0.1	0
44058	Trail mix, regular	0.25 cup	37.5	173	5	17	2	11	2.1	0
SOUPS										
50398	Beef barley, canned/Progresso Healthy Classics	1 cup	241	142	11	20	3	2	0.7	19
50081	Chicken noodle, chunky, canned	1 cup	240	175	13	17	4	6	1.4	19
50085	Chicken rice, chunky, ready to eat, canned	1 cup	240	127	12	13	1	3	1	12
50088	Chicken vegetable, chunky, canned	1 cup	240	166	12	19	0	5	1.4	17
90238	Chicken, chunky, canned	1 cup	240	170	12	17	1	6	1.9	29
50697	Cup of Noodles, ramen, chicken flavor, dry/Nissin	1 ea	64	296	6	37	14	6.3		
50009	Minestrone, canned, made w/water	1 cup	241	82	4	11	1	3	0.6	2
92163	Ramen noodle, any flavor, dehydrated, dry	0.5 cup	38	172	4	25	1	6	2.9	0
50043	Tomato vegetable, from dry mix, made w/water	1 cup	253	56	2	10	1	1	0.4	0
50028	Tomato, canned, made w/water	1 cup	244	85	2	17	0	2	0.4	0
50014	Vegetable beef, canned, made w/water	1 cup	244	78	6	10	0	2	0.9	5
50013	Vegetarian vegetable, canned, made w/water	1 cup	241	72	2	12	0	2	0.3	0
DESSERTS										
62904	Brownie, commercially prepared, square, lrg, 2-3/4″ × 7/8″	1 ea	56	227	3	36	1	9	2.4	10
46062	Cake, chocolate, homemade, w/o icing	1 pce	95	340	5	51	2	14	5.2	55
46091	Cake, yellow, homemade, w/o icing	1 pce	68	245	4	36	0	10	2.7	37
71337	Doughnut, cake, w/chocolate icing, lrg, 3 1/2″	1 ea	57	270	3	27	1	18	4.6	35
45525	Doughnut, cake, glazed/sugared, med, 3″	1 ea	45	192	2	23	1	10	2.7	14
47026	Animal crackers/Arrowroot/Tea Biscuits	10 ea	12.5	56	1	9	0	2	0.4	0
90636	Chocolate chip cookie, commercially prepared 3.5″ to 4″	1 ea	40	196	2	26	1	10	3.1	0
47006	Chocolate sandwich cookie, creme filled	3 ea	30	140	2	21	1	6	1.1	0
62905	Fig bar, 2 oz	1 ea	56.7	197	2	40	3	4	0.6	0
90640	Oatmeal cookie, commercially prepared, 3-1/2″ to 4″	1 ea	25	112	2	17	1	5	1.1	0
47010	Peanut butter cookie, homemade, 3″	1 ea	20	95	2	12	0	5	0.9	6

MDA CODE	FOOD NAME	AMT	WT (G)	ENER (KCAL)	PROT (G)	CARB (G)	FIBER (G)	FAT (G)	SAT (G)	CHOL (G)
62907	Sugar cookie, refrigerated dough, baked	1 ea	23	111	1	15	0	5	1.4	7
57894	Pudding, chocolate, ready to eat	1 ea	113	158	3	26	1	5	0.8	3
2612	Pudding, vanilla, ready to eat	1 ea	113	147	3	25	0	4	1.7	8
2651	Rice pudding, ready to eat	1 ea	142	231	3	31	0	11	1.7	1
57902	Tapioca pudding, ready to eat	1 ea	113	135	2	22	0	4	1.1	1
71819	Frozen yogurts, chocolate, nonfat	1 cup	186	199	8	37	2	1	0.9	7
72124	Frozen yogurts, flavors other than chocolate	1 cup	174	221	5	38	0	6	4	23
2010	Ice cream, light, vanilla, soft serve	0.5 cup	88	111	4	19	0	2	1.4	11
90723	Ice popsicle	1 ea	59	47	0	11	0	0	0	0
42264	Cinnamon rolls w/icing, refrigerated dough/Pillsbury	1 ea	44	150	2	24	5	1.2		
71299	Croissant, butter	1 ea	67	272	5	31	2	14	7.8	45
45572	Danish, cheese	1 ea	71	266	6	26	1	16	4.8	11
45593	Toaster pastry, Pop Tart, apple-cinnamon/Kellogg	1 ea	52	205	2	37	1	5	0.9	0
23014	Chocolate syrup, fudge-type	2 Tbs	38	133	2	24	1	3	1.5	1
510	Whipped cream topping, pressurized	2 Tbs	7.5	19	0	1	0	2	1	6
54387	Whipped topping, frozen, low fat	2 Tbs	9.4	21	0	2	0	1	1.1	0
FATS, OILS, AND CONDIMENTS										
90210	Butter, unsalted	1 Tbs	14	100	0	0	0	11	7.2	30
8084	Oil, vegetable, canola	1 Tbs	14	124	0	0	0	14	1	0
8008	Oil, olive, salad or cooking	1 Tbs	13.5	119	0	0	0	14	1.9	0
8111	Oil, safflower, salad or cooking, greater than 70% oleic	1 Tbs	13.6	120	0	0	0	14	0.8	0
44483	Shortening, household	1 Tbs	12.8	113	0	0	0	13	2.6	0
1708	Barbecue sauce, original	2 Tbs	36	63	0	15	0			
27001	Catsup	1 ea	6	6	0	2	0	0	0	0
53523	Cheese sauce, ready to eat	0.25 cup	63	110	4	4	0	8	3.8	18
54388	Cream substitute, powdered, light	1 Tbs	5.9	25	0	4	0	1	0.2	0
50939	Gravy, brown, homestyle, canned	0.25 cup	60	25	1	3	1	0.3	2	
23003	Jelly	1 Tbs	19	51	0	13	0	0	0	0
25002	Maple syrup	1 Tbs	20	52	0	13	0	0	0	0
44476	Margarine, regular, 80% fat, with salt	1 Tbs	14.2	102	0	0	0	11	1.8	0
8145	Mayonnaise, safflower/soybean oil	1 Tbs	13.8	99	0	0	0	11	1.2	8
8502	Miracle Whip, light/Kraft	1 Tbs	16	37	0	2	0	3	0.5	4
435	Mustard, yellow	1 tsp	5	3	0	0	0	0	0	0
23042	Pancake syrup	1 Tbs	20	47	0	12	0	0	0	0
23172	Pancake syrup, reduced kcal	1 Tbs	15	25	0	7	0	0	0	0
53524	Pasta sauce, spaghetti/marinara	0.5 cup	125	92	2	14	1	3	0.4	0

MDA CODE	FOOD NAME	AMT	WT (G)	ENER (KCAL)	PROT (G)	CARB (G)	FIBER (G)	FAT (G)	SAT (G)	CHOL (G)
53646	Salsa picante, mild	2 Tbs	30.5	8	0	1	0	0		0
504	Sour cream, cultured	2 Tbs	28.8	62	1	1	0	6	3.8	13
53063	Soy sauce	1 Tbs	18	11	2	1	0	0	0	0
53652	Taco sauce, red, mild	1 Tbs	15.7	7	0	1	0	0		0
53004	Teriyaki sauce	1 Tbs	18	15	1	3	0	0	0	0
8024	1000 Island, regular	1 Tbs	15.6	58	0	2	0	5	0.8	4
8013	Blue/Roquefort cheese, regular	2 Tbs	30.6	154	1	2	0	16	3	5
90232	French, regular	1 Tbs	12.3	56	0	2	0	6	0.7	0
44498	Italian, fat-free	1 Tbs	14	7	0	1	0	0	0	0
44696	Ranch, reduced fat	1 Tbs	15	33	0	2	0	3	0.2	3
8035	Vinegar & oil, homemade	2 Tbs	31.2	140	0	1	0	16	2.8	0
FAST FOOD										
6177	Baked potato, topped w/cheese sauce	1 ea	296	474	15	47		29	10.6	18
56629	Burrito w/beans & cheese	1 ea	93	189	8	27		6	3.4	14
66023	Burrito w/beans, cheese, & beef	1 ea	102	165	7	20	2	7	3.6	62
66024	Burrito w/beef	1 ea	110	262	13	29	1	10	5.2	32
56600	Biscuit w/egg sandwich	1 ea	136	373	12	32	1	22	4.7	245
66029	Biscuit w/egg, cheese, & bacon sandwich	1 ea	144	477	16	33	0	31	11.4	261
66013	Cheeseburger, double, condiments & vegetables	1 ea	166	417	21	35		21	8.7	60
56649	Cheeseburger, large, one meat patty w/condiments & vegetables	1 ea	219	563	28	38		33	15	88
15063	Chicken, breaded, fried, dark meat (drumstick or thigh)	3 oz	85.1	248	17	9	1	15	4.1	95
15064	Chicken, breaded, fried, light meat (breast or wing)	3 oz	85.1	258	19	10	1	15	4.1	77
56000	Chicken filet, plain	1 ea	182	515	24	39		29	8.5	60
56635	Chimichanga w/beef & cheese	1 ea	183	443	20	39		23	11.2	51
5461	Cole slaw	0.75 cup	99	147	1	13		11	1.6	5
56606	Croissant w/egg & cheese sandwich	1 ea	127	368	13	24		25	14.1	216
56607	Croissant w/egg, cheese, & bacon sandwich	1 ea	129	413	16	24		28	15.4	215
66021	Enchilada w/cheese	1 ea	163	319	10	29		19	10.6	44
66020	Enchirito w/cheese, beef, & beans	1 ea	193	344	18	34		16	7.9	50
66031	English muffin w/cheese & sausage sandwich	1 ea	115	393	15	29	1	24	9.9	59
66010	Fish sandwich w/tartar sauce	1 ea	158	431	17	41	0	23	5.2	55
90736	French fries fried in vegetable oil, medium	1 ea	134	427	5	50	5	23	5.3	0
56638	Frijoles (beans) w/cheese	0.5 cup	83.5	113	6	14		4	2	18
56664	Ham & cheese sandwich	1 ea	146	352	21	33		15	6.4	58
56662	Hamburger, large, double, w/condiments & vegetables	1 ea	226	540	34	40		27	10.5	122

MDA CODE	FOOD NAME	AMT	WT (G)	ENER (KCAL)	PROT (G)	CARB (G)	FIBER (G)	FAT (G)	SAT (G)	CHOL (G)
56659	Hamburger, one patty w/condiments & vegetables	1 ea	110	279	13	27		13	4.1	26
66007	Hamburger, plain	1 ea	90	274	12	31		12	4.1	35
5463	Hash browns	0.5 cup	72	151	2	16		9	4.3	9
66004	Hot dog, plain	1 ea	98	242	10	18		15	5.1	44
2032	Ice cream sundae, hot fudge	1 ea	158	284	6	48	0	9	5	21
6185	Mashed potatoes	0.5 cup	121	100	3	20		1	0.6	2
56639	Nachos w/cheese	7 pcs	113	346	9	36		19	7.8	18
6176	Onion rings, breaded, fried	8 pcs	78.1	259	3	29		15	6.5	13
6173	Potato salad	0.333 cup	95	108	1	13		6	1	57
56619	Pizza w/pepperoni 12" or 1/8	1 pce	108	275	15	30		11	3.4	22
66003	Roast beef sandwich, plain	1 ea	139	346	22	33		14	3.6	51
56671	Submarine sandwich, cold cuts	1 ea	228	456	22	51	2	19	6.8	36
57531	Taco	1 ea	171	369	21	27		21	11.4	56
71129	Shake, chocolate, 12 fl. oz	1 ea	250	317	8	51	5	9	5.8	32
71132	Shake, vanilla, 12 fl. oz	1 ea	250	369	8	49	2	16	9.9	57

Ener = energy (kilocalories); **Prot** = protein; **Carb** = carbohydrate; **Fiber** = dietary fiber; **Fat** = total fat; **Sat** = saturated fat; **Chol** = cholesterol.

This food composition table has been prepared for Pearson Education, Inc. and is copyrighted by ESHA Research in Salem, Oregon, the developer of the MyDietAnalysis software program.

PHOTO CREDITS

acquired immunodeficiency syndrome (AIDS) A disease of the immune system caused by human immunodeficiency virus (HIV); characterized by extremely low CD4 counts or susceptibility to opportunistic infections or illnesses that do not affect those with healthy immune systems

active listening Attentive and engaged listening that includes giving positive cues to the speaker, such as smiling and nodding

adaptation A change in a body system as a result of physical training

addiction Continued involvement with a substance or activity despite ongoing negative consequences

adrenocorticotropic hormone A hormone secreted by the pituitary gland that causes adrenal glands to secrete cortisol

aerobic Dependent on oxygen (oxidative)

agility The ability to rapidly change body position or body direction without losing speed, balance, or body control

aging A progressive decline in the maximum functional level of individual cells, whole organs, and entire organisms

alcohol abuse Use of alcohol that interferes with work, school, or personal relationships or that entails violations of the law

alcoholic hepatitis A condition resulting from prolonged use of alcohol in which the liver is inflamed; can result in death

alcoholism (alcohol dependence) A condition in which personal and health problems related to alcohol use are severe and stopping alcohol use results in withdrawal symptoms

allostasis The many simultaneous changes that occur in the body to maintain homeostasis

allostatic load The long-term wear and tear on the body that is caused by prolonged allostasis

anabolic steroids Artificial forms of the hormone testosterone that promote muscle growth and strength

anaerobic Without oxygen (nonoxidative)

android Body shape described as "apple-shaped," with excess body fat distributed primarily on the upper body and trunk

angina pectoris Chest pain due to ischemia, or reduction in blood flow to the heart muscle and surrounding tissues

angiogenesis Process in which malignant cells give off growth factors that induce new blood capillaries to grow toward the tumor; these supply the tumor's cells with oxygen and materials and carry off cellular waste

anorexia nervosa A persistent, chronic eating disorder characterized by deliberate food restriction and severe, life-threatening weight loss

antioxidant Compound in foods that helps protect the body against the damaging effects of oxygen derivatives called *free-radicals*. Includes vitamins C and E and the yellow, red, orange, and green plant pigments beta-carotene, lycopene, and lutein

aorta The artery that carries blood from the left ventricle to the rest of the body

appraisal The interpretation and evaluation of information provided to the brain by the senses

arrhythmia Irregular heartbeat; can involve abnormally fast or slow heartbeat or the disorganized, sporadic beat of fibrillation

arterial stenosis A narrowing of the inner channel of arteries and smaller arterioles due to the buildup of a sludgelike layer of fatty, waxy debris

arteries High-pressure blood vessels that carry blood away from the heart to the lungs or cells

arthritis An umbrella-term for over 100 conditions characterized by inflammation of a joint

asthma A condition in which air passages to and within the lungs "overreact" to smoke, allergens, or other triggers

atherosclerosis Hardening or stiffening of the arteries as plaque accumulates at injury sites in the inner linings of arteries

ATP Adenosine triphosphate; the cellular form of energy

atria Upper chambers of the heart that collect blood from the rest of the body

atrophy A decrease in muscle cross-sectional area

ballistic stretching Stretching characterized by bouncing, jerky movements and momentum to increase range of motion

barbell A long bar with weight plates on each end

barrier to change A stumbling block you may face in your efforts to alter a current behavior

barriers to physical activity Personal or environmental issues that hinder your participation in regular physical activity

basal metabolic rate Your baseline rate of energy use, dictated by your body's collective metabolic activities

behavior change An organized, deliberate effort to alter or replace an existing habit or pattern of activity

behavior change contract A formal document that clarifies the goals and steps you plan to take to change a current habit or habit pattern

benign Harmless; refers to a noncancerous tumor

binge eating disorder A variation of bulimia that involves binge eating but usually no purging, laxatives, exercise, or fasting

bioelectrical impedance analysis (BIA) A technique that distinguishes lean and fat mass by measuring the resistance of various body tissues to electrical currents

biofeedback A stress-management technique that teaches you to alter automatic physiological responses such as body temperature, heart rate, or sweating; uses a machine to monitor such responses and measure the success of conscious control attempts

biopsy Microscopic examination of tissue to determine if a cancer is present

blood alcohol concentration (BAC) The ratio of alcohol to blood volume; used as a measure of intoxication

blood pressure The pressure that blood in the arteries exerts on the arterial walls

Bod Pod An egg-shaped chamber that uses air displacement to determine total body volume, total body density, and percent body fat

body composition The relative amounts of fat and lean tissue in the body

body dysmorphic disorder A psychological syndrome characterized by unrealistic and negative self-perception focusing on a physical defect such as nose size

body mass index (BMI) A number calculated from a person's weight and height that is used to assess risk for possible present or future health problems

bulimia nervosa An eating disorder characterized by frequent bouts of binge eating followed by purging (self-induced vomiting), laxative abuse, or excessive exercise

caliper A handheld and spring-loaded instrument with calibrated jaws and a meter that reads skinfold thickness in millimeters

calisthenics A type of muscle endurance and/or flexibility exercise that employs simple movements without the use of resistance other than one's own body weight

calorie A measure of the amount of chemical energy that foods provide. One calorie (lowercase *c*) can raise 1 gram of water 1 degree C.

Calories (capital *C*). Nutritionists use kcal or *C* when they refer to specific foods. A medium-sized apple provides 50 Calories.

cancer The name given to a large group of diseases characterized by the uncontrolled growth and spread of abnormal cells

carbohydrate Member of a class of nutrients containing sugars and starches, which supply most of the energy that sustains normal daily activity

carbon monoxide A gas found in cigarette smoke that binds at oxygen receptor sites in the blood

carcinogen A cancer-causing agent

carcinomas Solid tumors that occur in epithelial tissues (the tissues covering body surfaces and lining most body cavities)

cardiac output The volume of blood ejected from the heart in 1 minute; expressed in liters or milliliters per minute

cardiorespiratory fitness The ability of your cardiovascular and respiratory systems to supply oxygen and nutrients to large muscle groups in order to sustain dynamic activity

cardiovascular disease (CVD) A disease of the heart and/or blood vessels

cardiovascular system The body system responsible for the delivery of oxygen and nutrients to body tissues and the delivery of carbon dioxide and other wastes back to the heart and lungs

chancre An open sore most frequently located at the site of an initial syphilis infection

chemotherapy The use of drugs to kill cancerous cells

chlamydia The most common bacterial STI in the United States, caused by the bacterium *Chlamydia trachomatis*

cholesterol A waxy lipid in the steroid class that is an important component of cell membranes and is transported in the blood by carriers called *LDL* and *HDL*. Some cholesterol in the blood comes from the diet; most is made in the liver.

chronic bronchitis A type of COPD characterized by inflammation of the main air passages (bronchi) in your lungs

chronic disease A medical condition that persists for a long period of time

chronic obstructive pulmonary disease (COPD) A group of lung diseases that cause swelling of the airways. COPD includes emphysema and chronic bronchitis

circuit training A workout where exercisers move from one exercise station to another, after a certain number of repetitions or amount of time

cirrhosis The last stage of liver disease associated with chronic heavy use of alcohol, during which liver cells die and damage becomes permanent

cohabitation Living intimately together without being married

collagen The primary protein of connective tissues (cartilage, tendons, ligaments, skin, bones) throughout the body

commitment Making choices and taking actions over time that perpetuate the well-being of the other person, oneself, and the relationship

complex carbohydrate Important energy-storage compound and structural building material in plants and animals. Also called *polysaccharides*, the complex carbohydrates are made up of long chains of sugar molecules and deliver "timed release" energy

concentric A muscle contraction with overall muscle shortening

congenital heart disease Heart disease present at birth

congestive heart failure (CHF) A cardiovascular disease in which the heart muscle is damaged or overworked, the pumping chambers are often taxed to the limit, and the heart lacks the strength to keep blood circulating normally through the body

contraindicated Not recommended for everyone

cool-down The ending phase of a workout where the body is brought gradually back to rest

core muscles Musculature that supports the trunk (back, spine, abdomen, and hips)

coronary artery disease (CAD) Atherosclerosis (the buildup of plaque deposits) in the main arteries that supply oxygen and other materials to the heart muscle. Also called *coronary heart disease (CHD)*

cortisol Your body's main stress hormone, secreted by the cortex or outer layer of the adrenal glands located on top of the kidneys. Stimulates the sympathetic nervous system; can also damage or destroy neurons

countering Substituting a desired behavior for an undesirable one

creatine phosphate A molecule that is stored in muscle cells and used in the immediate energy system to donate a phosphate to make ATP

cross-training The practice of using different exercise modes or types in your cardiorespiratory training program

dehydrated Depleted of normal, necessary levels of body fluids

dehydration A process that leads to a lack of sufficient fluid in the body, affecting normal body functioning

designer (club) drugs Synthetic versions of existing illicit drugs; includes Ecstasy, Rohypnol, GHB, and Special K

detoxification The process by which addicts end their dependence on a drug

diabetes mellitus A disorder characterized by inadequate secretion or utilization of insulin, excessive urine production, excessive amounts of sugar in the blood and urine, and thirst, hunger, and weight loss

diastole The relaxation phase of the heart cycle

diastolic blood pressure Blood pressure during the diastole phase of the heart cycle

diastolic pressure The pressure applied to the walls of the arteries during the heart's relaxation phase

disk herniation A permanent bulging of an intervertebral disc out of its normal space

disordered eating Atypical, abnormal food consumption that diminishes your wellness but is usually neither long-lived nor disruptive to everyday life

distress Stress based on negative circumstances or events, or those perceived as negative; can diminish wellness

downshifting Forging new values that include stepping back to a simpler life

drug abuse Excessive use of a drug

drug misuse Use of a drug for a purpose for which it was not intended

dual-energy X-ray absorptiometry (DXA) A technique using two low-radiation X rays to scan bone and soft tissue (muscle, fat) to determine bone density and to estimate percent body fat

dumbbell A weight intended for use by one hand; typically one uses a dumbbell in each hand

DVs (Daily Values) A list of all the important nutrients from two less inclusive government lists—the RDIs (Reference Daily Intakes) and the DRVs (Daily Reference Values). DVs are printed on all nutrition labels

dynamic flexibility The joint range-of-motion limits with muscular contraction applied

dynamic stretching Stretching characterized by controlled, full-range-of-motion movements that mimic exercise session movements

eating disorders Disturbed patterns of eating, dieting, and perceptions of body image that have psychological, environmental, and possibly genetic underpinnings, and that lead to consequent medical issues

eccentric A muscle contraction with overall muscle lengthening

emotional wellness The ability to control emotions and express them appropriately at the right times; includes self-esteem, self-confidence, self-efficacy, and other emotional qualities

emphysema A chronic lung disease in which the tiny air sacs in the lungs are destroyed, making breathing difficult

energy balance The relationship between the amount of calories consumed in food with the amount of calories expended through metabolism and physical activity

environmental tobacco smoke (ETS) Smoke from tobacco products, commonly called "secondhand smoke"

environmental wellness An appreciation of the external environment and an understanding of the role one plays in preserving, protecting, and improving the world and its dwindling resources

enzyme Protein that facilitates chemical reactions but is not permanently altered in the process; biological catalyst

epinephrine Also called *adrenaline*; one of two stress hormones released by adrenal glands that readies your body for quick action by stimulating sympathetic nerves

ergogenic aid Any nutritional, physical, mechanical, psychological, or pharmacological procedure or aid used to improve athletic performance

ergogenic drugs Substances believed to enhance athletic performance

essential amino acid One of 9 of the 20 types of amino acids, or building blocks, that our bodies cannot manufacture and that we must consume in our foods

essential fat Body fat that is essential for normal physiological functioning

essential fatty acid Lipid components, including linolenic acid, EPA, DHA, and linoleic acid, which the body cannot manufacture and which we must obtain in polyunsaturated oils

essential nutrient A nutrient necessary for normal body functioning that must be obtained from food

ethanol (ethyl alcohol) An addictive drug produced by fermentation and found in many beverages

eustress Stress based on positive circumstances or events; can present an opportunity for personal growth

exercise Physical activity that is planned or structured and involves repetitive bodily movement, done to improve or maintain one or more of the components of fitness

external exercise rewards Rewards for exercise that come from outside of a person (trophy, compliment, day at the spa)

family of origin The people present in one's household during the first years of life

fast-twitch muscle fiber Muscle fiber type that contracts with greater force and speed but also fatigues quickly

fat A lipid such as butter, lard, and bacon grease, all of which are solids at room temperature

fat mass Body mass that is fat tissue

fatty acid The most basic unit of triglycerides

fetal alcohol syndrome (FAS) A disorder that may affect the fetus when the mother consumes alcohol during pregnancy; among its effects are mental retardation, small head, tremors, and physical abnormalities

fiber Indigestible carbohydrates in the diet that speed the passage of partially digested food through the digestive tract. Fiber helps control appetite and body weight by creating a feeling of fullness without adding extra calories

fibrillation A sporadic, quivering heartbeat pattern that results in very inefficient pumping of blood

fight-or-flight response A physiological reaction induced by nervous and hormonal signals that readies the heart, lungs, brain, muscles, and other vital organs and systems in ways that promote survival: fleeing from or confronting a threat

FITT formula A formula for designing a safe and effective exercise program that specifies frequency, intensity, time, and type

flexibility The ability of a joint (or joints) to move through a full range of motion

flexible diets Weight-loss regimens that focus on portion size and make allowances for variations in daily routine, appetite, and food availability

folate A form of vitamin B that is vital for spinal cord development and helps break down homocysteine as the body digests proteins

general adaptation syndrome (GAS) A historical model proposed by Hans Selye attempting to explain the body's stress response, consisting of alarm, resistance, and exhaustion stages

genital warts A small, fleshy growth on the cervix, vagina, vulva, penis, scrotum, or anus; also called *venereal wart* or *condyloma*

global warming An increase in Earth's overall temperature

glycemic index A measurement of the rate at which foods raise levels of glucose in the blood, and in turn, trigger the release of insulin and other blood-sugar regulators

golgi tendon organs Muscle tension receptors located in tendons that are responsible for triggering muscle relaxation to relieve excessive muscle tension

gonorrhea The second most common bacterial STI in the United States, caused by the bacterium *Neisseria gonorrhoeae*

greenhouse gases Gases that contribute to global warming by trapping heat near the Earth's surface

gynoid Body shape described as "pear-shaped," where excess body fat is distributed primarily on the lower body (hips and thighs)

hallucinogens (psychedelics) Substances capable of creating auditory or visual distortions and heightened states

hangover A physiological reaction to excessive drinking, including symptoms such as headache, upset stomach, anxiety, depression, diarrhea, and thirst

health-related components of physical fitness Components of physical fitness that have a relationship with good health

heart rate The number of beats of the heart in 1 minute

heart rate reserve (HRR) The number of beats per minute available or in reserve for exercise heart rate increases; maximal heart rate minus resting heart rate

heat cramps Severe cramping in the large muscle groups and abdomen caused by high fluid and electrolyte loss in sustained exertion in the heat

heat exhaustion An elevated core body temperature, headache, fatigue, profuse sweating, nausea, and clammy skin brought on by sustained exertion in the heat with dehydration and electrolyte losses

heatstroke A core body temperature above 104 degrees, headache, nausea, vomiting, diarrhea, rapid pulse, cessation of sweating, and disorientation resulting from extreme exertion in very hot conditions

heavy episodic (binge) drinking Drinking for the express purpose of becoming intoxicated; five drinks or more at one sitting for men; four drinks or more at one sitting for women

hemoglobin A four-part globular, iron-containing protein that carries oxygen in red blood cells

hepatitis B virus (HBV) One of seven forms of the hepatitis virus; hepatitis B is the most common sexually transmitted form

herpes A condition characterized by sores or eruptions on the skin, caused by *herpes simplex virus 1* (HSV-1) or *herpes simplex virus 2* (HSV-2)

high-density lipoprotein (HDL) A form of lipoprotein sometimes called "good cholesterol." HDL levels rise in response to polyunsaturated fats and prevent and reduce plaque deposits in the blood vessels

homeostasis A stable, constant internal environment

human immunodeficiency virus (HIV) The virus that causes AIDS, transmissible through direct sexual contact or exchange of saliva, semen, vaginal fluid, blood, or other bodily fluids

human papillomaviruses (HPV) A group of viruses that causes *genital warts*

hydrostatic weighing A technique that uses water to determine total body volume, total body density, and percent body fat; a greater difference between out-of-water and in-water weight indicates more body fat

hypertension Sustained high blood pressure

hypertrophy An increase in muscle cross-sectional area

hypnosis A medical and psychiatric tool that trains people to focus on one thought, object, or voice and to become unusually responsive to suggestion

hypothermia A condition where the core temperature of the body drops below the level required for sustaining normal bodily functions

immunotherapies Therapies that stimulate the body's own immune system to combat cancer cells

individuality Refers to the variable nature of physical activity dose-response or adaptations in different persons

inhalants Products that are sniffed or inhaled in order to produce a high

intellectual wellness The ability to think clearly, reason objectively, analyze, and use your brain power to solve problems and meet life's challenges

intensity The resistance level of the exercise

internal exercise rewards Rewards for exercise that are based upon how one is feeling physically and mentally (sense of accomplishment, relaxation, increased self-esteem)

interval workout A workout that alternates periods of higher-intensity exercise with periods of lower-intensity exercise or rest

iron-deficiency anemia A disease in which the body takes in too little iron and makes too little oxygen-carrying hemoglobin

ischemia A damaging reduction in the blood (and therefore the oxygen supply) to a region of the heart, brain, or other organ

isocaloric balance A state in which the amount of calories consumed in food is approximately the same as the amount of calories expended through metabolism and physical activity

isokinetic A muscle contraction with a constant speed of contraction

isometric A muscle contraction with no change in muscle length

isotonic A muscle contraction with relatively constant tension

joint The articulation or point of contact between two or more bones

journaling Keeping a personal journal

kilocalorie (kcal) One thousand calories. Also designated

lactic acid An end-product of the nonoxidative breakdown of glucose that can increase acidity in muscles and the blood and cause muscular fatigue

lean body mass Body mass that is fat-free (muscle, skin, bone, organs, and body fluids)

legume Fruit or seed of plants of the legume family. Legumes include beans, peas, peanuts, and seeds. Soy products are derived from soy beans, which are legumes

leukemias Nonsolid cancers characterized by an increase in the number of white blood cells in blood-forming parts of the body, particularly the bone marrow and spleen

lifetime risk The probability that a person will develop cancer at some point during his or her lifetime

lipid A category of compounds including fats, oils, and waxes that do not dissolve in water

lipoprotein A lipid plus protein transport particle that can move along easily in the bloodstream; carries triglycerides or cholesterol

locus of control Your belief in whether control over your life events and changes comes primarily from outside of yourself (external locus of control) or from within yourself (internal locus of control)

low-density lipoprotein (LDL) A form of lipoprotein sometimes called "bad cholesterol." LDL levels rise in response to saturated fats in the diet and can contribute to plaque deposits inside blood vessels

lymphomas Tumors that develop in lymph nodes, lymph vessels, or related infection-fighting regions of the body

mainstream smoke Smoke emitted from a smoker's mouth

major mineral A mineral needed in relatively large amounts, including sodium, calcium, phosphorus, magnesium, potassium, and chloride

malignant Very dangerous or harmful; refers to a cancerous tumor

malignant melanoma An invasive cancer of the pigment-producing cells of the skin

marijuana Chopped leaves and flowers of a *Cannibus* plant; a psychoactive stimulant

maximal heart rate (HRmax) The highest heart rate you can achieve during maximal exercise

maximal oxygen consumption (VO$_2$max) The highest rate of oxygen consumption your body is capable of during maximal exercise; expressed in either liters per minute (L/min) or milliliters per minute per kilogram of body weight (ml/kg·min)

MET The standard metabolic equivalent used to estimate the amount of energy (oxygen) used by the body during physical activity; 1 MET = resting or sitting quietly

metabolic syndrome A medical condition characterized by a combination of high blood cholesterol, high blood pressure, abdominal fat deposits and large waist circumference, and insulin resistance or type 2 diabetes

metastasis Process by which cancer spreads from one area to different areas of the body

mineral An element such as calcium or sodium that allows vital physiological processes, including nerve transmission, heartbeat, oxygen delivery, and absorption of vitamins

mitochondria Cellular structures where oxidative energy production takes place

mode The specific type of exercise performed

monounsaturated fatty acid (MUFA) Lipid whose fatty acid chains have just one kinked (unsaturated) region. Olive oil, canola oil, and cashew oil are high in monounsaturated fatty acids

motivation One's inducement to do something such as change a current behavior

motor unit A motor nerve and all the muscle fibers it controls

municipal solid waste Solid wastes from residential, commercial, institutional, and industrial sources

muscle fiber The cell of the muscular system

muscle power The ability of a muscle to quickly contract with high force

muscle spindles (stretch receptors) Muscle length receptors located within muscle fibers that trigger muscle contractions in response to rapid, excessive muscle lengthening

muscular endurance The ability of a muscle to contract repeatedly over an extended period of time

muscular fitness The ability of your musculoskeletal system to perform daily and recreational activities without undue fatigue and injury

muscular strength The ability of a muscle to contract with maximal force

myocardial infarction (MI) Medical term for a heart attack; involves permanent damage to an area of the heart muscle brought on by a cessation of normal blood supply

myofibril Thin strands within a single muscle fiber that bundle the skeletal muscle protein filaments and span the length of the fiber

negative caloric balance A state in which the amount of calories consumed in food falls short of the amount of calories expended through metabolism and physical activity

nicotine The primary stimulant chemical in tobacco products

nicotine poisoning Symptoms often experienced by beginning smokers, including dizziness, diarrhea, light-headedness, rapid and erratic pulse, clammy skin, nausea, and vomiting

non-exercise activity Routine daily activities like standing up and walking around that use energy but are not part of deliberate exercise

norepinephrine One of two stress hormones secreted by adrenal glands that readies your body for quick action by increasing arousal

nutrient A chemical in food that is crucial for growth and function; includes proteins, carbohydrates (starches and sugars), lipids (fats and oils), vitamins, and minerals

nutrient-dense food Food or beverage that provides a high level of nutrients and thus maximizes the nutritional value of each meal and snack consumed

nutrition The study of how people consume and use the nutrients in food

obese In an adult, having a BMI of 30 or more, or a body weight more than 20 percent above recommended levels

oil A lipid such as corn and olive oil, which is usually a golden liquid at room temperature

omega-3 fatty acid A lipid in a class of lipid components that includes linoleic acid, EPA, and DHA; abundant in polyunsaturated oils from flaxseeds, walnuts, and certain fish. Found in lesser amounts in canola and soybean oils. The fatty acids are double-bonded at three sites, including one at the third carbon along the chain

omega-6 fatty acid A lipid in a class of lipid components that includes linoleic acid; abundant in polyunsaturated oils such as canola oil, corn oil, soybean oil, and sunflower oil. The fatty acids are polyunsaturated and have doubled-bonded carbons at two sites, including one at the sixth carbon along the chain

oncogenes Suspected cancer-causing genes present on chromosomes

oncologist A doctor who specializes in cancer detection and treatment

one repetition maximum (1 RM) The maximum amount of weight you can lift one time

opiates A class of drugs derived from the parent drug opium, characterized by the ability to relieve pain, induce drowsiness, and cause euphoria

osteoarthritis A type of arthritis characterized by stiffness, aching, swelling, or permanent deformation and dysfunction of a joint, caused primarily by wear and tear

osteoporosis A chronic degenerative bone disease characterized by diminished bone mass and porous, brittle bones

overload Subjecting the body or body system to more physical activity than it is used to

overtraining Excessive volume and intensity of physical training leading to diminished health, fitness, and performance

overweight In an adult, having a BMI of 25 to 29. Also defined as having a body weight more than 10 percent above recommended levels

Pap smear A procedure in which cells taken from the cervical region are examined for abnormal cellular activity

passive stretch A stretch that involves an outside force (such as a partner, your arms, weight, or gravity) to stretch targeted muscle groups. In contrast, an **active stretch** involves the contraction of the opposing muscle groups to stretch targeted muscle groups

pelvic inflammatory disease (PID) An infection of the female reproductive tract that can result from an untreated sexually transmitted infection

percent body fat Percentage of total weight that is comprised of fat tissue

physical activity Any bodily movement produced by skeletal muscles that results in an expenditure of energy

physical fitness The ability to perform moderate to vigorous levels of physical activity without undue fatigue

physical wellness A state of physical health and well-being that includes body size and shape, body functioning, measures of strength and endurance, and resistance to disease

plaque A pinpoint area of fatty, waxy debris that accumulates at a site (usually of an injury) along the inner wall of an artery or arteriole. As immune system cells and inflammation enlarge the mass, plaque can pile up, bulge inward, and partially or fully block blood flow through the channel.

plasma The yellow-colored fluid portion of blood that contains water, proteins, hormones, ions, energy sources, and blood gases

plyometric exercise An exercise that is characterized by a rapid deceleration of the body followed by a rapid acceleration of the body in the opposite direction

polyunsaturated fatty acid (PUFA) Lipid whose fatty acid chains have two or more kinked (unsaturated) regions. Corn oil, safflower oil, and cottonseed oils are high in polyunsaturated fatty acids

positive caloric balance A state in which the amount of calories consumed in food exceeds the amount of calories expended through metabolism and physical activity

post-traumatic stress disorder (PTSD) An acute stress disorder caused by experiencing an extremely traumatic event

pre-diabetes A condition that raises a person's risk of developing type 2 diabetes, marked by blood glucose levels that are higher than normal but not yet diabetic

principles of fitness General principles of exercise adaptation that guide fitness programming

progression A gradual increase in a training program's intensity, frequency, and/or time

progressive muscle relaxation (PMR) A stress-management technique that identifies tension stored in the muscles and releases it, one muscle group at a time

proof A measure of the percentage of alcohol in a beverage

proprioceptive neuromuscular facilitation (PNF) Stretching that is facilitated or enhanced by the voluntary contraction of the targeted muscle group or contraction of opposing muscles

protein Biological molecule composed of amino acids. Proteins serve as crucial structural and functional compounds in living organisms

psychoneuroimmunology (PNI) Science of the interaction between the mind and the immune system

pubic lice Tiny sucking insects that lay eggs at the base of pubic hairs and can be transmitted from partner to partner during sexual contact; also called "crabs"

pulmonary artery The artery that carries blood from the right ventricle to the lungs

pulmonary circulation Blood circulation from the heart to the lungs and back

pulse The pressure wave felt in the arteries due to blood ejection with each heartbeat

radiation Powerful, targeted beams of ionizing energy that can kill cancerous cells

range of motion The movement limits of a specific joint or groups of joints

rating of perceived exertion (RPE) A subjective scale of exercise intensity

RDAs (Recommended Dietary Allowances) A listing of the average daily nutrient intake level for a list of vitamins and minerals that meets most people's daily needs

relapse Resumption of behavior that one is attempting to cease

relative risk A measure of how likely a person is to develop cancer while engaging in known risk behaviors compared to people who abstain from these behaviors

relaxation breathing Inhaling deeply and rhythmically, and expanding then relaxing the abdomen; this breathing technique can help relieve tension and increase oxygen intake

repetitions The number of times an exercise is performed within one set

resistance The amount of effort or force required to complete the exercise

resistance training Controlled and progressive stressing of the body's musculoskeletal system using resistance (i.e., weights, resistance bands, body weight) exercises to build and maintain muscular fitness

respiration The exchange of gases in the lungs or in the tissues

respiratory system The body system responsible for the exchange of gases between the body and the air

resting heart rate The number of times your heart beats in a minute while the body is at rest; typically between 50 to 90 beats per minute

resting metabolic rate Basal metabolic rate plus the energy expended in digesting food

reversibility The concept that training adaptations will revert toward initial levels when training is stopped

rheumatoid arthritis A type of arthritis characterized by chronic inflammation, swelling, and pain in a joint brought about by an autoimmune attack of the body's own immune system on joint tissues

RICE Acronym for *r*est, *i*ce, *c*ompression, and *e*levation; a method of treating common exercise injuries

rigid diets Weight-loss regimens that specify strict rules on calorie consumption, types of foods, and eating patterns

sarcomas Solid tumors that occur in middle layers of tissue—for example, in bones, muscles, and connective tissue

sarcopenia The degenerative loss of muscle mass and strength in aging

saturated fat A lipid, usually a solid fat like butter, in which most of the chains of carbon atoms are loaded (or "saturated") with as many hydrogen atoms as the chain can carry. Saturated chains are straight, allowing them to pack together and act like a solid

sedentary Physically inactive; exerting physical effort only for required daily tasks and not for leisure-time exercise

self-care Knowing your body and taking appropriate action to stop progression of illness or injury

self-disclosure The process of revealing one's inner thoughts, feelings, and beliefs to another person

self-efficacy The degree to which you believe in your own ability to achieve something

set A single attempt at an exercise that includes a fixed number of repetitions

set point A preprogrammed weight that your body returns to easily when you gain or lose a few pounds

sexually transmitted infection (STI) A microbial infection spread through intimate contact with another person's skin or body fluids

sidestream smoke Smoke emitted from the burning end of a cigarette

simple carbohydrate Carbohydrate made up of one or two sugar subunits and that delivers energy in a quickly usable form. Glucose, a *monosaccharide*, has one sugar subunit. Table sugar, a *disaccharide*, has two sugar subunits.

skill-related components of fitness Components of physical fitness that have a relationship with enhanced motor skills and performance in sports

skinfold A fold of skin and subcutaneous fat tissue that is measured with calipers to determine the fatness of a specific body area; multiple skinfold measures are combined to estimate total body lean and fat masses

slow-twitch muscle fiber Muscle fiber type that is oxygen-dependent and can contract over long periods of time

social wellness A person's degree of social connectedness and skills, leading to satisfying interpersonal relationships

specificity The concept that only the body systems worked during training will show adaptations

speed The ability to rapidly accelerate; exercises for speed will increase stride length and frequency

spiritual wellness A feeling of unity or oneness with people and nature and a sense of life's purpose, meaning, or value; for some, a belief in a supreme being or religion

spotter A person who watches, encourages, and, if needed, assists a person who is performing a weight-training lift

stages of behavior change From the transtheoretical model, a set of states most people pass through in their awareness of, determination to alter, and efforts to replace existing habits or actions

static flexibility The joint range-of-motion limits with an external force applied

static stretching Stretching characterized by slow and sustained muscle lengthening

stimulants An agent, especially a chemical one, that temporarily arouses or accelerates physiological activity

storage fat Body fat that is not essential but does provide energy, insulation, and padding

stress A term used to describe a physical, social, or psychological event or circumstance that disturbs the body's "normal" state and to which the body must try to adapt. Also used to describe the disturbed physical or emotional state experienced as a result of such events/circumstances

stressor A physical, social, or psychological event or circumstance to which the body tries to adapt; stressors are often threatening, unfamiliar, disturbing, or exciting

stress response A set of physical and emotional reactions initiated by your body in response to a stressor

stretch reflex The reflex contraction of a muscle triggered by stretch receptors (muscle spindles) in response to a rapid overextension of that muscle

stretching Exercises designed to improve or maintain flexibility

stroke A sudden loss of function in a region of the brain caused by blockage in or rupture of a blood vessel, leading to oxygen deprivation, cell damage, or death

stroke volume The volume of blood ejected from the heart in one heartbeat; expressed in liters or milliliters per beat

sustainable choices Lifestyle choices that preserve and protect the planet's resources

syphilis A sexually transmitted disease caused by the bacterium *Treponema pallidum*

systemic circulation Blood circulation from the heart to the rest of the body and back

systole The contraction phase of the heart cycle

systolic blood pressure Blood pressure during the systole phase of the heart cycle

systolic pressure The pressure being applied to the walls of the arteries when the heart contracts

20 repetition maximum (20 RM) The maximum amount of weight you can lift 20 times in a row

talk test A method of measuring exercise intensity based on assessing your ability to speak during exercise

target behavior One well-defined habit chosen as your primary focus for change

target heart rate The heart rate you are aiming for during an exercise session; often a range with high and low heart rates called your *training zone*

tendon The connective tissue attaching a muscle to a bone

tendons Connective tissues that attach muscle to bone

trace mineral An element the body needs in very tiny amounts; includes iron, zinc, copper, iodine, selenium, fluoride, and chromium

training effect An increase in physical fitness as a result of overload adaptations in body systems

trans fat An unsaturated lipid or oil with hydrogen atoms added to cause more complete saturation and make the oil function as a solid. Margarines and vegetable shortenings are examples of *trans* fats

trichomoniasis An infection of the genitals caused by a protozoan; symptoms include foamy, yellowish discharge and unpleasant odor; also called "trich"

triglyceride Lipid molecule made up of three fatty acid chains or "tails" attached to one glycerol "head" containing a three-carbon backbone. Common form of fats in foods and in organisms

tumor A clumping of cells that grows more rapidly than surrounding tissue

type 1 diabetes An autoimmune disease that destroys the insulin-producing cells of the pancreas, compromising the body's ability to make insulin and to properly regulate blood sugar

type 2 diabetes A disease linked to obesity and inactivity in which the body loses its ability to respond to insulin and cannot properly regulate blood sugar

underweight In an adult, having a BMI below 18.5, or a body weight more than 10 percent below recommended levels

unprotected sex Sexual intercourse (vaginal, oral, or anal) without a condom or other method of protection

unsaturated fat A lipid, usually a liquid oil, in which most carbon chains lack the maximum load of hydrogen atoms. Unsaturated chains are kinked and can't pack tightly, thus they can slip past each other and act like liquids

urinary tract infection (UTI) An infection of the urethra or bladder caused by microorganisms; can be sexually transmitted or autoinoculated

Valsalva maneuver The process of holding one's breath while lifting heavy weight. This practice can increase chest cavity pressure and result in light-headedness during the lift; excessively increased blood pressure can result after the lift and breath are released

veins Low-pressure blood vessels that carry blood from the cells or lungs back to the heart

ventricles Lower chambers of the heart that pump blood to the rest of the body

vitamin Organic compound in foods that we need in tiny amounts to promote growth and help maintain life and health

waist-to-hip ratio (WHR) Waist circumference divided by hip circumference

warm-up The initial 5-to-20-minute preparation phase of a workout

weight cycling The pattern of repeatedly losing and gaining weight, from illness or dieting

weight management A lifelong balancing of calories consumed and calories expended through exercise and activity to control body fat and weight

wellness continuum A spectrum of wellness states from average to optimal in one direction and from average to premature death in the opposite direction

wellness The achievement of the highest level of health possible in physical, social, intellectual, emotional, environmental, and spiritual dimensions

whole foods Dietary items produced and consumed with the minimum of processing, such as refining, adding preservatives, or altering form for quick preparation

yo-yo dieting A series of diets followed by eventual weight gain. Yo-yo dieting can lead to weight cycling

Page number followed by *f* indicates figure, page number followed by *t* indicates table, and page number followed by *p* indicates photo.